Contents

Answers to the Check your knowledge quizzes are available at
www.pearsonfe.co.uk/Level2Beautyanswers

Acknowledgements

The publisher would like to thank the following for their kind permission to reproduce their photographs:

(Key: b-bottom; c-centre; l-left; r-right; t-top)

Alamy Images: Chris Cheadle 15, Dmitry Goygel-Sokol 91, foodfolio 85, ICP 76b, Jeffrey Black 108, Jonathon Tennant 162, medical-on-line 213/3, 213/4, Mira 221b, moodboard 212/3, Peter Banos 399l, Scott Camazine / Phototake 211/3, Stephen Jakub 175; **Aramis:** Aramis 216b; **BeautyExpress.co.uk:** BeautyExpress.co.uk 357, 374, 374/2, 374/3, 374/4, 374/5, 374/6, 374/7, 374/8, 380, 381, 399, 428t, 428b, 429, BeautyExpress.co.uk 357, 374, 374/2, 374/3, 374/4, 374/5, 374/6, 374/7, 374/8, 380, 381, 399, 428t, 428b, 429; **Camera Press Ltd:** camera press 147; **Carlton:** Carlton 301; **Carlton Professional:** Carlton Professional 38; **Ciate:** Ciate 133, 133c, 133b; **Corbis:** bridge 453; **cut2white:** cut2white 84, 173, 191, 220, 226, 274/3, 343, 421, 426, 459/1, cut2white 84, 173, 191, 220, 226, 274/3, 343, 421, 426, 459/1; **Dermalogica:** 17, 282, 283, 284, 285, 286, 287, 289, 289b, 290; **Image courtesy of The Advertising Archives:** Advertising Archive 392b, 486, Advertising Archives 392; **Getty Images:** Adam Gault 127, ariel skelley / stone 109c, Bloomberg 224, Bruce Talbot , Datacraft Co Ltd 456, David Woolley 329, Jupiterimages 117, martin barraud / stone 109t, Stockdisc 13; **MediSwab:** MediSwab 39t; **Minx Inc:** Brandon Wiggins 152l; **Pearson Education Ltd:** gareth boden 12, 37, 167b, 203b, 302l, 302r, 320b, 321, 330, 340, 415t, 415c, 415b, 435, 440/1, 440/2, 440/3, 440/4, 440/5, 440/6, 441/1, 441/2, 441/3, 441/4, 441/5, 441/6, 446/1, 446/2, 446/3, 446/4, 446/5, 446/6, 446/7, 446/8, 461b, 465/2, 465/3, 465/4, 465/5, 465/6, Image source 9, John Foxx Collection 187, Lord and Leverett 87, mind studio 18, 48/3, 48/4, 49, 54, 76, 76t, 83, 100, 102l, 102r, 108cl, 108cr, 113, 129, 157, 169, 215, 217b, 228, 269, 272, 272b, 279/1, 279/2, 279/3, 279/4, 279/5, 279/6, 279/8, 279/9, 291t, 295t, 295b, 300t, 300b, 309/1, 309/2, 309/3, 309/4, 309/5, 309/6, 310/7, 310/8, 310/9, 310/10, 310/11, 310/12, 311, 311/2, 311/3, 311/4, 311/5, 311/6, 312/1, 312/2, 312/3, 312/4, 312/6, 312/23, 313/1, 313/2, 313/3, 313/4, 313/5, 313/6, 314/1, 314/2, 314/3, 314/4, 314/5, 314/6, 315/1, 315/2, 317c, 317r, 320tl, 320tr, 335t, 335c, 335b, 336, 338, 338t, 338b, 341t, 341b, 342, 344/1, 344/2, 344/3, 344/4, 361, 363, 393/1, 393/2, 393/3, 393/4, 393/5, 393/6, 394/1, 394/2, 394/3, 394/4, 394/5, 394/6, 395/1, 395/2, 395/3, 396/1, 396/2, 396/3, 396/4, 396/5, 396/6, 397/1, 397/3, 397/4, 397/5, 397/8, 437/1, 437/2, 437/3, 437/4, 437/5, 437/6, 437/7, 437/8, 437/9, 438/1, 438/2, 438/3, 438/4, 438/5, 438/6, 438/7, 442/2, 442/3, 442/4, 442/5, 443/2, 443/4, 443/5, 443/6, 443/7, 443/8, 464t, 464b, 465/1, 466t, 466b, 468/3, 468/4, 468/5, 468/6, 469/1, 469/3, 469/5, 469/6, 469/8, 469/10, 470/1, 470/2, 470/3, 470/4, 470/5, 470/6, 471/1, 471/2, 471/3, 471/4, 471/5, 471/6, 472/1, 472/2, 472/3, 472/4, 472/5, 472/6, 472/7, 472/8, 473, 474, mind studio 18, 48/3, 48/4, 49, 54, 76, 76t, 83, 100, 102l, 102r, 108cl, 108cr, 113, 129, 157, 169, 215, 217b, 228, 269, 272, 272b, 279/1, 279/2, 279/3, 279/4, 279/5, 279/6, 279/8, 279/9, 291t, 295t, 295b, 300t, 300b, 309/1, 309/2, 309/3, 309/4, 309/5, 309/6, 310/7, 310/8, 310/9, 310/10, 310/11, 310/12, 311, 311/2, 311/3, 311/4, 311/5, 311/6, 312/1, 312/2, 312/3, 312/4, 312/6, 312/23, 313/1, 313/2, 313/3, 313/4, 313/5, 313/6, 314/1, 314/2, 314/3, 314/4, 314/5, 314/6, 315/1, 315/2, 317c, 317r, 320tl, 320tr, 335t, 335c, 335b, 336, 338, 338t, 338b, 341t, 341b, 342, 344/1, 344/2, 344/3, 344/4, 361, 363, 393/1, 393/2, 393/3, 393/4, 393/5, 393/6, 394/1, 394/2, 394/3, 394/4, 394/5, 394/6, 395/1, 395/2, 395/3, 396/1, 396/2, 396/3, 396/4, 396/5, 396/6, 397/1, 397/3, 397/4, 397/5, 397/8, 437/1, 437/2, 437/3, 437/4, 437/5, 437/6, 437/7, 437/8, 437/9, 438/1, 438/2, 438/3, 438/4, 438/5, 438/6, 438/7, 442/2, 442/3, 442/4, 442/5, 443/2, 443/4, 443/5, 443/6, 443/7, 443/8, 464t, 464b, 465/1, 466t, 466b, 468/3, 468/4, 468/5, 468/6, 469/1, 469/3, 469/5, 469/6, 469/8, 469/10, 470/1, 470/2, 470/3, 470/4, 470/5, 470/6, 471/1, 471/2, 471/3, 471/4, 471/5, 471/6, 472/1, 472/2, 472/3, 472/4, 472/5, 472/6, 472/7, 472/8, 473, 474, MindStudio 27, 39b, 40t, 40bl, 41, 48/1, 202b, 279/7, 288, 288b, 315cl, 315cr, 315bl, 315br, 317l, 409, 442/1, 443/1, 443/3, 455, 468/1, 468/2, *Nigel Riches.Image Source Ltd* 36, Peter Morris 364/1, 364/2, 364/3, 364/4, 364/5, 364/6, 364/7, 364/8, 364/9, 364/10, 459/2, 459/3, 459/4, 459/5, 460/1, 460/2, 460/3, 460/4, 460/5, 461t, stuart cox 101, 103, 107, 112, 126, 305, 473c, 473b, 484, studio8 201, 215b, studio8 Clark Wiseman 219c; **PhotoDisc:** Kevin Peterson 218, 367; **Photolibrary.com:** trinette reed / blend images 109b; **Science Photo Library Ltd:** 213, Alain Dex Publiphoto Diffusion 208l, Biophoto Associates 32/6, Dr Chris Hale 274/1, Dr H C Robinson 211/4, Dr P Marazzi 32/2, 209/1, 209/3, 209/6, 210/2, 210/3, 210/4, 210/6, 211/2, 213/1, 213/2, 213/6, 274/4, 332/3, 332/4, 332t, Dr P. Marazzi 32/5, 32/7, james stevenson 212/1, jane shemilt 210/1, science photo library 32, 32/4, 208br, 209/2, 209/5, 212/2, 213/5, 274/2, 332/5, science photo library 32, 32/4, 208br, 209/2, 209/5, 212/2, 213/5, 274/2, 332/5, st bartholomew's hospital 32/3, 274/5, st bartholomews hospital 208, 210/5, 211, western ophthalmic hospital 209/4, 332/2; **Shutterstock.com:** AISPIX 185, Alexander Bark 185b, AlexAnnaButs 495t, archana bhartia 218c, blend images 152, Brenda Carson 223, Danny E Hooks 51, grublee 128, Hadk 418, iofoto 110, 457, Ivanova Inga 10, 350, Ivanova Inga 10, 350, karoline cullen 493, Leegudim 355, Luba V Nel 227, Martin Allinger 308, martina ebel 219b, Mayer George Vladomirovich 181, Monkey Business Images 182b, NemesisINC 495b, omkar.a.v 204, Pan Xunbin 33, photobank.ch 277, Picsfive 375c, PonomarenkeNataly 481, *Poznyakov* 317, R. Gino Santa Maria 400, rj lerich 202, ruslan kudrin 463, *russ witherington* 20, sakala 30, 122, Serghei Starus 268, Stephen Coburn 156, Tania Zbrodko 291b, Tasha Lavigne 375t, Valua Vitaly 67, 99, 221t, 356, VladGavriloff 267, Vladimir Kozieiev 406, yuri arcurs 16, 182, 197, 218bl; **Skinlogic.co.uk:** Skinlogic.co.uk 205; **www.imagesource.com:** Image Source 135, 405, Image source Ltd 155, Nigel Riches 203

Cover images: *Front:* **Corbis:** Sonja Pacho

All other images © Pearson Education

Every effort has been made to trace the copyright holders and we apologise in advance for any unintentional omissions. We would be pleased to insert the appropriate acknowledgement in any subsequent edition of this publication.

Work-Based Learning

BEAUTY THERAPY

Jane Hiscock

Frances Lovett

Lindsey Anderson

Lisa Kniveton

ALWAYS LEARNING

PEARSON

Published by Pearson Education Limited, Edinburgh Gate, Harlow, Essex, CM20 2JE.

www.pearsonschoolsandfecolleges.co.uk

Heinemann is a registered trademark of Pearson Education Limited

Text: The following units © Pearson Education Ltd 2011: Client care and communication in
beauty-related industries; Display stock and promote products and services to clients; Working
in beauty-related industries; Provide manicure and pedicure services; Create an image based on
a theme. All other units © Jane Hiscock and Frances Lovett, Fareham College 2010, 2012
Edited by Liz Cartmell
Designed and produced by Kamae Design
Original illustrations © Pearson Education 2010, 2012
Illustrated by Hardlines, Oxford Illustrators, Maurizio De Angells and Kamae Design
Cover design by Pearson Education Ltd
Picture research by Susi Paz
Cover photo/illustration © Corbis/Sonja Pacho
Index compiled by Indexing Specialists (UK) Ltd., Hove

The rights of Jane Hiscock, Frances Lovett, Lindsey Anderson and Lisa Kniveton to be identified
as authors of this work has been asserted by them in accordance with the Copyright, Designs
and Patents Act 1988.

First published 2012

15 14 13 12
10 9 8 7 6 5 4 3 2 1

British Library Cataloguing in Publication Data
A catalogue record for this book is available from the British Library

ISBN 978 0 435 07489 0

Printed in Spain by Grafos S.A

Every effort has been made to contact copyright holders of material reproduced in this book.
Any omissions will be rectified in subsequent printings if notice is given to the publishers.

Websites
Pearson Education Limited is not responsible for the content of any external internet sites. It is
essential for tutors to preview each website before using it in class so as to ensure that the URL
is still accurate, relevant and appropriate. We suggest that tutors bookmark useful websites
and consider enabling students to access them through the school/college intranet.

Introduction

Why choose a career in beauty therapy?

A career in beauty therapy is varied and diverse, offering lots of opportunities to learn and develop skills in a range of different areas. Ultimately beauty therapy is a service industry and its main, and most rewarding, aim is to help others to feel good about their appearance and be the very best they can be.

A career in beauty therapy offers you the opportunity to tailor a job most suited to your personal circumstances or passion, whether that be travelling, working in a spa, working for yourself or specialising in one particular field, such as make-up design. With a Level 2 (VRQ) Diploma in Beauty Therapy, you have a firm foundation.

What is a VRQ?

VRQs (Vocationally Related Qualifications) are skills-based qualifications that prepare you for work by providing knowledge and understanding in Beauty Therapy. They are preparation for work qualifications, i.e. you will have the knowledge and understanding needed for the workplace once you have completed the course. Assessment of the qualification is through tests or assignments to check that you have met all the essential knowledge and understanding requirements. You will also undergo practical observations where you will need to demonstrate your skills.

How do I gain a VRQ Certificate/Diploma?

The qualification is gained by showing lots of evidence of what you have learnt within each unit and is practically based, so you will get a very good grounding in all the skill areas. This means that when you go into a salon, you have dealt with most client requests and have lots of confidence to perform the service that the client is paying for.

How do I get my evidence?

Many forms of evidence are acceptable and your trainer/lecturer will be able to guide you through the best options for your individual learning programme. Each of the different types of evidence is valid. These include:

- observed work
- witness statements
- assessment of prior learning and experience (APL)
- oral questions
- written questions and/or assignments.

These will be recorded on **evidence sheets** provided and will form a **portfolio**. A portfolio is just a collection of all the evidence together. It should be indexed and easy to follow.

Why index my evidence?

An assessor will observe or guide you through the types of evidence listed above. This person will have had special training for a specific qualification designed to help you present your evidence in a format suitable for your awarding body.

For quality control and fairness across the subject areas, an internal verifier will check the assessor and the portfolio instruction. This will be performed within your place of training and should happen on a regular basis.

The Awarding Organisation also has an external verifier who will visit your training establishment regularly and check that both assessors and internal verifiers are giving the correct information to you, the candidate. Then your portfolio can be accredited with a certificate. This can be achieved a unit at a time, or applied for all at once. It's essential that you keep your portfolio organised and present your work in an easy-to-view format.

What evidence do I need?

You should ask your assessor about the most suitable method for the work you are doing. Most portfolios have a mixture of evidence.

If you have previous experience (APL) — perhaps gained whilst working — or recent qualifications, they can also be counted. For example, if you work part-time in a shop, and have experience using the till, dealing with customers and handling complaints, then a witness statement from your employer that is current, valid, signed and dated is acceptable evidence.

This evidence would cover some of the reception units, as well as some communication units and the interpersonal skills required. It also covers some of the ranges required in your assessment books.

Other valid evidence could be photographs, project work, videotape or client record cards.

Standards

Your training establishment will register you with its awarding body. The awarding body will then issue you, the candidate, with your assessment book. Take care of it; it is very precious. It will become your only source of evidence for all your hard work.

Within your assessment book you will be given guidance on how to achieve each unit. There are conditions and terms that you must follow.

Performance criteria

You must perform these in the course of your assessed treatment. They are numbered and your assessor will tick them off as they are observed. For example, the Provide Facial Skincare unit has performance criteria including 'use consultation techniques to identify treatment objectives'.

Ranges

These must be covered through the various methods of assessment previously discussed — observed performance, oral question or simulation, written question, project or through APL.

How to use this book

This book has been designed with you in mind. It has a dual purpose:

1 To lead you through the Level 2 (VRQ) Diploma in Beauty Therapy, providing background, technical guidance with suggested evidence collection and key skill information.

2 As a reference book that you will find useful to dip into, long after you have gained your qualification.

To reinforce your learning process and get you thinking, there are several features to help you.

Key terms
These highlight terms that are central to your understanding of the topic that you may not have come across before.

Think about it
These activities will get you to think about applying theory to a practical situation. They will give you an opportunity to stop and think about what you are doing when you are carrying out treatments to ensure that you are striving for and achieving best practice.

Salon life
This covers a key issue or problem, including an account of a therapist's experience in the salon and expert guidance on the issue or problem covered.

My story
Short, real-life accounts from people working within the industry with tips and suggestions designed to get you to think about the things you may encounter and need to think about in your day-to-day life as a beauty therapist.

Frequently asked questions
Expert advice and answers to some of the most commonly asked questions on each practical topic – questions that may come up as you work through the practical units.

Check your knowledge
This is a list of multiple choice and/or short-answer questions provided at the end of each unit to help you check your knowledge and understanding of that unit. Answers are available at www.pearsonfe.co.uk/Level2Beautyanswers

For your portfolio
These are tasks or activities which encourage learning through research and investigation. They are designed to help you to gather and generate evidence for your portfolio and key skills.

Getting ready for assessment
At the end of each unit you will find helpful information and advice about how that unit is assessed and guidance on what you will need to be able to demonstrate to your assessor in terms of skills and competencies.

Section

1

Professional skills

Essential professional knowledge

What you will learn

- You – as a therapist
- You and your client
- You, your client and the law

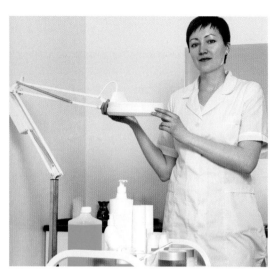

Introduction

Essential professional knowledge is literally everything you need to know about the skills you will require to become a qualified beauty therapist.

Before you can decide upon the most suitable treatment for your client, or prepare **treatment plans**, you need to have a clear understanding of the basic essential principles of what you are doing.

This section covers the underpinning knowledge you will need before you start working through any practical unit. You will need to refer back to this section each time you start a new practical unit.

You – as a therapist

In this outcome you will learn about:

- your professional presentation
- professional ethical conduct
- how to prepare to work
- salon services
- treatment planning and preparation
- effective teamwork and relationships
- record keeping
- safe working practices and legislation.

Key terms

Treatment plan – an outline of the most suitable skincare and treatment programme for a client to get maximum benefit.

Your professional presentation

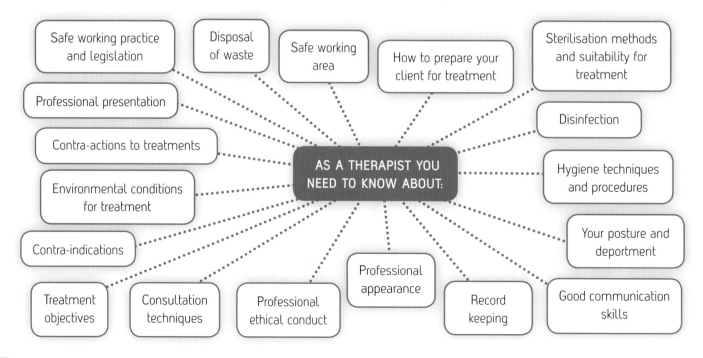

Safe working practice and legislation

Disposal of waste

Safe working area

How to prepare your client for treatment

Sterilisation methods and suitability for treatment

Professional presentation

Contra-actions to treatments

Environmental conditions for treatment

Contra-indications

AS A THERAPIST YOU NEED TO KNOW ABOUT:

Disinfection

Hygiene techniques and procedures

Your posture and deportment

Treatment objectives

Consultation techniques

Professional ethical conduct

Professional appearance

Record keeping

Good communication skills

All **Awarding Organisations**, clients and employers will expect you to have a professional appearance, not only to achieve your assessments but also to set the standards within your working life as a fully qualified therapist.

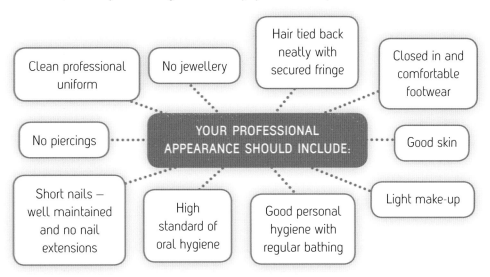

Awarding Organisation – your examination board which dictates and monitors the quality of the training you receive and issues you with your certificate when you have achieved your award.

Hygiene – conditions and good practices that promote and preserve health by preventing cross-infection.

A professional appearance helps you feel the part and gives the client confidence in your ability as a therapist. The expected standards of personal appearance are described below.

Hair

Hair needs to be clean, tidy and professional looking. It should be tied back away from the face. Your hairstyle should not interfere with the treatment. It is very distracting for clients if you have to keep flicking hair out of your eyes, and they may find this irritating. Equally important, by constantly touching your hair you will be breaking hygiene rules. You'll read more about **hygiene** on pages 34–40.

Nails

Nails should be clean, short and unvarnished (unless the employer states that, as a nail technician, you can have varnish on). Clients may develop an allergy to varnish, and chipped nail varnish is not a good advert for your trade! Unvarnished nails can also be seen to be clean. Long nails may scratch the client's skin when performing massage. Rough cuticles, bitten or dirty nails set a poor example and will not inspire confidence in your skills.

Jewellery

Hygiene and professional ethics state that the only jewellery permitted is a plain wedding band and small unobtrusive earrings. Rings could scratch the client and carry germs. Remember that other body piercing may cause offence to some clients and does not reflect a professional image. It is also a good idea not to take precious jewellery to work – this will reduce the risk of losing it.

Uniforms

Most salons and training establishments require a professional uniform to be worn. This should be clean, pressed, and of a suitable length to work in. It is advisable to go up a size to allow free movement, or at least try it on with arm movements tested!

Essential professional knowledge

It is also advisable to have several uniforms in order to allow one to be in the wash, and to prevent one uniform getting too soiled. Regular washing is essential to prevent body odour build-up as this can give off an unpleasant stale smell to the client.

Your training establishment will probably have a uniform policy and tell you the recommended supplier to go to — you should receive a good discount for bulk purchase as you are in a college or training establishment. Wear your uniform with pride — it will help you to feel professional and look the part!

Make-up

Subtle make-up may be worn, but heavy or stale-make-up (e.g. left over from last night) is not professional. If the skin is clear and the eyebrows tidy, the therapist may decide not to wear make-up at all — this is personal choice. The key should be how the therapist feels and looks on the day. Light make-up can hide minor blemishes and help tired eyes. If you need a 'pick me up', use it wisely.

Perfume

Remember that strong perfume may be as unpleasant to the client as body odour. Choose a light fragrance that does not overpower, and remember that stale perfume can be very off-putting.

Also bear in mind that perfume cannot hide body odour, so the use of anti-perspirants and deodorants is recommended, as well as daily bathing to prevent an accumulation of smells. An anti-perspirant will prevent perspiration building up, and a deodorant will help prevent odour. Most of the products available do both jobs.

Think about it

Personal presentation not only includes a professional appearance – good grooming and a smart uniform. Follow health and safety practice in the salon specifically covers personal hygiene, clothing and accessories suitable for the workplace as well as what to avoid, e.g. anything with the potential for an accident, such as very high heels, or dangling jewellery.

My story

Salon life

Hi. My name is Sam and I have just completed my Level 3 Diploma in beauty treatments. I have just got my first job in a well known spa in the New Forest in Hampshire, near to where I live. I thought my professional standards were good and my professional appearance was fine. However, as part of the interview procedure I was given the Code of Conduct for all therapists — they are part of the employment contract.

Hair must be up in a bun at all times and I had to buy a sponge ring to use so that it is the right shape. A spare pair of tights must always be in my locker in case of a ladder in my tights and bare legs are not permitted. I am not allowed to wear my salon (closed-in) shoes outside. They must be worn in the salon only. My nails must be short with no free edge showing over my fingers and no jewellery is to be worn at all. No chewing is permitted and certainly no smoking is allowed at all. I thought college was strict about this, but working for a national chain of spas is even more exacting. However, I can appreciate that it ensures all employees look the same.

At first I thought it was really harsh but now I feel very professional; when the staff are together for photos or public relations events it looks great. I suppose it's like being in the armed forces or being an air stewardess where you wear your uniform to represent who you are and fly the flag for your company. My professional standards are now even higher than when I was at college — yours will be too.

Shoes

Your shoes should be clean and comfortable for a full day's work. If your shoes do not fit securely, you could have, or cause, an accident.

Check with your training establishment about your footwear — commercial companies that supply uniforms often supply shoes too. Although in adverts for uniforms you may see the model wearing flip flops or open-toe shoes, they are not practical for all treatments. They would not provide protection if, say, hot wax were to be spilt on your feet.

Remember high heels are for going out in; they are not suitable for long working days and can damage your posture. Leather shoes allow the feet to breathe and are therefore more hygienic, preventing a build-up of bacteria, which may cause odour problems and lead to athlete's foot. All people in occupations that involve long periods of standing would benefit from support tights — even the young — as these can prevent varicose veins forming and stop the legs from aching.

Oral hygiene

Regular dental care will prevent tooth decay and keep gums healthy, so stopping bad breath forming. Regular brushing, mouth sprays, sugar-free mints and breath fresheners are also advisable to prevent stale breath being passed over the client. Remember that bad breath can be a sign of illness, so it may be worthwhile getting a dental or medical check-up if you think you may have a problem.

It is only polite and courteous to your client to avoid strongly flavoured foods, such as curry, garlic and onions, especially at lunchtime. Smoking can also cause odours that cling to the breath — a good excuse to give up smoking, even if only at work.

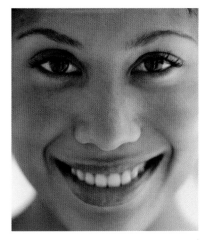

Oral hygiene

Think about it

It's not only on the breath that smoke lingers – it clings to clothing and hair, which can be off putting if you are delivering a treatment, say a facial, where you are in very close contact with your client. A mint cannot hide all of that! Smoking in public places has been banned since July 2007 so you will be liable to a heavy fine – £50 or a maximum of £200, if prosecuted – if you are found smoking in your workplace. For more on this, see You, your client and the law on page 42.

Benefits of professional presentation

For the therapist:

- Professional presentation helps you feel ready to take on a professional job role.
- It helps you feel part of a team as you all look the same.
- It encourages you to feel confident — you can take pride in looking proficient.
- It gives you self-assurance that you are meeting health and safety regulations.
- It gives you a self-belief and identity — you look as if you belong in the salon.
- It allows you to represent both yourself and the whole salon image.

For the client:

- A clean, tidy appearance gives a positive, lasting impression of both you as a therapist and the corporate image of the salon.
- Clients feel 'in safe hands' as you look competent and efficient.
- It gives clients encouragement with their treatments — clients often want to look like their therapist.
- It instils trust and a belief in you and your abilities because you look groomed and clients then realise that your treatments are effective.

Essential professional knowledge

Preparing to work

Personal presentation will take you only so far in your job role and dealing with clients — your attitude has to be right, too. Beauty therapy is a service industry. The general public are your clients and they pay for your service and expertise. Therefore they should also be entitled to your full attention and care.

It is not just the décor of a salon that creates atmosphere, it is the ambience created by the people within it. How the therapist mentally prepares for work goes a long way to producing the calm, relaxed feeling of a salon which allows the client to gain maximum benefit from the treatment.

Put on a smiling, caring expression when you are working — you may have lots of your own personal problems but passing them on to your client is not acceptable. Never gossip to your client about others: either staff or clients. Do not shout, swear or curse at work — you will develop the habit and not even realise when or to whom you are doing it.

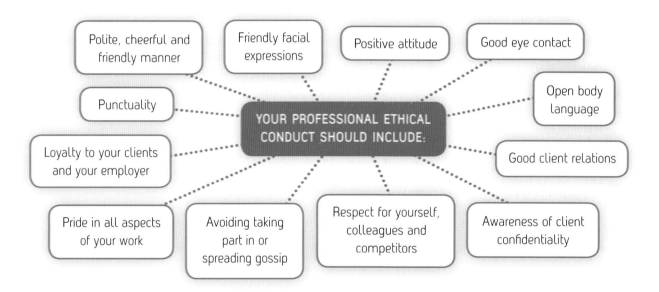

YOUR PROFESSIONAL ETHICAL CONDUCT SHOULD INCLUDE:

- Polite, cheerful and friendly manner
- Friendly facial expressions
- Positive attitude
- Good eye contact
- Open body language
- Punctuality
- Loyalty to your clients and your employer
- Good client relations
- Pride in all aspects of your work
- Avoiding taking part in or spreading gossip
- Respect for yourself, colleagues and competitors
- Awareness of client confidentiality

Think about it

Imagine going to a really grumpy therapist, who started late, rushed the consultation, didn't even remember your name and was generally rude. You just wouldn't go back again, would you?

It is said that you get out of life what you put in — and that is also true about a beauty therapy treatment. A quiet, relaxing facial should be as pleasurable to give as it is to receive. A good therapist will gain satisfaction from a tranquil hour and you will find that giving a facial massage is very soothing to both of you.

As a quality check after a treatment, a good therapist should ask herself:

- Would I like to be treated as I have just treated that client?
- Would I pay for the treatment I have just given to that client?
- Could I have improved upon the quality of my service?
- Was it as restful and as peaceful as it could have been?
- Has the client rebooked?

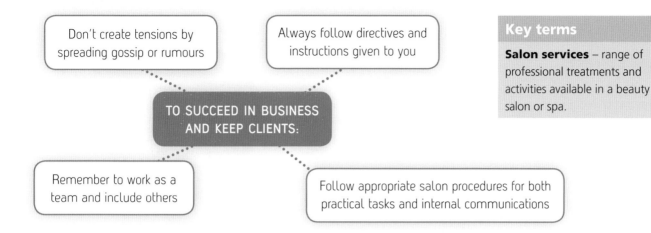

Don't create tensions by spreading gossip or rumours

Always follow directives and instructions given to you

TO SUCCEED IN BUSINESS AND KEEP CLIENTS:

Remember to work as a team and include others

Follow appropriate salon procedures for both practical tasks and internal communications

Key terms

Salon services – range of professional treatments and activities available in a beauty salon or spa.

Salon services

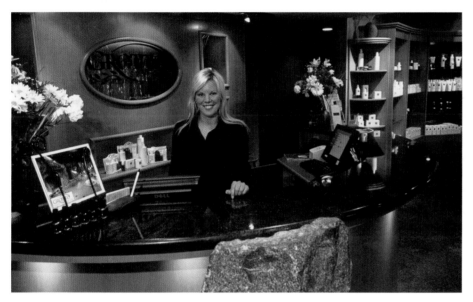

A good therapist is pleasant, patient and helpful to everyone who comes into the salon. The needs of each person will vary and you must be able to give correct information. If you do not know, you must be professional enough to admit your knowledge is not sufficient, and get a salon manager to help – rather than making something up.

Treatments offered

Even if you personally cannot perform the entire treatment list, it is important to be aware of all the treatments and sell them. A professional therapist will have a thorough knowledge of the treatment process, the advantages or disadvantages of each, and each of the topics mentioned below. The salon will lose business if you just shrug and say you do not know.

Think about it

Knowledge about your salon and the treatments and products it offers is key! Read through all new literature for the salon or new treatments when they are launched. Take responsibility to be up to date with all aspects of your salon, even if you cannot perform the treatments yet. For example, you could sit in on a training exercise or volunteer to be the model so that you can talk about what the treatment feels like and how it had a great effect on your skin. The same applies with products. Take home samples and try them so that you can talk with confidence about the feel, consistency or benefits of the product.

Essential professional knowledge

My story

Personal experience

Hi, my name is Sana. I am a first year Beauty Therapy student at a large college and when I first started I didn't know very much about other groups and what went on in other classes. The first term was all input for our manicure and pedicure and facial classes, so we were busy learning and didn't mix very much with the students in other years.

When we moved on to our practical assessments the external verifier said we could ask students from other classes to model for us and we could model for them. So far I have had a deep condition treatment on my hair for someone in the hair salon, I have had epilation on my face for a Level 3 student (I have quite dark skin, with facial hair) and I have had a full body massage for another group. This means I have had lots of different treatments and I now know what the other classes do – when I am on reception I can recommend treatments even though I don't do them myself. I feel more confident talking about all salon services now that I have experienced them and I would recommend that everyone does the same. I went home and raved about how lovely my massage treatment was and now my mum and older sister are coming in as assessment models for the other group.

It has really enabled me to get enthusiastic about what the college offers clients and I cannot wait to go on to Level 3 treatments and learn all about them.

Think about it

Do not guess the time it takes for a treatment: if you underestimate, it will disrupt the day's running order, and the therapist will be stressed trying to catch up; if you overestimate, the treatments will finish early and there will be gaps when the therapist is doing nothing, which is not cost-effective.

Key terms

Contra-action – an adverse physical reaction, as a result of treatment or products. This should be recorded on the record card.

Suitability of treatment

Not all treatments are suitable for every client. Some treatments require a sensitivity test, prior to the appointment, in order to assess the sensitivity of the skin or eyes. If a client has a treatment that was not entirely suitable for her, she will not be pleased. A customer who is not completely satisfied will not return and may spread bad publicity about the salon instead. Remember also to check for product suitability as clients may have allergies or intolerances.

Treatment timings

The timings of treatments should be accurately given. Do not mislead the client or underestimate how long a treatment may take, or your credibility will be undermined. In addition to this, the smooth running of the salon will be disturbed if timings are not given correctly. Learn the price list and treatment menu thoroughly so you can accurately book in a client, and not disrupt the running order for the whole day.

Time is money and in order to be cost-effective the timing of treatments must be accurate. Standard timings also help maintain the quality in the salon, so that all therapists offer the same time for each treatment. Clients are then all treated equally and get the same value for money.

The frequency of treatments given should also be negotiated with the client and will be dependent upon the time available, financial considerations of the client, the condition or suitability of the area of the body to be treated, and any **contra-actions** to the treatment.

If a deluxe manicure treatment with paraffin wax takes 45 minutes, and the receptionist has booked the client in for only 30 minutes, there is very little time to offer a relaxing treatment. So, either the treatment is modified (losing money for the salon), the treatment is rushed and the client is left dissatisfied, or the therapist overruns and keeps the next client waiting. All of this could so easily have been avoided, if the treatment time had been correct in the first place.

Prices

Prices will vary from salon to salon, and area to area. Price lists should always be on display. This allows the client to view the costs for herself and is also additional advertising.

Prices given should be truthful, with no hidden extras — no one likes to be conned.

Special offers

If the salon has any offers to pass on to the client, then the therapist needs to be aware of them. This helps to promote the offer and provides a chance to sell additional treatments that your client may not be aware of.

Most people like a bargain, or offer, and if they get to hear about it after the offer closes they may not be pleased.

Remember that there is legislation in place regarding sale prices (refer to the Sale of Goods Act, page 58, in the legislation section) so be careful when advertising a sale in your window.

Retail sales

Retail sales form an important part of any busy salon, and can help boost a therapist's pay at the end of the week.

Many salons offer a full retail sales service to complement the products used in the treatment. The therapist needs to be aware of what the salon sells, whether it is in stock, and what the benefits and features of each product are.

Money will be lost if you ignore the customer who wants to buy the product that has just been used within the treatment. Most suppliers provide large sizes of product for use in the treatment room, with a smaller retail size for the client. During the consultation, the therapist will ask the client about her homecare routine and which products she uses. Continuous care at home with the right products boosts the benefits of a salon treatment and good results can be seen.

The Beauty Salon

Face and eyes

Express facial (30 minutes)	£25
Radiance boost facial (30 minutes)	£32
Anti-ageing facial (60 minutes)	£45
Deep-cleansing facial (75 minutes)	£60
Eyebrow shape	£10
*Eyelash tint	£12
*Eyebrow tint	£10
*Eyelash and brow tint	£20

Patch test required 24hrs before treatment

Clients need to know what the different treatments and services are and the cost involved

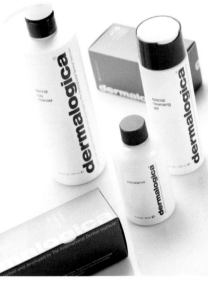

Retail sales are an important part of any business

For your portfolio

Carry out a comparison between two local salons in your area – are the prices and treatments offered the same or very different? Do they have a similar client base or do they cater for different tastes?

Think about it

Learners are sometimes hesitant about what they regard as 'hard selling', but it should be viewed as part of the aftercare given to a client, which involves recommending products that will enable the client to support the treatments carried out in the salon. It's a difficult skill to get right, and there is a fine balance between putting off a client with a hard-selling approach and not actually recommending anything! The skill comes with experience, confidence and belief in your products.

For your portfolio

When you sell retail-size salon products, keep a copy of the till receipt or daily taking sheet. This will be excellent evidence for your portfolio and shows you have communicated and listened to your client's needs.

If you are employed in a salon, also keep a copy of the salon price list and all the advertising materials the salon may have. You need to be aware of what your salon offers, regardless of whether you can perform the treatment or service, and you should understand what each involves.

Complaints

Realistically, a busy salon will encounter complaints. It is therefore important for the salon to have a complaints procedure, which staff are aware of and have been trained to follow. This will mean that when a complaint does arise, however minor, the correct salon policy can be followed. Here is an example of a complaints procedure.

1 Deal with any complaints pleasantly in a professional manner.
2 Calm the client and remove her from the reception desk to a more private area.
3 Listen to her. Be objective and not defensive – the complaint may be valid.
4 Be prepared to apologise if you are in the wrong and offer some form of compensation – a free treatment perhaps.
5 Try to reach a mutually satisfactory outcome. This will minimise the damage that a complaint may have on other customers, and prevent further legal action being taken.
6 Should the complaint be about another person, speak to the staff member later in a calm manner. Do not blame others in front of the customer.
7 Record the complaint in the customer comments book.
8 Be aware of the legal implications of further action (refer to the section on insurance on page 60–61).

Treatment planning and preparation

Treatment planning is essential for the smooth organisation of a salon where there is more than one therapist working. Through good organisation, the relaxed, calm atmosphere that a salon should have will be in place, and that will be reflected in the mood of both customers and staff. Even if there is only one therapist employed, treatment planning will help with time management in order to ensure that money is not lost.

Remember the old saying:

Time = money

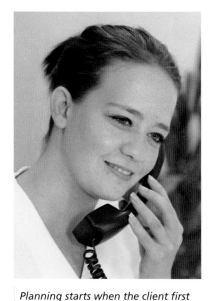

Planning starts when the client first books in for a treatment

Treatment planning should be viewed as an investment. The more planning carried out 'behind the scenes', the more professional the treatment becomes. The key is to be organised.

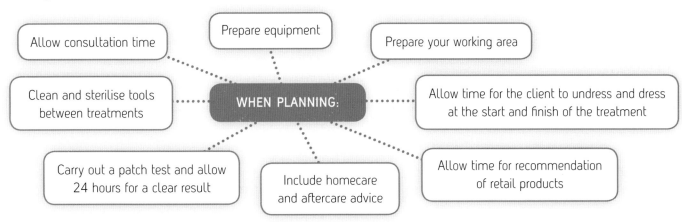

Good working relationships between staff should also be part of the planning for the salon manager or owner. Teamwork is very important and regular training and team building is essential.

The receptionist

A good receptionist is worth their weight in gold. They are the first person the client comes into contact with – often called 'front of house' as in a theatre. They represent everyone else within the business and should create a welcoming and excellent first impression. Their planning also needs to be first rate. A good receptionist will plan the whole day's running order for all therapists, with the right time allowances to ensure the day runs smoothly.

All the planning for the treatment starts with the receptionist and the initial booking of treatments. The receptionist needs to know:

- what treatments are being offered through the day and therefore which preparations can begin early, e.g. turning on the wax heaters
- what any treatment involves and therefore how much time should be booked out
- if this is a first treatment for the client or the middle of a course
- if a full consultation is needed, therefore requiring more time
- the 'before' and 'after' time required for the treatment, that is undressing/dressing, removing/putting on shoes, etc.

Extra time should be included so that a client relationship can be built up.

Last-minute alterations

An organised therapist will make the receptionist aware of any alterations to the day, any time out of the salon, and any change of plans, well in advance.

Obviously, the uncontrollable factor is sickness. If you have a full column of clients booked in and are unable to attend work because of illness, there is very little that can be done. Therefore, the earlier you notify the salon, the better.

The receptionist should be able to rearrange some clients for another day, or at least notify them, as they may wish to cancel. The other therapists in the salon then have

Think about it

Treatment planning and being on reception should be done in a calm and organised manner – if you are hurried and anxious, you will pass those feelings on to the client, who may be agitated and consequently not enjoy her treatment. Business may be lost.

Essential professional knowledge

the task of covering all the clients who cannot be contacted. This is dependent upon the goodwill of the other staff members, and a good relationship is vital for the health, growth and atmosphere of the salon.

It is useful to be aware of what the establishment policy is regarding illness and sick cover, as well as sick pay.

Good working relationships between staff should also be part of the planning for the salon manager or owner. Teamwork is very important and regular training and team building is essential.

Reliability is a valuable quality and helps to build goodwill among team members. If you are constantly relying on others to counter the effects of your bad planning or time management, then tensions may increase in the workplace.

Think about it

To obtain evidence of your salon reception duties, you will need to spend time acting as the salon manager on a rota basis. This puts you in charge of allotting treatments and managing the bookings for the day. If you are trying to fit in a full page of treatments and half of your team is off sick, it will involve a lot of swapping about and possible cancellation of clients. You will certainly see the other side of the coin and how disappointed clients are when their treatments are cancelled.

Sickness in the salon – what it may mean

For the therapist:

- spreading of germs or disease in the salon to both clients and staff members, especially something that is highly contagious such as sickness or diarrhoea
- unhygienic practice – even if it is a minor complaint such as a running nose, you cannot afford to 'drip' all over the client!
- lost wages – especially if you have a high sickness rate for odd days off
- lost business.

For the client:

- a cancelled appointment, which can be very disappointing
- exposure to additional germs and illness if a therapist with a contagious condition comes into work
- delays and rescheduling into another therapist's column
- the decision to take her business elsewhere.

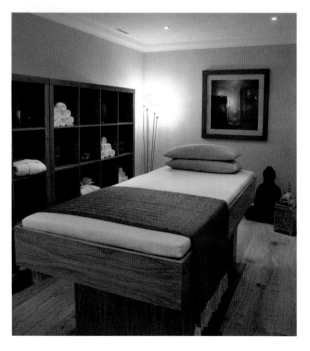

Environmental conditions

Treatment planning and preparation should also include the salon environmental conditions for both the client and therapist. More of the legislation requirements can be found in You, your client and the law on page 42 and in Follow health and safety practice in the salon. However, a general overview of what is acceptable to set the room ambience and to give a relaxing treatment is outlined opposite.

The room should not only look professional but must also be the right temperature, with soft lighting and gentle music to set the tone for relaxation

Suitable environmental conditions should include:

- heating — warm but not too stuffy or so hot that you and your client break into a sweat

- soft lighting — sufficient so that you can see what you are doing but the client can close their eyes and relax. Do not use overhead strip lighting which will hurt the client's eyes

- noise levels — avoid loud noises and sudden banging or loud music. Pick appropriate soft music and ensure that the client is not agitated by heavy metal or rock music. Your choice of music can wait until your drive home in the car — don't assume that what you like is suitable for the salon or the client

- ventilation — the treatment room should be sufficiently well ventilated to allow airflow. If it is too stuffy, both you and your client will get a headache — too draughty and the client will be too cold

- pleasant aroma — avoid heavy scents either from candles, air fresheners or the smell of food. The aroma in the treatment room should be pleasant and not overwhelming or too sickly sweet

- privacy of working area — regardless of the type of treatment, the area should be private and not in the main thoroughfare. The client should feel relaxed and not worried that they might be seen or disturbed. A closed salon room is ideal as long as you do not make yourself vulnerable and can easily gain help should your client behave in an inappropriate or abusive manner

- hygiene — a clean and hygienic working area will always set the tone of a professional and capable therapist and instil confidence. A client entering a working area which is still dirty from the previous treatment may not wish to wait (nor should they) for you to clean up and begin their treatment. You will have lost the business

- client comfort — go the extra mile with your client care and it will reap rewards for you — add a blanket or extra bedding for warmth, check the client is comfortable, provide a knee prop to aid with back problems, use a pillow for support and use hot towels or flannels for make-up and mask removal; generally pamper the client to make sure they feel special. They are paying for your time and expertise so make it such a special experience that they cannot wait to return!

Develop and improve personal effectiveness within the job role

You must prepare for the working day ahead and contribute to the planning of the salon. Remember, however, that treatment planning is not just about appearance and personal presentation as discussed on pages 10–13. Just as important is your approach or mind-set. Most organisational skills develop from having the right attitude.

Being organised and planning ahead can become second nature and almost part of your personality at work. Being prepared, tidy and forward thinking are very good habits to cultivate!

Benefits of personal effectiveness and organisation

The therapist will learn to ask themselves these questions:

- At home:

  Is my appearance professional and as good as it could be?

  Do I have everything I need for the day: money, lunch, keys, handbag, loose change for parking or the bus?

  Have I allowed enough time for my journey, public transport, or time to walk?

- At work:

  What treatments do I have booked in?

  Am I prepared for them? Have I got enough of the right equipment, stock and tissues, sponges and cotton wool?

  What time is my first appointment?

  Do I need to organise a float, till roll or fill up tea/coffee?

  Is my working area clean, tidy and welcoming for the client?

  Mind-set/mental approach:

  Am I calm and relaxed to greet my client?

  Am I focused on the client and not on my own problems?

  Am I confident in what I am doing?

  Am I fully prepared?

For the client:

- They will feel calmed by the tranquil atmosphere in the salon.

- Their pace will match the therapist's relaxed approach and they can begin to unwind.

- They will feel cosseted and pampered by the therapist's undivided attention.

- Their tension will drain away as they realise their treatment is hassle-free.

- They will want to repeat the experience — and will book another appointment!

Think about it

You will be given an appraisal at work to see how well you are doing and you will be expected to review your own performance at work. Ask yourself the following as you go through the day:

- What went right today and why?
- Did anything go wrong and why?
- Did I keep my clients waiting for their treatment or service to begin?
- Have I allowed enough time to give full attention to each client?
- Are my clients totally satisfied with my service?
- Is all my equipment to hand?
- Have I left my client unattended to go and get equipment?
- Can I help colleagues with their set up, or do I need help with mine?
- Would I pay for the treatments I have carried out today?
- How could I improve upon my performance tomorrow at work?

By continually evaluating your answers to the above questions you will be able to recognise and improve upon your working pattern. If being disorganised is a habit that you have fallen into, with the attitude that 'it really doesn't matter, because someone else will do it', then bad habits need breaking.

Effective teamwork and relationships

During your practical sessions, to enable assessments to take place, you will be asked to run a realistic working environment (RWE), with fee-paying customers booked in, just as in the industry. These sessions will involve you acting as salon manager for a day. You need good teamwork and an excellent relationship with your peers to be able to plan and run an RWE session effectively. How you organise the session affects everyone, and you need to be aware of what is expected of a salon manager.

The salon manager plays a vital role and it is important that you understand how what he or she does affects how the salon operates.

The manager

The role of the salon manager is vital to the treatment planning and preparation of the working day. A good manager will organise the salon, the staff and take responsibility for the wellbeing and safety of the clients.

For the salon, the manager will:

- have a set system in place for morning and evening preparation and jobs to be done (these should be on a rota basis for all to do)
- have procedures and rules for everyone to follow – this will provide a consistent standard of service
- have clear guidelines on treatment times and expected preparation time
- provide realistic times for specific treatments.

For the staff, the manager will:

- hold regular training sessions for everyone so that all members of staff know what is expected of them
- praise and reward those who perform well
- hold regular **appraisals** and direct those who are not organised
- instruct clearly and without favour
- instruct clearly with regard to being cost-effective, not wasting products and being uneconomical
- lead by example and be professional at all times.

For the client, the manager will:

- ensure that systems and procedures are in place for the health and wellbeing of all clients and visitors, including risk assessments on the salon and equipment, upholding the law on health and safety and holding regular fire evacuation practices (see pages 43–55 for more health and safety information)
- hold a first aid certificate that is up to date and valid
- protect the client with regular sensitivity testing for potential allergy-related products and ensure all staff are trained in these procedures
- take responsibility for complaints and refunds.

> **Key terms**
>
> **Appraisal** – a one-to-one meeting between an employee and their line manager to discuss how the job role is going and identify further training required. It may involve a considered opinion, estimation or judgement of an individual or an estimate of value.

Record keeping

Good record keeping is absolutely essential to any beauty salon. You should create and use good systems in order to keep track of your work and the clients.

Record cards

The functions of a record card are:

- to record relevant contact details so as to be able to contact the client if necessary
- to provide full and accurate information about the client to ensure client safety
- to ensure consistency of treatment — regardless of who performs the treatment
- to record the number of treatments in a course and the date of each — this is so that if the client changes therapists for any reason, there is a complete record of what they have had and when
- to note changes to the treatment programme or contra-actions if they occur
- to record the progress of the condition or treatment success
- to safeguard the salon and the therapists — to prevent clients taking legal action for damages or negligence.

The record card should be filled out in full for every treatment or service the client has. It should be written accurately, neatly and legibly.

Think about it

A record card can also be used to record information that will enable you to develop a better relationship with your client and perhaps to avoid saying something embarrassing. For example, a note that says 'recently widowed' or 'newly married' will not only be a good jog for your memory, but if you are off sick, and another therapist treats your regular clients, they will know whether to handle the client with extra sensitivity or enquire about her honeymoon — it doesn't take much to add a personal touch to a client's day!

Record systems

Most salons have a number system in place (see page 25), or keep records on computer. This is both for safekeeping and for easy retrieval. Most software packages for computers have a database system for easy recovery of names and storage. A computer system is a large cost to start with, but can be very easy to use, with the correct training. It is ideal for use in a larger salon, with a wide client base. However, the Data Protection Act 1998 needs to be upheld (see You, the client and the law, page 42).

If the data is set up in a database or spreadsheet, it is easy to print labels with client names and addresses so that you can post them details of promotions and special offers.

Think about it

The record card should be signed and dated, every time, to show the client gives written consent to the treatment. If the client is under 16 you must also obtain parental or guardian written consent. Some Awarding Organisations do not allow assessments to take place on minors, so do always check the age of the client when booking the treatment. The more detailed your record card, the safer and easier the treatment for all concerned.

For your portfolio

Some Awarding Organisations will require a parent/guardian's signature on a consent form for clients less than 16 years of age, and this should be attached to the record card. You will need to make sure a copy is in your portfolio if you are treating a young person.

Think about it

The personal information on record cards should always be kept private and confidential. Under the Data Protection Act you are not permitted to pass on names, addresses and other information about your client. If the salon or therapist does so, they may be liable to prosecution.

The storage of record cards should be given consideration. They need to be accessible to the receptionist or therapist, but not so open that others can view them. A locked filing cabinet or drawer is most common, with limited access to the keys.

The two most common ways of filing names are:

- a number system – client 1, client 2, etc.
- an alphabetical system – A, B, C, etc.

Alphabetical systems tend to use the first letter of the surname and if two names begin with the same letter, then the second letter is used, and so on.

Dermologica include a detailed skin mapping diagram on their facial treatment record card (Source: Dermologica)

Essential professional knowledge

Benefits of record cards

For the therapist:

- It provides a complete picture of the client. This will include: personal details, lifestyle, occupation, any medical conditions and minor health issues that may impact upon treatment.
- It gives an immediate view of potential problems: allergies to products, adverse reactions to products or treatments (known as contra-actions) and medical considerations which may affect the treatment, such as pregnancy.
- It tracks the treatments the client has and if she has had a course of specific treatments, providing a record of what the client has paid to date and how many treatments she has had – so avoiding any possible disputes.
- It provides a chart of the progress made and provides an opportunity to boost the client's morale and state how well she is doing.
- It protects the therapist against any accusation of misconduct, malpractice or negligence if filled out correctly and signed by the client – the client will have given her consent to the treatment being carried out.

For the client:

- It ensures the client's protection by providing a record of her medical history, so regardless of which therapist treats the client, all are aware of any medical problems.
- It provides a record of the client's improvement and allows her to see progress being made.
- It makes the client feel special, and it personalises the treatment – the client isn't just a number, she matters to the salon.

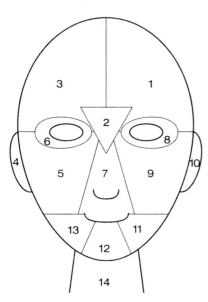

Skin mapping diagram (source Dermologica)

Subject specific record cards

Obviously, each client record card will be different and be personal to the clients: recording their treatment plan, skin problems, and personal history. Most product houses supply their own record cards which can be purchased in bulk. These offer a thorough checklist of contra-indications, the client's health, skin type, previous products used, retail sales history and so on. They also include a detailed line drawing of the face and body so that you can accurately highlight the problem areas – you must be as detailed as possible for both the continuity of the treatments and so that other therapists are aware of the treatment programme.

Think about it

Whichever treatment you are performing, the client will need a subject specific record card, so if she has a manicure, facial and eye treatments, she will need to have all three in her record file. You will need to fill out all of them as evidence for your assessments and as a written record to show her consent to having these treatments performed.

You and your client

In this outcome you will learn about:

- consultation techniques and questioning the client
- contra-indications
- contra-actions
- hygiene and avoiding cross-infection
- treatment objectives and client expectations

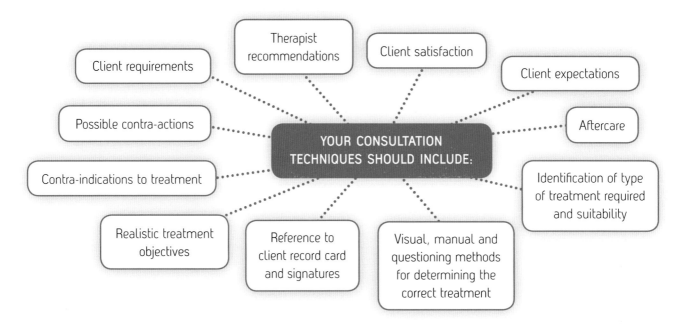

Client requirements

Therapist recommendations

Client satisfaction

Client expectations

Possible contra-actions

Aftercare

Contra-indications to treatment

YOUR CONSULTATION TECHNIQUES SHOULD INCLUDE:

Identification of type of treatment required and suitability

Realistic treatment objectives

Reference to client record card and signatures

Visual, manual and questioning methods for determining the correct treatment

Consultation techniques and questioning the client

This is a vital part of your role as a successful therapist. All treatments and services are based upon what you discover within the initial consultation. The only way to make a correct diagnosis of the client's needs is through questioning and then tailoring your plan to the information you receive. All practical assessments are based upon successful client consultations and recognising the client's needs.

All thriving salons earn their reputation by providing an excellent personal service. Care and attention to the client is the key to good business. The consultation should be carried out in privacy, and the service should be free. It is standard practice to link a consultation with a treatment plan.

The consultation also provides the initial bonding process between client and therapist. You can get to know the client a little better as well as gaining a clear picture of her for the treatment, including: contra-indications, her current skincare regime and how effective it is, and what she hopes to gain from the treatment or service. Managing a client's expectation is often a hard part of the consultation — a facial will make the skin look better and clearer, but it will not change the shape of the face, or turn the client into her favourite celebrity!

A good therapist will use all the skills mentioned and follow the client's body language to help obtain the information required for a good effective treatment plan. It must be agreed mutually that the time and money involved and the results suit both your client and yourself. If the plan is unrealistic, the client will not stay with the salon; she will go elsewhere.

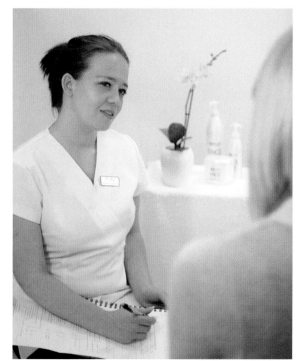

A successful consultation leads to a good treatment or service

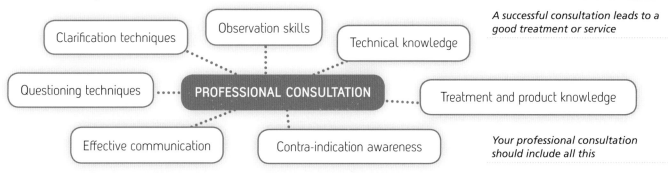

Clarification techniques

Observation skills

Technical knowledge

Questioning techniques

PROFESSIONAL CONSULTATION

Treatment and product knowledge

Effective communication

Contra-indication awareness

Your professional consultation should include all this

Questioning techniques

Asking questions is a skilled task. If you really want to find out what the client thinks and needs from you, you need to ask her. How you ask, what you ask and the type of question will dictate the reply you get. So, it is important that you give some care to your questioning technique.

If you ask the right questions and listen carefully to the answer, the treatment almost plans itself. All information should be included on the record card, which you will be filling out as you discuss details during the consultation. Use the record card as your guide. As already stated, verbal questioning will determine all the personal details — refresh your memory by looking at record cards on page 24. There are two types of questions: closed and open.

Closed questions

Closed questions usually need only one-word answers. They do not allow conversation to flow, but they are good for confirming information, so they have their place. For example, 'Have you ever had high blood pressure?' will enable you to confirm or eliminate information when the client responds with 'Yes, I have' or 'No, I have not'. Sometimes you have to use a closed question if you just require facts, but try to keep them to a minimum.

Open questions

Open questions provide a hook for the other person to respond in more detail than a simple 'yes' or 'no' answer. For example, 'How did you get to the salon today?' requires the client to give a more detailed answer, so such questions are good to break the ice. They help build a rapport with the client and put them at their ease.

A professional therapist will use open or leading questions to help put her new client at ease and draw them out ahead of the consultation. For example, the following open questions could be asked as she greets the client at the door.

- What's the weather doing out there now?
- How far have you come?
- Where did you manage to park the car?
- How did you hear about us?

It is better to use open questions than closed questions, such as the following.

- Is it still raining?
- Have you been here before?
- Did you get the bus?
- Is this your lunch hour?

Open questions are also a good means of recommending products, as you can start a dialogue about which products they have used, how they found them, how long they lasted, and so on.

A mixture of both open and closed questions will need to be used in the consultation process, but try to use them in the appropriate context — then they will become a great tool towards a thorough and professional consultation.

Observation skills

Diagnosis of the client's wellbeing is not only discovered by the consultation questions but also through observation. It can reveal as much as, and sometimes more than, questioning alone. You will be carrying out detailed observations on the specific areas of the client to be treated — these are covered in the individual practical units. However, it is not just about looking at the skin, or the area to be treated, it is about seeing the client as she first walks into the salon. The unconscious body language of the client can speak volumes about her general attitude and state of mind.

Think about it

We are all different. One client may be quite open and talk freely about herself and what she hopes to get from the treatment or service; others may be shy, and it may be some time before you fully gain the client's trust and confidence. As in life in general, relationships take time to build.

Never assume something about the client and listen carefully to the answers given.

It's a good idea to have a practice run – ask a close family member, or someone you know really well, whether you can carry out a full consultation on them. Although you know the person, try to view them as a client. Ask about lifestyle, skincare regime, diet, and so on, to build up a good picture of them.

A dropped pair of shoulders and dragging feet will indicate that she is nervous, a bit low in self-esteem or worried or anxious about something. A confident client will have more direct body language, more eye contact, with a spring in the step and an upright posture. So, when your client arrives it is important to observe:

- How they walk in — what does the body language say: confident or hesitant?
- How they stand
- How they sit
- If there is a mobility issue or disability to be aware of, or any other special consideration.

In addition to this, you may be able to look at some of the area to be treated (if on the face or hands), the condition of the client's skin, the amount of care and attention previously given to the area and how well the client is groomed — her hair, nail varnish, make-up.

If the client doesn't wear nail varnish or make-up, it may mean that she does not know how to use them, or perhaps considers them too expensive or time-consuming to bother with. She might also prefer a more natural look. All this will give you an indication of which treatments are likely to best suit the client's needs.

The other important factor to look at is, of course, your client's reactions to you.

Clarification techniques

Clarification means checking the details given by the client to ensure the information that she gives you is recorded correctly. You need to do this whenever information is being passed on to you. It will happen at all stages of client contact. The following are examples.

1   When the client makes a telephone booking, all information regarding date, time, the nature of treatment or service, and the client's name and number should be repeated back as confirmation. Avoid saying what the treatment is too loudly, as it could be of a sensitive nature, e.g. if the client is booked in to have a bikini wax, she may not appreciate everyone in reception knowing about it.

2   When the client arrives at reception for the appointment, the time of the booking and the name of the therapist can be repeated to the client.

3   When the client is having the consultation.

Repetition of details will enable the correct treatment plan to be prescribed and reinforces what the therapist may already know. For instance: 'So, Mrs Lakhani, your skin has been dry for most of the winter months. What products are you using?' This also gives the client lots of opportunities to respond to your open questioning techniques and therefore builds up a rapport between you.

Technical knowledge

It is very important that you fully understand the treatments you are talking about. Do not make anything up — this is very unprofessional. Always refer to the manufacturer's instructions and product information if you are unsure.

Think about it

Try to use straightforward language when talking to your client. Use words that she will recognise and avoid jargon: for example, refer to blackheads not comedones. The client will want to know what the treatment or service can do for her and the results. Resist the temptation to show off your knowledge of technical terms — they will only confuse her.

Essential professional knowledge

You should always have a copy of your salon's price list at hand to refer to. You could give it to the client to take home to look at later, as she may not take in everything you say during the consultation and might like to book a further treatment.

A good price list should have the treatment description, time of the treatment and the cost, along with a brief description of what happens and how it feels: for example, waxing should be highlighted as being slightly uncomfortable, like a plaster being ripped off the skin, and a deep facial massage could be described as 'total relaxing bliss'!

Product knowledge

Products, like treatments, require some time and effort so that you fully understand what they can do and how to use them properly. Be sure the information, benefits and effects you are claiming are true. It is also professional to ensure that the product you wish to sell to your client is appropriate and in stock. Selling an unsuitable product just to close the sale is very bad practice. You will lose the client as they can no longer trust you – you may have gained a sale in the short term but lost a client in the long term.

Regular training and visits from manufacturers will ensure that your information is up to date and accurate. Many companies are happy to visit training establishments to introduce their product. It is a good idea to volunteer to model for product training so that you can talk about what the treatment/product feels like and keep experimenting with the products. It is common for therapists to have their favourite products and just stick to those, as they feel confident with them. Because they use the same products all the time, they keep on recommending them, never extending their knowledge to other products. Often it is only when a product is discontinued that the therapist is forced into trying something new – so try to keep an open mind.

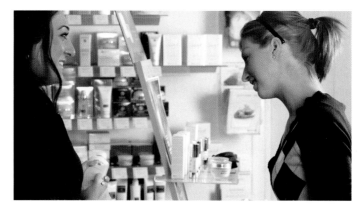

Treatment and product advice

The client has come to you (and is paying) for your skill and expertise. Some of her issues may be of a personal or sensitive nature. Be gentle with her and treat her kindly. Treat her as you would wish to be treated.

When giving advice remember never to patronise or talk down to your client. All clients should be treated with the same respect and courtesy, regardless of how trivial their problems or questions may seem. Be both honest and realistic with aims and objectives in the treatment plan, especially with courses of treatment.

Make sure the client realises that results may take some time and are often not instant. Perhaps some small treatments that do have instantly visible results could be used as a morale booster, such as a nail varnish with a manicure or an eyebrow tidy.

Think about it

Under the Trade Descriptions Act 1968 it is a crime to sell goods falsely, or to sell, or offer for sale, goods that have a false claim made about them. So, you cannot claim a cream will remove wrinkles or make you look 20 years younger. Look at skin product advertisements in magazines and on television: while they may say that the product can make the skin appear smoother or reduce the appearance of fine lines, they will not claim that the product will make fine lines disappear, as this would be a false claim. So, be very careful with regard to the law when putting together adverts or promotion materials for your treatments.

Get to know your products well and recommend them with confidence

Contra-indications

A contra-indication is the presence of a condition which makes the client unsuitable for treatment. A contra-indication means that treatment should not take place at all because it will be harmful to the client or make the condition worse, or it is a risk to others in the salon. A treatment is normally unsuitable because the client has a medical condition which may be external and/or visible, or it may be 'hidden' and discovered during the consultation.

Refer to individual practical units for full details of relevant contra-indications specific to the treatment or service. You should refer to them prior to commencing any treatment.

It is important that you do not treat the client because:

- the disease could be contagious and there is a risk of cross-infection to both therapist and other clients
- the condition may be made worse by a treatment
- there may be a reaction later, which puts the client's health at risk.

This is why it is essential to complete a thorough consultation, prior to any treatment being given.

If the contra-indication is small and localised in one area, treatment may take place with some adaptation. For example, a minor cut would be covered with a plaster. But a larger problem, such as a leg with open, weeping eczema, would be a definite contra-indication and further advice should be sought from the client's GP.

Be aware that some GP's surgeries request a small fee to cover administration costs which must be paid by the client. The salon provides a short letter outlining the treatments to be undertaken and the GP can just sign this. Most doctors are very open to their patients having beauty treatments and massage, as they recognise the health benefits – and some doctors refer clients to salons, for treatments such as electrolysis and massage.

The cost of a permission slip is preferable to risking a reaction to drugs taken, and a possible court case for negligence. The GP's permission slip could then be placed in the client's record card so that all therapists are aware of medical problems for that client and therefore all therapists are protected.

Anyone receiving chemotherapy or radiotherapy would be unsuitable for treatment as would anyone with a history of deep vein thrombosis. Always check with your Awarding Organisation with regard to its contra-indications policy.

Be very careful not to cause undue alarm when talking to your client about contra-indications. You are not medically trained and cannot offer an opinion on a possible contra-indication or medication taken and you may offend the client. Simply refer the client to their own GP and suggest they have the condition checked. You may be in a good position to notice a change in the skin or a mole – especially if it is on the client's back – but under no circumstances are you able to diagnose a possible skin cancer, or any other major condition.

Think about it

Remember – it is not just contra-indications that may prevent the treatment from taking place – some minor cosmetic procedures may also stop the treatment. If the client has just had any form of injected in-fills, e.g. collagen or dermal fillers around the mouth or eyes, recent plastic surgery, or is having strong medical level skin peels or taking large doses of steroids for a medical condition, then the treatment should not take place for 3–6 months afterwards.

Essential professional knowledge

General contra-indications

To help you remember different contra-indications, try to visualise looking from the outside of the body and work inwards, as shown in the table below. What you may see on the skin comes first, then muscles, bone, blood, and so on.

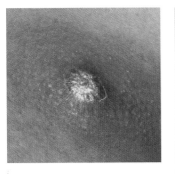
Boil

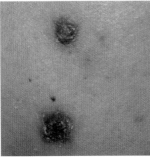
Impetigo

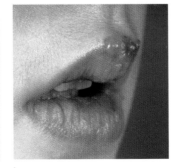
Cold sore

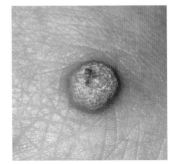
Wart

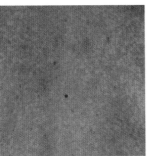
Measles

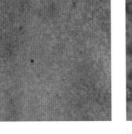
Chickenpox

Oral thrush

Skin	Muscles	Bones	Body systems
• Skin infections, disease or disorders • Open wounds or weeping sore • Cuts, bruising or abrasions • Raised or hairy moles or moles with uneven edges which have bled or weep • Unknown swellings • Recent scar tissue – do not treat until GP approval is agreed • Varicose veins or phlebitis • Medicines which impair the skin's healing properties or increase its fragility: e.g. Accutane given for acne may cause severe dryness and further treatments may exacerbate the condition; or antibiotics which can result in oversensitivity to sunlight and cause rashes or pigmentation. (Refer to You and the skin, pages 186–87, for a full list of medications and vitamins which affect the skin.)	• Dysfunctional muscular conditions, such as Parkinson's disease or multiple sclerosis • Loss of sensation to the area • Spastic muscle conditions • Dysfunction of the nervous system which affects the muscles, such as motor neurone disease • Dropped muscular tone, such as Bell's palsy (recognised as one side of the face being lower than the other) • Recent procedures, such as Botox® injections which freeze the facial muscles and may impair sensation • Collagen infill injections around the eyes or mouth	• Broken bones • Recent dental work, implants in the jawbone or cosmetic surgery such as rhinoplasty	• High or low blood pressure • Heart conditions • Diabetes • Epilepsy • Severe asthma • High fever, colds and flu • Hormone imbalances • Any systemic disease such as chronic liver conditions • Disorders of the endocrine system affecting any of the glands, such as thyroid • All types of cancer

It is very important you follow these guidelines when dealing with contra-indications:

◉ As a therapist, it is not your place to mention specific conditions to the client, because you are not medically trained. You can recommend that the client see her GP, but do not name the condition, nor offer any diagnosis or cure.

◉ It is important that the contra-indication is discovered prior to the treatment or service starting, rather than half way through. This stops the client being disappointed in not getting the full treatment and keeps your professionalism in place. It will also stop the condition from spreading to others, or putting them at risk.

◉ Some contra-indications if they are minor will not prevent the treatment from taking place, either because they can be covered over, or are not in the area to be treated. A client with a bruised big toe having a facial can obviously continue with the treatment.

◉ Clients may be forgetful and omit to mention they have a condition, such as high blood pressure, but may list the medication they are taking, often not remembering what it is for. Stop the treatment until you do know what conditions they have and ensure you get a GP's approval for treatment in writing and the client signs the consent form.

Contra-actions

A contra-action is the unfavourable reaction of a client to a treatment. Some treatments do cause some slight reaction, which is normal and to be expected: for example, a waxing treatment will cause the skin to go red, and there may be some blood spotting. It is a normal reaction to the slight trauma that the skin has undergone. However, an abnormal reaction to a treatment would be a severe response, such as that shown in the photograph.

It is up to the therapist to respond quickly to any adverse reaction that happens within the salon, in order to minimise the problem and not make it worse. The client must also be informed of what to look for after the treatment has finished and what action to take at home.

Contra-actions can occur with the application of any product — even one your client has used for years can suddenly produce a reaction not seen before.

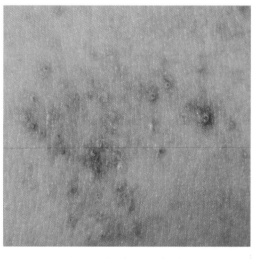

A contra-action on the skin can be burning, heat rash or general irritation

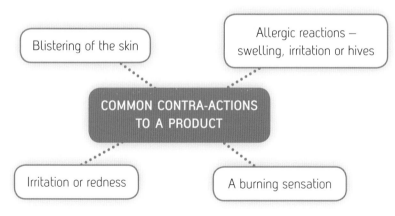

Blistering of the skin

Allergic reactions — swelling, irritation or hives

COMMON CONTRA-ACTIONS TO A PRODUCT

Irritation or redness

A burning sensation

Refer to individual practical units for specific contra-actions.

Essential professional knowledge

Think about it

During the consultation remember to ask your client whether she has any allergies. An allergy to anything can appear at any time, even if the client has been using the same products for years.

Nut allergies are more common than ever and lots of beauty products have nuts or nut extracts in them – exfoliators have groundnuts in them, almond oil is found in massage creams and there are also 'hidden' nut ingredients which may cause an irritation. Be very careful about using carrier oils for massage with nut additives in them.

Labels that claim a product is 'dermatologist-tested' carry no guarantee that the client won't have a reaction and what you have in a bottle is not necessarily what stays on the skin, as alcohol and water evaporate quite quickly, leaving behind a different compound for the skin to absorb.

Allergies

One common reaction to a product used within the treatment may be an allergic reaction. Clients can develop an allergy to a product they have been using for years. It can literally occur overnight. It may be a reaction to a food, a cleaning substance or an airborne droplet such as someone's perfume. Refer to You and the skin, page 214, for a full explanation of how an allergy occurs and how it affects the body.

Some allergies can be life-threatening and the client may go into anaphylactic shock, a condition of extreme hypersensitivity, which is an emergency condition requiring urgent medical attention. Symptoms include breathlessness, fever and, in extreme cases, the person falls unconscious and the heart stops.

Clients with a severe allergy will carry an EpiPen® which administers a dose of adrenalin to counter the effects of the allergy. Allergies to shellfish, bee stings and nuts are very common, but it can be a reaction to any substance such as house dust, pet hairs, and so on.

Hygiene and avoiding cross-infection

Hygiene may be defined as: 'The science concerned with the maintenance of health; clean or healthy practices or thinking.' So for you, as a professional therapist, hygiene could be described as good practice to maintain your own health, your clients' health and your colleagues' health.

However, there is no such thing as a completely sterile environment; perhaps the closest to it would be an operating theatre within a hospital. Germs are all around us and, while some are beneficial to humans, many of them are not. Beauty therapy treatments demand close human contact, so care must be taken to provide the maximum protection against cross-infection.

Think about it

The World Health Organisation is warning about the emergence of a new breed of superbugs which are resistant to antibiotics. The most common of them are methicillin-resistant staphylococcus aureus (MRSA) and clostridium difficile (C. difficile) and they are the most widely reported. MRSA causes infection, boils and abscesses and can be fatal if it enters into the blood stream. C. difficile is found in the gut and rarely causes problems in healthy people but when the balance of bacteria in the gut is impaired it causes diarrhoea and severe inflammation of the bowel, which can prove fatal.

Many superbugs live on or in the body quite harmlessly and only cause problems when the immune system is weakened by illness (or if they enter via an open wound in the skin, mouth, nose or urinary tract). This is why it is more common to pick up a superbug in a hospital where patients' immunity is already low. They spread in the same way as any other bacteria – through touching contaminated surfaces and then touching a vulnerable person, such as a baby, the elderly or someone who is already ill.

Good salon and personal hygiene should prevent any infections spreading: washing hands well after using the toilet, before eating and before and after treating each client.

Expert advice on hygiene can be confusing. There have been conflicting reports in the media regarding AIDS and hepatitis, and the resistance of some bacteria, such as MRSA, commonly found in hospitals, to antibiotic treatment. The most valuable up-to-date information can be gained from your Awarding Organisation's code of ethics or practice (refer to it for more details). These guidelines have been established after a great deal of research on behalf of the beauty industry, and are most likely to be current.

It is important to understand the responsibilities we each have under the Health and Safety at Work etc Act 1974, and under the COSHH (Control of Substances Hazardous to Health) regulations. Refer to the legislation section on pages 42–58 for extra guidelines.

Micro-organisms

In order to understand how to maintain the highest hygiene standards it is important to know how infection can occur. Micro-organisms are organisms that are too small to be seen by the naked eye. These micro-organisms are ever-present in the environment and can cause different types of infection.

Micro-organism	Diseases they cause
Bacteria	Boils, impetigo, sore throats, meningitis, pneumonia, diphtheria, tuberculosis, typhoid fever, tetanus (lock jaw), whooping cough
Viruses	Common cold, flu, cold sores (Herpes simplex) warts, measles, rubella, mumps, chicken pox, Hepatitis A, B and C, HIV
Fungal/yeast infections	Ringworm of the foot, body, head and nails, thrush, infection to the heart and lungs, which may prove fatal
Protozoa	Diarrhoea, malaria, amoebic dysentery

Micro-organisms enter the body using any route they can:

- through damaged, broken skin
- through the ears, nose, mouth and genitals
- into hair follicles
- into the blood stream via a bite from blood-sucking insects (e.g. malaria).

So, disease is spread by:

- direct contact with a person who has a disease or infection
- infection from droplets in the air, as when someone sneezes near you
- indirectly — when you touch an infected item such as a towel or cotton wool.

Think about it

Disposable gloves

There are a wide variety of disposable gloves on the market and therapists must ensure that health and safety legislation is adhered to, to protect themselves and their clients from cross-contamination. Most Awarding Organisations also specify that gloves should be worn for treatments in which there is a possibility of contact with bodily fluids and/or if the skin is being pierced, for example epilation, intimate waxing and microdermabrasion.

- Always buy medical-standard, single-use only disposable gloves from a reputable manufacturer and use within the expiry dates.
- Gloves should be chosen to fit snugly on the hands.
- Do not apply talc to the hands prior to use as this may cause an allergic reaction.
- Always wash and dry hands thoroughly before and after using gloves.
- Do not use the gloves if they are damaged, smell or have holes in them.
- Latex gloves should be avoided as they may cause an allergic reaction.

Essential professional knowledge

Think about it

All good hygiene practices should be continuously carried out to ensure that no cross-infection takes place – starting with preparation of the work area, the treatment itself, through to leaving the work area and equipment clean and tidy ready for the next treatment. The client will then have total confidence in the salon and it ensures you are following all the required health and safety regulations.

The symptoms and severity of the infection or disease will depend on the type of invasion, the strength of the person's immune system, whether it is able to defend the body, and their general health. If a person is run-down, then the micro-organisms have more chance of multiplying rapidly. They also thrive in poor hygiene. The best ways of avoiding these are prevention – through good hygiene practices.

Some of these diseases are life threatening, but many are not and can be prevented by good hygiene. For example, protozoa can be transmitted from contaminated food and water, which grow and infect the bowel causing ill health with diarrhoea.

Many of these diseases are also radically reduced by vaccination. Precautions can be taken against both Hepatitis B and tetanus – recommended for beauty therapists. Most school children are given immunisation against measles, mumps and rubella, unless there are medical reasons not to have the injections. Whooping cough has been dramatically reduced by the same method of immunisation.

Refer to Contra-indications, pages 31–33, for recognition of the common diseases that may prevent the treatment from taking place.

My story

Cleaning your tools

Hi, my name is Anya. We were learning pedicures and had to swap partners with someone we had never worked with before. Unfortunately, although the tutor told everyone to make sure they followed the correct sterilisation procedures, the student didn't sterilise her equipment properly, and I'm fairly certain I got athlete's foot from her tools – I didn't see her put them in the autoclave, but I couldn't prove anything. I told my tutor about it, and she reminded everyone in the group how important it is to clean and sterilise tools properly. Too late for me though!

Good hygiene practices

How do you maintain good hygiene practices in a beauty salon?

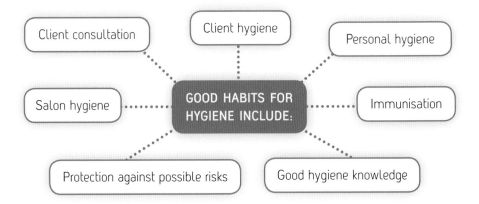

GOOD HABITS FOR HYGIENE INCLUDE:
- Client consultation
- Client hygiene
- Personal hygiene
- Salon hygiene
- Immunisation
- Protection against possible risks
- Good hygiene knowledge

A guide to controlling micro-organisms

Alcohol

Alcohol-based disinfectants are very good for soaking metal instruments such as small manicure equipment. The usual dilution is 70 per cent isopropyl alcohol – or a surgical spirit base. Once it has been used, the disinfectant should be thrown away and a fresh solution made up for every client.

Isopropyl alcohol is an antibacterial solvent used in many different products, from aftershave to hand lotions and cleaners. It is made from propylene, which is obtained during the cracking of petroleum. It is a good cleaner, but the fumes can be an irritant, so surgical spirit, commonly bought over the counter at the chemist or local wholesale supplier, can be used instead.

Ammonia

Ammonia is commonly used as a base for trade liquids used to kill bacteria, e.g. barbicide that is used to soak suitable instruments in salons. The drawback with using ammonia is its strong smell!

Antibiotics

An antibiotic is a chemical substance that destroys or inhibits the growth of micro-organisms. Antibiotics are usually used to treat infections that will respond well to them, such as fungal or bacterial infections, and are given to humans and some animals for treatment. They can be taken as tablets, or as a cream applied to the area, or in an injection, or, if in hospital, they can be administered in a drip form straight into the blood stream. They are not available over the counter to buy. They are only issued on prescription from a doctor.

Antiseptic

An antiseptic is a chemical agent which destroys or inhibits the growth of micro-organisms on living tissues, thus helping to prevent infection when placed on to open cuts and wounds.

Autoclave

An autoclave is a piece of equipment rather like a pressure cooker, used to sterilise small metal equipment, such as eyebrow tweezers and manicure items. It works by heating distilled water under pressure to a temperature higher than 100°C, so creating an environment where germs cannot survive.

Ideally, the autoclave should heat up to 121°C for 15 minutes. There is a stacking system of baskets in the base so that lots of small tools can be put in together, but they should be washed and clean prior to sterilisation. If several therapists use the autoclave at one time, be sure that the equipment is easily identifiable – perhaps with a blob of nail varnish, otherwise you will not know which tools belong to whom. The autoclave is most suitable for small metal tools. Refer to the individual manufacturer's instructions for use.

Bactericide

This is a chemical that kills bacteria but not necessarily the spores, so reproduction may still take place. It can also be called biocide, fungicide, virucide or sporicide.

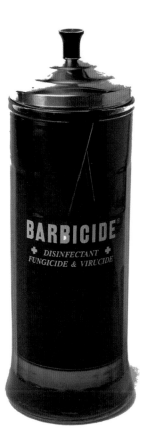

A Barbicide® disinfecting jar

Chlorhexidine

Trade names for chlorhexidine include Savlon and Hibitane. Chlorhexidine is widely used for skin and surface cleaning and some sunbed canopies. Check the individual manufacturer's instructions for cleaning.

Detergent

A detergent is a synthetic cleaning agent that removes all impurities from a surface by reacting with grease and suspended particles, including bacteria and other micro-organisms. Detergents need to be used with water but are ideal for cleansing large surface areas.

Disinfectant

This is a chemical that kills micro-organisms but not spores – most commonly used to wash surfaces and to clean drains. Disinfectants can only work against bacteria and fungi. They reduce the number of organisms, minimising the risk of infection. In medicine, disinfectants (e.g. Triclosan) are used to clean unbroken skin. Hypochlorous acid is a weak unstable acid, occurring only in solution, which can be used as a bleach and disinfectant. Products containing sodium or calcium hypochlorite can be used on large surfaces, such as floors and walls, as they are relatively inexpensive to buy. They can however be corrosive and are not suitable for soaking metal instruments or applying directly on to the skin.

Phenol compounds

Phenol compounds are ideal for large areas that need cleaning, but phenol does have a chlorine base and should not be used on the skin. It is used in industrial cleaning preparations and the old-fashioned carbolic soap.

Sanitation

Sanitation is a generic term relating to health and the measures for the protection of health, that is to be free of dirt and germs, and to be hygienic. The word comes from the Latin *sanitas*, meaning health.

Sterilisation

Sterilisation is the complete destruction of all living micro-organisms and their spores.

Surgical spirit

Surgical spirit is widely used and easily available from chemists. It can be used for skin cleansing, and to remove grease on the skin. Surgical spirit comes in varying strengths of dilution. A 70 per cent alcohol base concentration is acceptable for cleansing.

Ultraviolet boxes

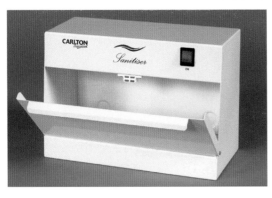

Some salons use an ultraviolet (UV) light box to destroy bacteria. UV rays are generated from a quartz mercury vapour lamp (similar to a mini sunbed) with a low rate of penetration. The tools have to be thoroughly clean and dry before they go into the box, otherwise germs will cling to the dirt or dead skin cells on the surface and form a barrier preventing sterilisation from fully taking place. The tools also need to be turned around after 15 minutes because the rays only clean the surfaces of the tools. Only metal tools such as cuticle nippers are suitable for UV sterilisation and, of course, once you touch them taking them out of the box, they are no longer sterile.

UV rays are harmful to the eyes, so the box should be switched off before you open it. UV bulbs have a limited life, so a log of usage should be kept and the bulbs replaced when recommended by the manufacturer. Always follow manufacturers' instructions.

For your portfolio

Investigate the recommendations of beauty wholesalers and suppliers for cleaning and sterilisation products. Look at the advantages/disadvantages of each. Which is the most effective? Which has the most pleasant smell? Which is the best value for money? Which is the most versatile and can be used on lots of surfaces? Which ones would you use if you had your own salon?

Use the internet to research advice on cleaning and sterilisation, e.g. the Health and Safety Executive, your Awarding Organisation and Habia websites.

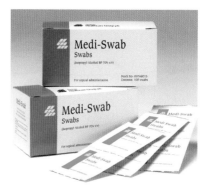

Medi-wipes

There are a great many commercial products on the market for cleaning and sterilisation — with lots of different trade names. This is merely a general guide. Please consult the manufacturer's instructions for each individual piece of equipment. Most companies have their own particular favourites that they recommend.

Your personal hygiene

- Always wash your hands — ideally with bactericidal gel — before and after every treatment.
- Wear disposable gloves for treatments if there is a possibility of an exchange of body fluids, e.g. waxing.
- Wear protective clothing for protection and to ensure a professional appearance, e.g. an apron for waxing.
- Cover cuts or broken skin with a waterproof plaster.
- Keep nails short and scrub under them with a nail brush.
- Do not come into work if you know you have an infection or disease likely to put anyone else at risk, e.g. impetigo.
- Wash hands thoroughly after every visit to the toilet.
- Follow the guidelines given in the section on professional presentation (pages 10–13) for clean uniform, etc.
- Attend training programmes about hygiene and the use of sterilising equipment.
- Do not use equipment that is cracked or broken, as germs will be present. This includes chipped cups, plates or glasses.

Salon hygiene

- Sanitise used equipment as fully as possible. This means following the manufacturer's instructions for individual equipment, such as using the recommended cleaner for make-up brushes so that the bristles do not fall out. Some cleaners will dissolve the glue that holds them in place.
- Tools should always be washed in hot, soapy water, rinsed well and dried thoroughly, before using a sterilising fluid or a UV box.
- Invest time and correct training in the use of sterilisation equipment, such as an autoclave or sanitising unit.

Think about it

Germs and disease can be found in all sorts of unlikely places. Even a cracked cup will contain germs, so if you give the client coffee in a chipped mug, or water in a cracked glass, you are not upholding good hygiene practices. Always dispose of chipped or cracked cups/mugs/glassware.

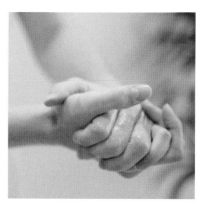

Thorough handwashing is essential to good hygiene

Essential professional knowledge

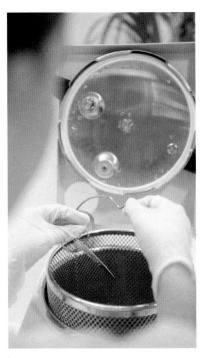

An autoclave can be used to sterilise metal instruments by using a very high temperature to kill bacteria

- Clean the treatment area or room thoroughly. Clean it daily and also wipe generally after each treatment has taken place. There are many preparations on the market for use on walls, floors and work surfaces, trolleys and couch and stool.
- All work surfaces should be cleaned regularly with hot water and detergent.
- Couch roll and towels can be used as a barrier between blankets and the clients – they can then be disposed of, and fresh ones put on for each client.
- Tissues tucked into the headband or turban can be disposed of after use, so keeping the headband/turban looking fresh.
- Towels should be washed after use – so your salon needs to invest in plenty of towels to ensure you do not run out.
- The same applies to towelling robes for clients. Big fluffy robes are very luxurious, but the image would soon be spoilt if dirty ones were given to clients. Soft cotton robes are easier to wash and keep clean.
- When carrying out a facial and wrapping the client up in blankets, for hygiene purposes use a cotton sheet as a barrier between the blanket and the client. The sheet can be washed on a boil wash, therefore washing and drying times and costs are saved as you do not have to keep drying heavy blankets. Some salons use duvets to cover clients and the covers can be easily replaced.
- Disposable brushes for applying make-up will prevent cross-infection from lips and eyes.
- Make-up pencils should be wiped clean with spirit and re-sharpened to get rid of any contamination.
- Powder eye shadows and blushers need to be scraped on to a palette and then applied to the client, to avoid contamination.
- Creams and oils need to be decanted into a smaller bowl, using a spatula, and any excess should be thrown away. Never pour back into the original container any product that has been in contact with your hands or the client. In order to be cost-effective, be careful not to pour out too much, as it may be wasted.
- Disposable spatulas should be used for waxing, that is one use from pot to client, to avoid contamination.

Client hygiene

- It is a good idea to have some form of notice in the reception area asking clients to inform staff if they are suffering from any contagious diseases.
- Always carry out a full consultation to discover any contra-indications.
- Always perform a physical check of the area to be treated for infection, etc.
- Do not treat if any unrecognised problems are present.
- Ask the client to sign the declaration on the record card stating that all medical and other information is correct to date, to avoid possible repercussions later.
- Before you start, always wipe the area to be treated with the appropriate lotion, e.g. surgical spirit, Hibitane or the recommended choice of your establishment.
- Provide all possible protection for the client and insist that clients use the recommended procedure, e.g. treading on the couch roll with bare feet to avoid touching the floor surface.
- Discourage the client from having a treatment if she has the beginnings of an illness – she may really want the treatment but spreading a cold or flu to you and to other clients and therapists is not sensible.

Think about it

Most commercial washing powder manufacturers now make a washing powder which is antiseptic/bacterial at a 40-degree wash – use it for all linens and you will be safeguarding the clients' hygiene.

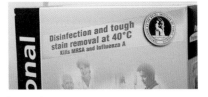

A good washing powder keeps laundry disinfected and is also eco-friendly as it washes at a low temperature

Client modesty

Whatever treatment your client is having, remember to preserve her modesty and dignity. This is especially important on the first treatment, as the client may be very unsure of the procedures.

- Explain fully to clients how they will be positioned and how much clothing they will need to take off – a facial would not require the removal of the lower garments, but a wax treatment would. Make sure clients understand this.

- Always allow clients to get undressed and into a robe in privacy behind the curtains.

- Cocoon the client in a blanket and towels, with couch roll if required for treatment, and only expose the area of the body being treated. This will not only ensure the client is cosy and secure, but will also preserve modesty and provide warmth.

- Provide full instructions and a modesty towel if carrying out a more intimate treatment, such as a bikini wax. Ask the client to place protective couch roll in the panty line rather than just assuming she won't mind you doing it.

- Ensure your working area or cubicle is private and that others are not able to see in. No one having a bikini or leg wax wants to feel that they can be seen by the general public. Even a facial is not a very relaxing treatment if the client feels exposed.

- Respect clients' modesty by keeping personal details, information and record cards confidential and private. It is a privilege to be a party to certain information – do not abuse the clients' trust by sharing information with others unless it is necessary for a professional referral.

- Allow the client time and personal space to dress and prepare to meet the outside world after the treatment. Do not pull back the curtains and tell her to get up as your next client is waiting – this is very bad practice.

- Finally, treat your client as you yourself would wish to be treated – with dignity, respect and as a valued customer.

Treatment objectives and client expectations

It is important to explain the treatment thoroughly to the client. It is equally important that the client understands what the treatment involves. This will help to ensure client satisfaction, avoid misunderstandings, dispel any unrealistic expectations and give the client confidence in the salon and the therapist.

Honesty between therapist and client is part of the ethical conduct that is expected of all beauty therapists in order to maintain high professional standards. The table below gives some examples of unrealistic and realistic expectations.

Treatment aim	True	False
Waxing is a permanent method of hair removal		✓
Regular waxing makes the hairs grow back weaker		✓
All hairs grow back at the same time		✓
Waxing does not hurt		✓
Waxing does not change the hair colour	✓	
Tinting makes the eyelashes thicker		✓
Tinting the eyelashes is permanent		✓
Regular facials make the skin grow older faster		✓

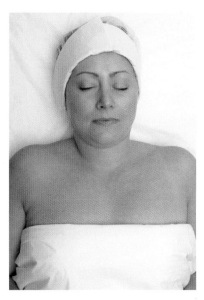

Make sure your client feels secure and relaxed before you start

Think about it

It is important to give the client aftercare advice on hygiene practices to be carried out following treatments such as comedone or milia extraction, waxing or eyebrow shaping where there may be blood spotting. There is a risk of infection occurring if the client does not follow simple hygiene rules such as keeping the area clean, covering it with a plaster and avoiding picking at the skin.

Think about it

A satisfied customer will return and will also tell everyone else about how good their salon experience was – word-of-mouth advertising is invaluable and free! A good reputation starts with positive feedback and grows from there.

Be truthful with your clients and they will always respect and trust you.

Essential professional knowledge

The client must also be aware of:

- the time involved in a treatment
- the total cost of the treatment or course of treatments
- the position she will be in – on the couch, seated, etc.
- the expected outcomes
- the length of time the treatment should last
- the possible contra-actions to the treatment
- the aftercare and home care for the treatment
- the cost of items that may be purchased
- the cost of maintenance, e.g. for artificial nail structures
- how often the treatment should be given for maximum effect
- the reasons for a sensitivity test, consultation and record cards.

The entire list above has a part to play in creating the complete picture for the client, so that the therapist gains the client's full trust and confidence.

You, your client and the law

In this outcome you will learn about:

- legislation
- local by-laws
- insurance
- independent regulators
- industry codes of practice
- salon guidelines.

There are many regulations and lots of **legislation** covering you and your work in the salon. Any person dealing with members of the public and working with other people has to be aware of the law, and how to use it to be safe. You do not need to know all the regulations in detail, but you do need to know what your responsibilities are.

Legislation

All businesses are covered by laws as set down by the government in Acts of Parliament. These Acts of Parliament are continually being updated to fit into modern society, so you will find that Acts have dates after their title stating when they were updated, such as Trade Descriptions Act 1968 (amended 1987).

These Acts are the law of the land. Breaking or ignoring them is therefore an offence, and can lead to punishment. You could be fined, your business could be closed or you could go to prison.

As well as UK law, there is European Union law to follow, too. The European Union (EU) is currently made up of 27 countries, including the UK, which joined the EU in 1993. EU laws are decided in Brussels, where the European courts are based, and all EU member states follow the same legislation.

Key terms

Legislation – laws passed by parliament.

Think about it

None of us can get away with claiming ignorance about the law. We should each take responsibility for our deeds and actions and must face the consequences if we act recklessly or endanger others. Insurance cover may be null and void if you are proven to be negligent or if legislation or establishment rules have been broken or ignored. An accident or injury to others could be the result with serious implications to you personally and your employers.

In order to be fully competent in employment it is essential that you have a sound knowledge of the basis of consumer protection and health and safety legislation. You need to understand how these laws protect you, your colleagues and your clients. The specific legislation that you need to know is given on the following pages.

Health and Safety at Work etc Act 1974

This requires all employers to provide systems of work that are, as far as is reasonably practicable, safe and without risk to health.

The employee has a duty to herself/himself, to other employees and to the public.

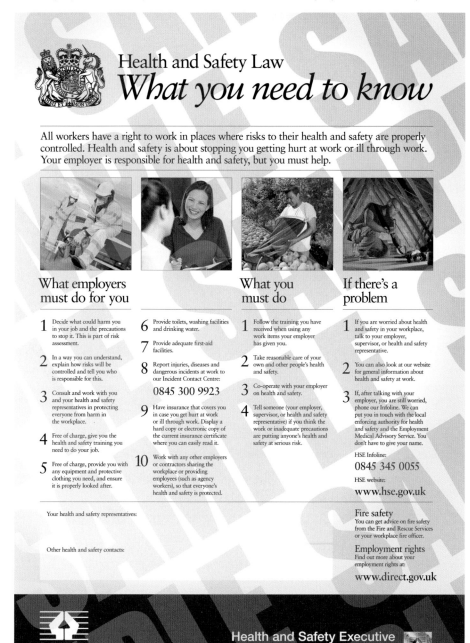

(Source: Health and Safety Executive)

The employer must:	The employee must:
Identify health and safety risks and hazards	Be aware of risks and hazards and not endanger others
Provide information and training for employees on services and equipment	Participate in regular training sessions, follow manufacturers' instructions and use, handle, store and dispose of products correctly
Provide storage for products and equipment	Store products and equipment correctly
Provide and maintain PPE	Comply with PPE regulations and use the equipment provided
Organise regular scheduled maintenance and checks of the salon and equipment by a competent person	Report faulty equipment and perform checks before use
Provide the correct environmental conditions	Maintain the correct environmental conditions
Observe and remove any obstructions	Ensure walkways and doorways are not obstructed
Provide the correct waste and recycling bins	Dispose of waste correctly
Ensure scheduled and regular breaks occur and are catered for	Take regular breaks and actively participate in organisation of rotas for fair working conditions
Provide eyesight tests when requested	Inform the employer if a sight test is required
Provide workstations, stools, desks and couches at the correct height and size	Use equipment for its intended purpose only and work safely
Provide staff training on how to correctly lift and carry objects	Lift and carry objects safely
Provide a designated first aider and a full first aid box	Identify the first aider and the location of the first aid box
Report injuries, diseases and dangerous occurrences to the HSE	Inform a manager of any injuries, diseases or dangerous occurrences
Display safety signs	Observe and follow safety signs
Provide fire fighting equipment and fire evacuation training	Participate in fire fighting equipment and evacuation training and only use in an emergency
Carry out risk assessments and ensure accident report forms are completed	Ensure risk assessments and accident report forms are completed in full
Provide amenities for staff	Use amenities safely
Provide safety glass and locks on windows and doors	Ensure window and doors are locked at the end of the day
Hold valid and current liability insurance	Work within the guidelines of their professional body to ensure insurance is valid and safe
Have salon policies and procedures in place and have regular meetings	Attend training and follow salon policies and procedures
Provide the opportunity to keep safe and valid client records	Keep accurate records and follow data protection law
Consult experts and implement knowledge within all aspects of the business	Participate in training sessions and implement any updates

Employers' and employees' health and safety responsibilities

The Act allows various regulations to be made, which control the workplace. It also covers self-employed persons who work alone, away from the employer's premises.

Employers' responsibilities	Shared responsibilities	Employees' responsibilities
Planning safety and security	Safety of all individuals in the workplace	Correct use of systems and procedures
Providing information about safety and security	Safety of the working environment	Reporting flaws or gaps in the system or establishment procedures
Updating systems and procedures with five or more employees	Never knowingly endangering anyone	Taking reasonable care of themselves and others
Regular training and information for all staff	Following all Health and Safety at Work Act directives	Cooperating with employers in the discharge of their obligations

In 1992 EU directives updated legislation on health and safety management and widened the existing acts. These came into force in 1993. There are six main areas:

- provision and use of work equipment
- manual handling operations
- workplace health, safety and welfare
- personal protective equipment at work
- health and safety (display screen equipment)
- management of health and safety at work.

Some provisions of the EU directives are:

- the protection of non-smokers from tobacco smoke
- the provision of rest facilities for pregnant and nursing mothers
- safe cleaning of windows.

The Management of Health and Safety at Work Regulations 1999

These regulations place responsibility firmly on the employer to make significant risk assessments for the health and safety of employees and others working in the salon, record any significant findings, and instruct and train employees in the correct way to ensure all are protected. Codes of practice and systems need to be monitored, reviewed and adjusted to suit. All employees should be informed of these, and a statutory poster for health and safety displayed in the workplace.

The regulations cover a great deal of information for employers including:

- risk assessment
- principles of prevention to be applied
- health and safety arrangements
- health surveillance
- health and safety assistance
- procedures for serious and imminent danger and dangerous areas
- contact with external services
- information for employees
- cooperation and coordination
- persons working in host employers or self-employed person undertaking work

- capability and training
- employer's duties
- temporary workers
- risk assessments for new or expectant mothers
- protection of young persons
- exception certificates
- provisions of liability
- exclusion of civil liberties
- extension out of Great Britain
- amendments to the Health and Safety (First Aid) Regulations 1981.

Employment Rights Act 1996

This Act covers all aspects of an employee's terms and conditions after they have been employed for a month or more. After two months' employment, an employee should have a written contract with their conditions of work including:

- details of payment, along with commission and incentives
- hours of work and expected holiday entitlement
- the amount of notice an employee is expected to give
- the amount of notice the employer expects the employee to give
- the date the employment started
- a full job description
- the employee's workplace location.

If an employee does not receive a contract of employment in writing, they can apply to an industrial tribunal and the employer is obliged by law to provide one.

The Workplace (Health, Safety and Welfare) Regulations 1992

The employer should ensure the workplace complies with the requirements of these regulations by:

- maintaining the workplace and all equipment and systems used there
- ensuring adequate ventilation
- keeping the workplace at a reasonable temperature (minimum 16°C)
- making sure employees have sufficient light to work comfortably
- keeping the workplace clean and tidy
- ensuring employees have enough space to work comfortably
- keeping floor and 'traffic routes' in a reasonable condition (no holes, slopes or uneven surfaces)
- ensuring workstations and seating are suitable
- providing suitable washing and toilet facilities (with soap and a means of drying hands)
- making sure employees have accommodation for clothing (worn at work) and changing facilities
- providing employees with facilities for resting and eating (if meals are to be eaten on the premises)

- providing clean drinking water and cups
- regularly removing waste materials
- keeping employees safe from falling objects
- making sure all doors and gates are suitably constructed and fitted with any necessary safety devices
- making sure windows are protected against breakage and signs (or similar) are incorporated where there is a danger of someone walking into them
- making sure escalators and moving walkways have safety devices fitted so they can be stopped in an emergency.

Think about it

In most settings separate toilet facilities must be available for men and women. However, in small, mostly female salons, men and women can use the same facilities as long as the toilet is a separate cubicle and it can be locked. In larger health clubs and spas the toilet and locker facilities would be separate.

Heat stress

The Health and Safety Executive draws attention to heat stress at work. The best working temperature in beauty therapy is between 15.5 and 20°C.

Humidity (the amount of moisture in the air) should be within the range of 30 to 70 per cent, although this will vary if your salon has a sauna and steam area. These should be in a well-ventilated area away from the main workrooms, while still being accessible to clients. There should also be sufficient air exchange and air movement, which must be increased in special circumstances, such as chemical usage. Treatment rooms used for nail art, aromatherapy, bleaching or eyelash perming will need specialist ventilation methods.

- Mechanical ventilation – extractor fans, which can be adjusted at various speeds.
- Natural ventilation – open windows are fine, but be careful of a draught on the client.
- Air-conditioned ventilation – passing air over filters and coolers brings about the desired condition, but of course this is the most expensive method!

Physical effects	Psychological effects
Headaches	Irritability
Sweating	Aggressive behaviour
Palpitations	Fatigue – resulting in mistakes being made
Dizziness	Lethargy
Nausea, vomiting	Lack of concentration
Feeling faint	

The effects of heat stress

A build-up of fumes, or of strong smells (for example from manicure preparations), will cause both physical and psychological problems, which affect not only clients but staff, too!

The Manual Handling Operations Regulations 1992

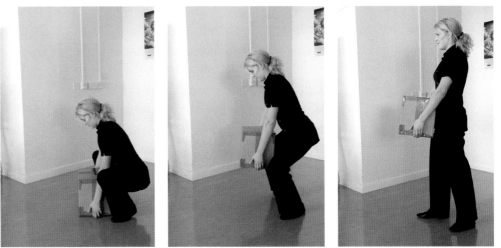

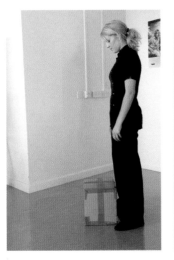

Safe lifting procedures should always be followed

The Health and Safety Executive (HSE) has drawn attention to skeletal and muscular disorders caused by manual handling and lifting, repetitive strain disorders and unsuitable posture causing low back pain. The regulations require certain measures to be taken to avoid these types of injuries occurring.

Think of all the situations that may apply in the salon:

- stock unpacking and storage – lifting heavy objects
- couch height adjustable for individual therapists
- chairs or stools used in the treatment rooms
- trolley height
- reception desk and chair
- rotation of job roles so that the therapist is not in the same position for every treatment
- height and size of nail art desk.

The Personal Protective Equipment at Work Regulations 1992

Every employer and self-employed person must ensure that suitable personal protective equipment is provided both for themselves and for their employees in situations where they may be exposed to a risk to their health or safety while at work. This is particularly relevant to waxing (refer to Remove hair using waxing techniques, page 407) and where there is a risk of contamination by body fluids (see also Environmental Protection Act 1990, The Controlled Waste Regulations 1992 and The Special Waste Regulations 1996 on page 54).

Protective clothing

This covers both equipment and protective clothing provisions to ensure safety for all those in the workplace. The regulations also provide that workplace personnel must have appropriate training in equipment use. Protective clothing, such as white overalls for work wear, ensures cleanliness, freshness, and professionalism. For certain treatments it may be advisable to wear extra disposable coverings. The client's clothing must also be protected.

Think about it

It is worth considering all of these factors when purchasing equipment, as you then have to work with the consequences!

When purchasing a couch for home or mobile use, it is worth pretending to carry out a facial, complete with client lying on the couch, to find the right height. Working at a couch at the wrong height is very bad for the back in the long term, and may cause considerable discomfort.

Think about it

Research what your Awarding Organisation states about protective clothing. It may invalidate your insurance if you do not follow the rules – and it may ruin your own clothing if tint or wax were to be spilt on your uniform or trousers, for example.

Protection against infectious diseases

It is essential to protect against all diseases that are carried in the blood or tissue fluids. Protective gloves should be worn whenever there is a possibility of blood or tissue fluid being passed from one person to another, that is through an open cut or broken skin. Two specific infectious diseases to mention are:

- AIDS (Acquired Immune Deficiency Syndrome) – this disease is caused by HIV (Human Immunodeficiency Virus). The virus is transmitted through body tissue. Most people are aware of AIDS because of media coverage. The virus attacks the body's immune system, and therefore carries a strong risk of secondary infection, such as pneumonia, which could be life threatening. As there is no known cure, prevention through protection is vital.

- Hepatitis variants (A, B and C) – hepatitis is an inflammation of the liver. It is caused by a very strong virus transmitted through blood and tissue fluids. This can survive outside the body, and can make a person very ill indeed; it can even be fatal. The most serious form is Hepatitis B and you can be immunised against this disease by a GP. For those who can prove they need this protection for their employment there is no cost involved. Most training establishments will recommend this.

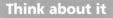

Always use protective clothing for hygiene and good client care

Think about it

Always cover cuts with a plaster to prevent cross-infection.

The Control of Substances Hazardous to Health (COSHH) Regulations 2002

The COSHH Regulations require employers to control exposure to substances that are hazardous to health in the workplace. Exposure can be prevented or reduced by:

- finding out what the health hazards are
- deciding how to prevent harm to health by carrying out a risk assessment
- providing control measures to reduce harm to health
- making sure they are used
- keeping all control measures in good working order
- providing information, instruction and training for employees and others
- providing monitoring and health surveillance in appropriate cases
- controlling exposure to hazardous substances in the workplace
- planning for emergencies.

Most products used in the salon are perfectly safe, but some products could become hazardous under certain conditions or if used inappropriately. All salons should be aware of how to use and store these products.

Employers are responsible for assessing the risks from hazardous substances and must decide upon an action to reduce those risks. Proper training should be given and employees should always follow safety guidelines and take the precautions identified by the employer.

The COSHH regulations require that the containers of hazardous substances are labelled with warning symbols. These symbols are shown overleaf.

For your portfolio

Take a look at 'Working with substances hazardous to health: What you need to know about COSHH' available on the HSE website. Look also at the HSE's COSHH essentials web tool.

Essential professional knowledge

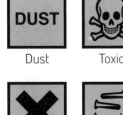

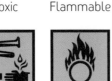

Dust	Toxic	Flammable
Irritant	Corrosive	Oxidising agent

COSHH symbols showing the different types of hazardous substances

Here are some examples of potential hazards.

- Highly flammable substances, such as solvents, nail varnish remover or alcohol steriliser, are hazardous because their fumes will ignite if exposed to a naked flame.

- Explosive materials, such as hairspray, air freshener or other pressurised cans, are also highly flammable and will explode with force if placed in heat, such as an open fire, or even on top of a hot radiator.

- Chemicals can cause severe reactions and skin damage – if chemicals are misused, vomiting, respiratory problems, and burning could be the result.

COSHH precautions

Employers must, by law, identify, list and assess in writing any substance in the workplace. This applies not only to products used for treatments in the salon but also to products that are used in cleaning such as bleach or polish. Potentially hazardous substances must be given a hazard rating, or risk assessment, even if it is zero.

It is essential that you read all of the COSHH sheets used in the salon, and be safe: follow what they say, never abuse manufacturers' instructions and attend regular staff training for product use. You never know when you might need it!

Think about it

Along with COSHH you may see MSDS (material safety data sheet management) or PSDS (product safety data sheets). In Britain we most commonly refer to COSHH sheets but the meaning is the same worldwide: it is a form containing data regarding the properties of a particular substance.

It is intended to provide workers and emergency personnel with procedures for handling or working with that substance in a safe manner, and includes information such as physical data (melting point, boiling point, flash point, etc.), toxicity, health effects, first aid, reactivity, storage, disposal, protective equipment and spill-handling. An MSDS for a substance is not really intended for use by the general consumer, focusing instead on the hazards of working with the material in an occupational setting in specific industries.

It is, however, important to use an MSDS specific to both country and supplier, as the same product (e.g. paints sold under identical brand names by the same company) can have different formulations in different countries. The formulation and hazard of a product using a generic name (e.g. sugar soap) may vary between manufacturers in the same country.

Think about it

- Manufacturers have to supply a COSHH sheet containing product data for each product. The COSHH sheets should be kept together in a central folder in the salon so that everyone can refer to them.

- A reaction can happen if a client has recently used a chemical at home and it reacts with the products used in the salon, e.g. home hair colours.

- Clients on long-term medication are more likely to have a reaction. Triggers include hormone replacement therapy, the contraceptive pill, heart and blood pressure medication – this should be recorded on the client's record card.

Health Act 2006

This law has been introduced to protect employees and the public from the harmful effects of 'second-hand' smoke inhalation (passive smoking). Below is a summary of its key points.

- From 1 July 2007 it has been against the law to smoke in virtually all enclosed and substantially enclosed public places and workplaces.

- Public transport and work vehicles used by more than one person should be smoke-free.

- Non-smoking signs should be displayed in all smoke-free premises and vehicles.

- Staff smoking rooms and indoor smoking areas are no longer allowed, so anyone who wants to smoke must go outside.

- Managers of smoke-free premises and vehicles have legal responsibility to prevent people from smoking.

- Anyone not complying with the smoke-free law is committing an offence and can be issued with a fixed penalty notice – up to a maximum of £200 if prosecuted and convicted by a court.
- Failure to display non-smoking signs carries a fixed penalty of £200, or a maximum fine of £1000 if prosecuted and convicted by a court.
- Failing to prevent smoking in a smoke-free place has a maximum fine of £2500.

The Gas Safety (Installation and Use) Regulations 1998

These relate to the use and maintenance of gas appliances. You may think that this does not apply to you as a therapist, but read on! The Gas Safety (Rights of Entry Regulations) 1996 & 2004 give gas and Health and Safety Executive (HSE) inspectors the right to enter premises and order the disconnection of any dangerous appliances. The inspectors themselves are not usually trained gas fitters, so they will instruct you to contact your local service engineer. Gas fumes are silent, with no smell, and deadly.

The Fire Precautions (Workplace) Regulations 1997 (as amended 1999)

The Fire Precautions (Workplace) Regulations bring together existing health and safety and fire legislation to form a set of dedicated fire regulations which aim to achieve a risk appropriate standard of fire safety for persons in the workplace.

The regulations were amended in 1999 in order to confirm the concept of employers having unconditional responsibility for the safety of employees. As a result, most workplaces are now subject to the legal requirements of the above regulations. They require small business owners to adequately assess the fire risks associated with their work activities and to decide what needs to be done to control these risks. The steps to be taken for a fire risk assessment are similar to those taken for general risk assessments, although the business also has a general duty to the public (refer to Follow health and safety practice in the salon, page 67).

Staff need to be aware of the procedures involved in the event of a fire, preferably through the displaying of a notice. It is recommended that every salon has some form of fire-fighting equipment – even if it is just a fire blanket. Contact the fire authority in your area, who will be happy to assist you.

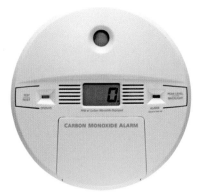

If you have a boiler on the premises you need a carbon monoxide detector – it can be a silent killer if fumes build up

The Provision and Use of Work Equipment Regulations 1998

The key points here are to ensure that all equipment at work is properly maintained, fit for purpose and in a good state of repair, as explained below.

Suitability of equipment

Employers must ensure that equipment is suitable for the purpose for which it is used or provided. When selecting equipment, they need to be aware of the working conditions, the risks to health and safety in the premises in which the work equipment is to be used and any additional risk posed by the use of the equipment.

Maintenance

Equipment must be maintained in efficient working order and good repair. Wherever possible, maintenance should take place when equipment is switched off to avoid risks to the person's health and safety; if maintenance can only take place when the equipment is switched on, precautions should be taken to protect the person carrying out the work. Where equipment has a maintenance log, this must be kept up to date.

Inspection

Where the safety of equipment depends on the installation conditions, it must be inspected after installation and before being put into service for the first time; or after assembly at a new site or in a new location, to ensure that it has been installed correctly and is safe to operate. This is also to ensure that health and safety conditions are maintained and that any wear and tear is detected and remedied in good time. Inspections that take place under this regulation should be recorded and kept until the next inspection takes place and is recorded.

Equipment should be used only for the purposes of the employer's business, and if equipment is obtained from another business, it should be accompanied by an inspection certificate.

Specific risks

Where the use of equipment is likely to involve a specific risk to health or safety, the equipment must only be used by staff trained to operate it. Where appropriate, employers need to provide training.

Any repairs, modifications, maintenance or servicing should only be carried out by a competent person.

Information and instructions

Staff operating equipment must be provided with adequate health and safety information and, where appropriate, written instructions on how to use it. This also applies to employees who supervise or manage the use of equipment.

Training

For health and safety reasons, staff should be given adequate training to operate equipment, including training in the methods which may be adopted when using the equipment, any risks involved and precautions to be taken. This also applies to employees who supervise or manage the use of equipment.

Protection against specified hazards

Employers are responsible for taking measures to ensure that staff using equipment should be protected from hazards that might endanger their health and safety. If it is not possible to prevent the risk, then it needs to be adequately controlled.

High or very low temperature

Where equipment, or any article or substance produced, used or stored in work equipment, is at a high or very low temperature, it needs to be protected so as to prevent injury to any person by burn, scald or sear.

Controls for starting equipment

Where appropriate, equipment should be provided with one or more controls for the purposes of starting it (including restarting after a stoppage for any reason).

Stability

Equipment should be stabilised by clamping, or another method, where necessary for health or safety purposes.

Lighting

The work area where equipment is to be used should have suitable and sufficient lighting.

The Electricity at Work Regulations 1989

These regulations affect the use of electrical equipment in every salon, clinic or health club. Regulation 4 of the Act states: 'All electrical equipment must be regularly checked for electrical safety.' In a busy salon this may be every six months. The check must be carried out by a 'competent person', preferably a qualified electrician. All checks must be recorded in a book kept for this purpose only.

Types of equipment to be checked include:

- wax heaters
- autoclaves
- thermal boots
- infrared lamps
- foot spas that plug in
- paraffin wax heaters
- fast nail UV dryer boxes.

A 'competent person' need not be a qualified electrician, but must be capable of attending to basic safety checks. Manufacturers often supply their own technical staff to attend to safety checks.

PAT Testing (Portable Appliance Testing)

All companies and organisations should comply with the Electricity at Work Regulations. Each electrical appliance should be comprehensively tested to meet the exacting requirements of the IET (Institution of Engineering and Technology) code of practice for In-Service Inspection and Testing of Electrical Equipment.

Ideally, the electrician or competent person should be a member of both NICEIC (National Inspection Council for Electrical Installation Contracting) and NAPIT (National Association of Professional Inspectors and Testers). All engineers should undertake a NAPIT technical assessment and be subject to regular inspection and monitoring of their work and records.

All electrical equipment to be tested has to be disconnected from the mains supply. This may be inconvenient so ideally it should be carried out of normal salon hours.

If electrical apparatus is found to be faulty, the equipment must be withdrawn from service and repaired. An electrical safety record book should be used to record dates, the nature of the repair and by whom it was done. It should also contain a list of tests carried out on the equipment under inspection, the results of those tests, and be signed by the competent person who carried them out.

This is essential for public liability insurance purposes and in case of legal action being taken for accidents due to negligence.

The Pressure Systems and Transportable Gas Containers Regulations 1989

Steam sterilising autoclaves fall under this Act. You are required to have a written scheme of examination carried out or certified by a competent person.

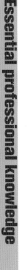

Essential professional knowledge

Environmental Protection Act 1990
The Controlled Waste Regulations 1992 (as amended in 1993)
The Special Waste Regulations 1996

These Acts require all clinical waste to be kept apart from general waste and to be disposed of to a licensed incinerator or landfill site, by a licensed company. This includes:

- waste which consists wholly or partly of animal or human tissue
- blood or other body fluids
- swabs or dressings
- syringes or needles.

The Reporting of Injuries, Diseases and Dangerous Occurrences Regulations (RIDDOR) 1995

These regulations cover the recording and reporting of any serious accidents and conditions to the local environmental health officer, whose remit covers beauty therapy and hairdressing salons. This officer will investigate the accident and make sure that the salon prevents the accident from happening again in the future. The officer can also assess the risk factors in each instance.

An accident or death at work must be reported within ten days. If the accident does not require a hospital visit, but the person is absent from work for more than three days, a report still needs to be made.

If an employee reports a work-related disease, a report must be sent. A work-related disease could include occupational dermatitis, asthma caused through work or even hepatitis. Accidents as a result of violence or an attack by another person must be reported. A car accident when on company business is reportable in the same way as an accident at work.

A dangerous occurrence in which no one was actually injured must also be reported: for example, if the ceiling of the salon collapses overnight.

If you are a mobile therapist working in someone's home and you have an accident yourself or you injure the client you must report it.

The Health and Safety (Display Screen Equipment) Regulations 1992 (amended 2002)

These regulations implement an EU Directive and were amended in 2002. They require employers to minimise the risks in visual display unit (VDU) work by ensuring that workplaces and jobs are well designed with specific thought given to position of the monitor and height of chair in relation to how the workplace station is set up.

There is no difference between a VDU, a VDT, a monitor and display screen equipment (DSE). All these terms mean the same thing: a display screen, usually forming part of a computer and showing text, numbers or graphics. Some users may get aches and pains in their hands, wrists, arms, neck, shoulders or back, especially after long periods of uninterrupted VDU work. Repetitive strain injury (RSI) is the term used to refer to these aches, pains and disorders, but can be misleading as it means different things to different people. A better medical name for this group of conditions is 'upper limb disorders'. Usually these disorders do not last, but in a few cases they may become persistent or even disabling.

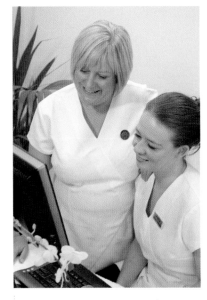

Many salons use computers for bookings and stock taking – ensure it is set up correctly for posture, good health and safety

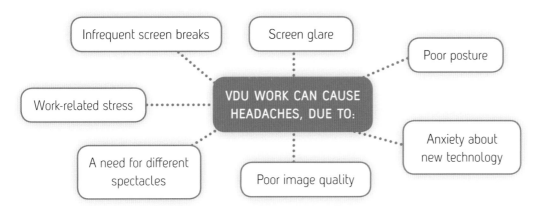

Problems can often be avoided by good workplace design, so that you can work comfortably, and by good working practices (like taking frequent short breaks from the VDU). Prevention is easiest if action is taken early, before the problem has become serious.

Extensive research has found no evidence that VDUs can cause disease or permanent damage to eyes. But long spells of VDU work can lead to tired eyes and discomfort.

Once the employer recognises these considerations to the positioning of screens, any problems can be easily put right. People who suffer from photo-sensitive epilepsy and are susceptible to flickering lights and striped patterns may be affected by the use of VDUs in some circumstances.

Employers have to analyse workstations, and assess and reduce risks. They should look at:

- the whole workstation including equipment, furniture, and the work environment — workstations need to meet minimum requirements
- the job being done
- any special needs of individual staff
- planning work so there are breaks or changes of activity
- arranging eye tests, on request, and provide spectacles if special ones are needed
- providing health and safety training and information, so that employees can use their VDU and workstation safely, and know how to make best use of it to avoid health problems, e.g. by adjusting the chair.

Employers' Liability (Compulsory Insurance) Act 1969

Employers and self-employed persons must by law hold employer's liability insurance. This will reimburse them against any legal liability to pay compensation to employees for bodily injury, illness or disease caused during the course of their employment.

Employers must insure for at least £2 million per claim, but check with your own salon's insurance company. Also follow the recommendations of your professional association.

It is worth remembering the following points.

- A legal claim made against your salon could result in very large financial losses and possibly the sale of the owner's business or even private home.
- Public prosecution results in a heavy fine for those not having this essential insurance cover.

◉ Damage to the salon could be so great that the business might never recover.

◉ Some cases can take up to ten years to come to court and with inflation the claim against you could be very much more than your original cover, if you only take the minimum requirements.

Consumer Protection Act 1987

This Act follows European laws to safeguard the consumer in three main areas: product liability, general safety requirements and misleading prices.

Before 1987 an injured person had to prove that a manufacturer was negligent before suing for damages. This Act removes the need to prove negligence.

An injured person can take action against:

◉ producers

◉ own brand manufacturers

◉ importers

◉ suppliers such as wholesalers or retailers.

In the salon this means that only reputable products should be used and sold. Care should be taken in handling, maintaining and storing products so that they remain in top condition.

It is important that all staff are aware of consumer protection laws when selling products and when using products in a treatment.

The Cosmetic Products (Safety) Regulations 2008

The Cosmetic Products (Safety) Regulations 2008 defined a cosmetic product as 'any substance/preparation that is used on the skin, teeth, hair, nails, lips ... with the intention to cleanse, perfume, and change the appearance of, to protect, keep in good condition or to correct body odours' — which covers just about everything that is found in a salon!

A cosmetic product must be clearly labelled with the following information:

◉ a list of ingredients — either on the outer packaging of the product, or if there is no outer packaging, on the container itself

◉ name and address of the manufacturer/supplier

◉ minimum shelf life — on both the outer packaging and the container itself

◉ storage instructions — to help the consumer to maintain the product at its best

◉ warnings and precautions — on the outer packaging and the container

◉ batch number or lot code — this would allow a manufacturer to recall a batch of products if necessary

◉ its function

◉ its weight.

Medicines Act 1968

This Act deals with the supply and use of topical anaesthetics and is enforced by the police and the Medicines and Healthcare product Regulatory Agency (MHRA). Product licence conditions are for medical application only and not for cosmetic use, therefore their use by a beauty therapist can be unlawful.

Misuse of Drugs Act 1971

This act is intended to prevent the non-medical use of certain drugs. For this reason it controls not just medicinal drugs (which will also be in the Medicines Act) but also drugs with no current medical uses. This includes illegal use of magic mushrooms, all class A drugs, some alcohols (certainly for the underage user) and some drugs available on prescription, such as codeine, if not used for a medical condition and if sold, imported or exported for profit.

Trade Descriptions Act 1968

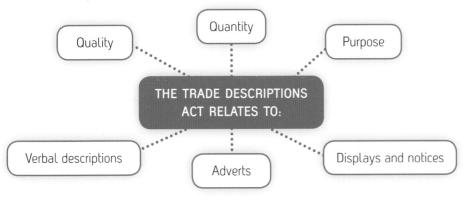

Quality

Quantity

Purpose

THE TRADE DESCRIPTIONS ACT RELATES TO:

Verbal descriptions

Adverts

Displays and notices

This Act is concerned with the false description of goods. It is important to realise its relevance. It is illegal to mislead the general public. This also applies to verbal descriptions given by a third party and repeated. So, if a manufacturer's false description of a product is repeated you are liable to prosecution. The law states that the retailer must not:

- supply information that is in any way misleading
- falsely describe or make false statements about either a product or a service on offer.

The Consumer Protection from Unfair Trading Regulations 2008

The European Union adopted the Unfair Commercial Practices Directive (UCPD) in May 2005 in order to strengthen laws on trade descriptions within Europe, as these varied from country to country. In the UK, the directive was implemented as The Consumer Protection from Unfair Trading Regulations, which came into force on 26 May 2008.

The regulations maintain good practice and are specific about what retailers may or may not do. The retailer may not:

- make false contrasts between present and previous prices
- claim to offer products at half price unless they have already been offered at the full price for at least 28 days prior to the sale.

Be mindful of using statements saying something is 'our price'. Comparison of prices can be misleading and can be illegal — be sure that the product is identical in every way. You should also check that products are labelled with their country of origin.

Think about it

Linked to the Trade Descriptions Act for misleading advertising of products advice is the Advertising Standards Agency (ASA). The ASA is the UK's independent regulator of advertising across all media, now including marketing on websites. There was controversy when two advertisements for skin care products had to be withdrawn from use. The two major cosmetic companies involved were heavily fined because the images of the celebrities used to sell the products were so airbrushed in post production of the photographs that they looked much younger and their skin became completely flawless. The ASA upheld complaints that this was misleading to the general public and the adverts were withdrawn immediately.

Essential professional knowledge

Related acts: Supply of Goods and Services Act 1982 amended 2003; Sale and Supply of Goods Act 1994; The Sale and Supply of Goods to Consumers Regulations 2002.

- Wherever goods are bought they must 'conform to contract'. This means they must be as described, fit for purpose and of satisfactory quality (that is, not inherently faulty at the time of sale).

- Goods are of satisfactory quality if they reach the standard that a reasonable person would regard as satisfactory, taking into account the price and any description.

- Aspects of quality include fitness for purpose, freedom from minor defects, appearance and finish, durability, and safety.

- It is the seller, not the manufacturer, who is responsible if goods do not conform to contract.

- If goods do not conform to contract at the time of sale, purchasers can request their money back 'within a reasonable time'. (This is not defined and will depend on circumstances.)

- For up to six years after purchase (five years from discovery in Scotland) purchasers can demand damages (which a court would equate to the cost of a repair or replacement).

- A purchaser who is a consumer (that is they are not buying in the course of a business) can alternatively request a repair or replacement.

- If repair and replacement are not possible or too costly, then the consumer can seek a partial refund, if they have had some benefit from the good, or a full refund if the fault(s) have meant they have enjoyed no benefit.

- In general, the onus is on all purchasers to prove the goods did not conform to contract (e.g. were inherently faulty) and should have reasonably lasted until this point in time (that is perishable goods do not last for six years).

- If a consumer chooses to request a repair or replacement, then for the first six months after purchase it will be for the retailer to prove the goods did conform to contract (e.g. were not inherently faulty).

- After six months and until the end of the six years, it is for the consumer to prove the lack of conformity.

Disability Discrimination Act 1995 amended 2005; Equality Act 2006

This Act makes it unlawful to discriminate against disabled people in employment, the provision of goods, facilities and services, education, and the buying or renting of property or land. In 2007, the promotion of civil rights for disabled people became the responsibility of the new Equality and Human Rights Commission (EHRC).

It is illegal for an employer (employing 20 or more staff) to discriminate against a disabled person or prospective employee on the grounds of their disabilities. If a person is suitable for the job, it is up to the employer to make the necessary arrangements and adjustments in the workplace to ensure there is no disadvantage for the disabled person.

It is also unlawful to harass a person on the grounds of their disability. All employers must take positive steps to avoid harassment happening in the workplace.

The Working Time Regulations 1998

The Working Time Regulations (1998) merged with the European Working Time Directive into UK law. The regulations were amended with effect from 1 August 2003.

The regulations control how employers organise the average working week, minimum daily and weekly rest breaks, and paid holiday entitlement – which before the regulations were introduced, was left very much up to what the employer wanted to do. The law applies to full-time, part-time and casual workers. You should not work more than 48 hours in a week, with a rest period of 11 hours between each working day, with a minimum of one day off a week. If working for more than six hours, you are entitled to a 20-minute break.

Performing Rights – within Copyright, Designs and Patents Act 1988

This Act is designed to protect the people who write music but then do not get the royalty payments they should when the music is played. Any use of music in the treatment room, reception or in exercise groups is classed as a public performance.

PPL is the body that is responsible for collecting licence payments from people wishing to use music on behalf of artists and record companies. Under the Copyright, Designs and Patents Act 1988, PPL can take legal action against anyone who does not pay a licence fee to use music – and it does. This can mean a considerable fine for those who try to avoid paying. So all salons and exercise/aerobic instructors need to purchase music that has a built-in licence. Although more expensive to purchase in the first place (a CD price can vary from £10 up to about £30) it does save all the worry of a heavy fine, if caught.

Most good specialist music shops have a section of licensed music – just ask.

Data Protection Act 1998

The Act states that every organisation (data controller) that uses and processes personal information (personal data) must notify the Information Commissioner's office, unless they are exempt. Failure to do so is a criminal offence.

The main purpose of registration is to ensure that the eight principles of 'good information handling' are being followed – that data should be:

1 fairly and lawfully processed
2 processed for limited purposes
3 adequate, relevant and not excessive
4 accurate
5 not kept longer than necessary
6 processed in accordance with the person's rights
7 secure
8 not transferred to countries outside the European Economic Area (EEA) without adequate and proper protection.

The fee for notification and annual renewal of a register entry had been £35 for all data controllers, but from 1 October 2009, this was replaced by a two-tier payment charge: for businesses employing fewer than 250 staff the cost remains at £35; a higher fee of £500 is payable by businesses with more than 250 employees. The fee paid also relates to turnover – businesses with a turnover of £25.9 million will go into tier two, but this does not apply to charities and public authorities.

For your portfolio

To find out more about data registration visit the Information Commissioner's website, or contact the Information Commissioner's Office, Wycliffe House, Water Lane, Wilmslow, Cheshire SK9 5AF.

Any person can ask to see the information held by an organisation about him or her within 40 days for a fee that is now only £2. It is possible to gain compensation through a civil court action if you feel there has been any infringement of rights, in which information that was given for a specific purpose has been abused.

Local Government (Miscellaneous Provisions) Act 1982

This relates to the local authorities in your particular area. Section 8 of the Act is concerned with the registration of any practitioners who pierce the skin. This applies to:

- acupuncture
- tattooing
- ear and body piercing
- epilation.

It applies to both salons and mobile therapists.

The concern of most local authorities is that through registration they will be able to keep some control of hygiene regulations and ensure that people have recognised qualifications. The enforcement of these regulations will depend upon the individual authority, as does the amount of inspection that takes place, and the scale of fees for registration.

This does not include people working in hospitals.

Local by-laws

Local government **by-laws** are laws decided by the local authority or borough council of an area, and they can differ from region to region. Therefore, Manchester has different local by-laws from Birmingham. However, both these authorities have a register of salons offering body massage as a treatment. This is to maintain a professional, qualified salon base and to eliminate the 'massage parlour' image.

You need to investigate the by-laws in your own area from your borough council — these by-laws relate to hygiene, and the registration of ear piercing, and epilation salons, as well as tattoo parlours.

London Local Authorities Act 1995

This Act requires all premises in London that carry out treatments to be licensed by their local authorities. This is for any skin piercing treatments, acupuncture, tattooing and ear piercing — and some local authorities also expect salons to register if they offer massage, too. So contact your local authority to check whether you need a licence when you start your new salon.

Insurance

Professional indemnity insurance

Every single professional beauty therapist should have this **insurance** protection, regardless of how few or how many treatments they carry out.

The best deal for these kinds of insurance policies can usually be found via your professional body — professional bodies are often able to offer the best rates because they negotiate on behalf of members and get a considerable discount.

Key terms

By-laws – laws decided by the local authority for your area.

Key terms

Insurance – whereby the beauty therapist (or salon) pays an annual fee to an insurer (insurance company) to compensate them in case of loss incurred during the course of their work.

As an employee you need to check with your employer whether you are covered on the company's business insurance, or if you need to organise your own cover. A salon owner or employer should include this in the public liability policy, so that all employees are protected against claims made by clients.

Public liability insurance

This insurance is not compulsory, but it is certainly advisable. It will protect the employer should a member of the public be injured on the premises. This could be something as unexpected as a roof tile hitting the client on her way into the salon. If this results in the client being unable to work for a long period of time, the client can sue the salon owner for compensation.

Insurance is important – so protect yourselves and your clients. Contact your professional association for guidance on all aspects of insurance.

Think about it

Never assume anything when it comes to insurance cover.

Always check whether you have cover as a therapist working in a salon. Would you be personally liable if things go wrong?

Check you are covered if you are a mobile therapist entering clients' homes. What if you were to spill wax on their new bedroom carpet? Are you covered?

If you are running a business from home, do not automatically think your household insurance will cover your work and clients coming to your home. What if a client were to fall in the driveway, and hurt herself? Would you be covered?

Accidents can and do happen – and many clients have heard of these 'no win, no fee' solicitor firms willing to take legal action against you. Better to be safe than sorry! Be covered and you have security and peace of mind. One of the advantages of joining a professional association is that they negotiate better and reasonably priced insurance cover.

Independent regulators

Advertising Standards Authority (ASA)

The ASA is an independent body set up to regulate the content of advertisements, sales promotions and direct marketing in the UK.

It is responsible for maintaining the quality of advertising standards through codes of practice for television, radio and other types of adverts, such as interactive adverts. The ASA can stop misleading, harmful or offensive advertising, ensure that sales promotions are run fairly, and help to reduce unwanted advertising sent through the post, by email or by text message. It also deals with mail order problems. Part of its role is to investigate complaints made about advertising, sales promotions or direct marketing.

The advertising standards codes especially apply to beauty products. Advertisements must be careful not to mislead or misdirect the consumer into believing that wrinkles will disappear, that skin will look ten years younger or that lines can be permanently removed. Adverts may refer to temporary prevention of the skin drying out, but any long-term or permanent correction of the lines or wrinkles is not possible and therefore not allowed in advertising.

ACAS (Advisory, Conciliation and Arbitration Service)

ACAS is an independent organisation that offers impartial advice to individuals and organisations to help resolve disputes or disagreements at work. It aims to encourage better and more direct workplace communication and to help businesses improve their employment practices. Since April 2009, ACAS has concentrated less on how to manage disciplinary issues, grievances and dismissals and more on resolving problems in the workplace at an early stage, so saving businesses time and money.

BSI British Standards

BSI British Standards is the UK's national standards body, which brings together representatives from a range of organisations to develop formal standards for the benefit of UK business and consumers. Standards are there to help industry and society at large. So even if you are not involved in developing or manufacturing products, you are bound to come into contact with BSI Standards every day. The aim of the Standards is to:

- promote and share best practice, so designers can focus on developing better products
- set benchmarks for performance, quality and safety
- ensure similar products work together (e.g. making sure all CDs are the same dimensions)
- make technical requirements
- reduce risks
- reduce costs.

Industry codes of practice

Industry codes of practice or ethics are a guide to correct procedures and etiquette as dictated by professional therapists' associations, of which there are several. Which professional body you join is a matter of personal choice, and may depend upon the one favoured by your training establishment.

The cost involved in joining depends on your level of entry – a student membership is normally available and with your joining pack you will be given a code of ethics or a code of practice.

This code is a book of rules that the therapist agrees to abide by, as part of the contract of membership. If these rules are broken or ignored, membership can be withdrawn.

Being a member of a professional body brings benefits, which can include:

- a good insurance deal negotiated on the members' behalf
- support and advice upon leaving college
- a monthly magazine, with useful articles and adverts for jobs and equipment
- regular legal updates
- free legal helplines, for all aspects of your business
- discount cards for suppliers
- a business guide for setting up on your own.

The following is a typical set of rules and regulations for a professional therapist organisation.

Key terms

Industry code of practice
– a guide to correct procedures and etiquette within a particular industry.

Federation of Holistic Therapists Code of Ethics and Professional Practice

The Federation of Holistic Therapists (FHT) is the UK and Ireland's largest and leading professional association for beauty, complementary and sports therapists. Professional therapist members of the FHT agree to abide by the FHT Code of Ethics and Professional Practice and any amendments or additions that may be made in the future.

Duties as a professional therapist

The definition of a professional therapist concerns the welfare of clients and the protection of the public from improper practice. This includes:

- making the care of your client your first concern
- providing a high standard of care at all times
- clients being treated with respect, as individuals
- professional knowledge being kept up-to-date
- acting lawfully in your professional and personal practice
- personal accountability for your professional activity.

Failure to abide by this Code will result in disciplinary procedures being applied by the FHT Professional Conduct Panel ranging from a warning with sanctions according to conditions of practice, suspension until further training is completed, or termination of membership, depending on the nature of the breach. When an allegation is made against a professional therapist, the FHT will always take account of the standards set out in this Code when considering that allegation.

Guidelines to advertising your services

All advertising undertaken in relation to professional practice must be accurate, must not be misleading, false, unfair or exaggerated. Personal skills, equipment or facilities cannot be promoted as being better than anyone else's. Advertising any product or service requires promoting knowledge, skills, qualifications and experience in an accurate and professionally responsible way without making or supporting unjustifiable statements. Any potential financial rewards should be made explicit and play no part at all in the advice or recommendations of products and services that clients and users receive.

Limits of competence

A professional therapist must only carry out treatments and give advice within their area of training and competence. Clients' consent should be obtained before introducing new treatments into their existing treatment programme. A professional therapist has the right to refuse to treat a client if the treatment is outside of their competency level. In such circumstances they should refer to an appropriately qualified professional therapist or suggest that they contact their GP.

Regulation

Holistic therapies are not currently regulated by statute that provides protection of title. Protection of title prevents anyone calling themselves a 'doctor', physiotherapist, chiropodist, chiropractor, etc. without being registered with the relevant statutory regulator under the provisions of an act of parliament. Membership of a professional association for a therapy that is not regulated enables the therapist to demonstrate to clients that they are suitably qualified, insured and participating in Continuing Professional Development (CPD).

(Source: Federation of Holistic Therapists; www.fht.org.uk, January 2012)

Salon guidelines

All the legislation mentioned above should be considered within the normal working life of the beauty therapist. Working safely and following the correct legal procedure is very important.

It is also very important to follow the **salon guidelines** for the particular establishment you are in — be it a training establishment, salon or spa, ocean liner or renting a room in a health suite.

It is vital that you are aware of the policies on health and safety, safety training and what exactly is expected within the job role. Normally salon rules are very similar, regardless of where the salon is located, but the safety procedures to follow if your salon happens to be floating in the Caribbean Sea will be very different.

Essential professional knowledge

For your portfolio

Visit the Federation of Holistic Therapists' website and check out both their code of practice and membership information – you can also find out about insurance, products, and interesting articles.

Key terms

Salon guidelines – policies and procedures followed within the salon.

It is very important that the salon expectations and the required behaviour for therapists are set out at the beginning. This could be at your induction training, or even at the initial interview.

Regular reviews of policies and regular training for updates is essential, as is your attendance. If a member of staff continually ignores safety requirements, whether through negligence or through ignorance (if they have not attended training), this could form the basis for dismissal. Worse still, should an accident happen through negligence, injury may occur, and the person responsible may be found liable.

Health and safety rules

These will encompass all aspects of the Health and Safety at Work Act, plus COSHH guidelines and the Electricity at Work Act.

You should be in no doubt about:

- therapists' responsibilities
- salon procedures
- treatment safety
- equipment safety
- protection against cross-infection.

Client safety	Storage procedures	Stock regulations
Positioning of client	Electrical equipment	COSHH regulations followed
Minimum risk of hazard for bed height – getting on and off	Chemicals	First aid procedures in place
Correct use of equipment and products	Valuables	Stock rotation
Correct diagnosis for treatments	Stock	Spillage management
Correct evacuation procedures	Money	Correct storage and containers

Salon procedures for health and safety

Your employer or head of the training establishment should have all these standard procedures in place. If you are not instructed within your first few weeks of beginning your new post – then ask.

Check your knowledge

1 Which of the following statements is correct?
   a) All products should have a list of ingredients on them if they contain nuts.
   b) Products do not need any ingredients listed on the outside.
   c) Products only need a list of ingredients on them if they are bought at a chemist or through a salon.
   d) All products must have all ingredients listed on them.

2 The Data Protection Act states that:
   a) all information on the record card must be accurate and correct
   b) clients must be kept safe at all times
   c) all personal information must be kept private and confidential
   d) all consultation forms must be the same.

3 What does the Consumer Protection Act state?
   a) The consumer must be kept safe while on the premises.
   b) The consumer must be protected from unsafe products.
   c) The consumer must be protected against unfair prices.
   d) The consumer must be protected against disease.

4 What does the Health and Safety at Work Act state about responsibility?
   a) Both the employer and employees are responsible for health and safety in the workplace.
   b) It is the employer who is responsible for health and safety.
   c) It is the client who is responsible for their own health and safety.
   d) It is the salon owner who is responsible for health and safety.

5 The Trade Descriptions Act states:
   a) It is illegal to make false claims about a product or service.
   b) It is illegal to put an advert on television.
   c) It is illegal to employ a foreign person without a work permit.
   d) It is illegal to offer unsafe treatments.

6 An example of a viral infection is:
   a) athlete's foot
   b) a cold sore
   c) scabies
   d) impetigo.

7 A bacterial infection is the cause of:
   a) ringworm
   b) diarrhoea
   c) warts
   d) boils.

8 A contra-action is:
   a) a condition which is present and means the treatment cannot go ahead
   b) a condition that the client is born with
   c) a reaction which appears during or just after treatment
   d) a condition which means the treatment has to be adapted.

9 An autoclave is:
   a) a waxing pot
   b) an effective sterilisation method
   c) a hot towel heater
   d) a chemical sterilising agent.

10 Sterilisation is:
   a) the removal of dirt and being ultra clean
   b) the removal of bacteria
   c) the removal of viruses
   d) the removal of bacteria, spores and viruses.

Section

2

The workplace environment

Follow health and safety practice in the salon

What you will learn

- Maintain health, safety and security practices
- Follow emergency procedures

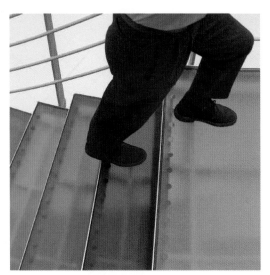

HSE — Health and Safety Executive

Five steps to risk assessment

Advice is available from the Health and Safety Executive (Source: Health and Safety Executive)

Introduction

A beauty salon should be a haven of tranquillity where the client can relax, unwind and enjoy her treatment, secure in the knowledge that she is in good hands and her professional therapist is in total control. Part of setting the scene is ensuring not only that the treatment is of the highest quality but also that the client is safe and not at risk.

Unfortunately, because of the very nature of its business a busy beauty therapy salon has the potential to be a dangerous place. Any business whose livelihood involves dealing with the general public, that is, the customer, could be viewed as an accident waiting to happen! The types of treatments involved in a salon are also a potential hazard: most equipment relies on electricity to work, we use chemicals when eyelash tinting and perming, we work with hot wax, and so on — each of the units carries its own potential hazards and risks.

It may not be obvious to the client that lying on a couch having a relaxing facial is potentially dangerous. In fact, it should not even cross the client's mind, but the therapist should view all treatments as a possible risk, and then minimise that risk. Your motto should be: 'Prevention is better than cure.'

This unit is for everyone at work, regardless of whether they are a paid worker, a volunteer, part-time or full-time employee or a self-employed therapist in a mobile business. Everyone within the workplace has an obligation by law to secure their own and others' health, safety and welfare. This unit is about identifying the factors that contribute to you becoming a responsible employee.

Think about it

There are three frameworks which you need to be aware of and work within as a therapist to work safely:

Legislation – the making of health and safety laws as an Act by both the British government and the European Parliament, for example the Health and Safety at Work Act.

Codes of practice – these are as drawn up by your professional body as a guideline of expected conduct and equipment use for the policies that insure you, for example the Federation of Holistic Therapies (FHT).

Workplace policies – the rules and regulations of your employer and the 'house rules' of your particular working establishment, e.g. in a spa, salon or cruise ship. These should be the same as legislation but may have bits added for specialist areas such as health and safety at sea.

The Health and Safety at Work etc Act 1974 covers the legal requirements of an employer. **The Health and Safety Executive (HSE)** gives lots of advice for those considering going into business and employing others.

But what about you? Who are you responsible for? As a professional therapist, you are as liable as your employer, perhaps more so as you have regular direct contact with the customer. You are just as accountable in legal terms should a client be able to prove you were negligent.

Key terms

Health and Safety Executive (HSE) – an enforcing authority responsible for health and safety regulations in Great Britain. It ensures that risks to people's health and safety from work activities are properly controlled.

Therefore, as a professional therapist you will be required to abide by various pieces of legislation, codes of practice and workplace policies. Individual salons usually have their own 'house rules' and favourite methods of doing things that are largely governed by the owners' preferences. The uniform, the décor and the daily running of the salon are personal and the working pattern will differ from salon to salon. The health and safety policies should not.

This unit is not a guide to completing a full risk assessment – that should be done by a trained professional who specialises in that field. The aim of this unit is to make you aware of the significant risks in the beauty salon, and to show you how to identify the risks and deal with them appropriately.

Be able to maintain health, safety and security practices

In this outcome you will learn about:

- how to conduct yourself in the workplace to meet with health and safety practices and salon policy
- dealing with hazards within your area of responsibility following salon policy
- maintaining a level of personal presentation, hygiene and conduct to meet with legal and salon requirements
- following salon policy for security
- making sure tools, equipment, materials and work areas meet hygiene requirements
- using required personal protective equipment (PPE)
- positioning yourself and the client safely
- handling, using and storing products, materials, tools and equipment safely to meet with manufacturers' instructions
- disposing of all types of salon waste safely and to meet with legal and salon requirements.

How to conduct yourself in the workplace

It is your responsibility to carry out your work in accordance with your **level of competence**, workplace instructions, suppliers' and manufacturers' instructions and legal requirements.

Refer to Professional skills on pages 10–64 for further advice on personal presentation and hygiene. In this section you will be looking at the safety aspect of your presentation and how it contributes to safety in the salon.

As the therapist, you must:

- be professional at all times
- have short nails, minimal jewellery, safe shoes and a clean, hygienic uniform
- follow the Health and Safety Act and be responsible in actions and consequences for both yourself and others
- go on regular training courses to be safe and competent

Key terms

Level of competence – the limits of a person's authority; usually the extent of a person's responsibility as set out in their job description and workplace policies.

Think about it

Never exceed your own level of competency as it may make any insurance claims invalid. It might also jeopardise your own or someone else's health or become a risk to safety in the salon.

- be knowledgeable and use your knowledge: know the correct person to inform in case of an accident, who to contact for first aid and the salon policies on health and safety
- be as hygienic and as thorough as possible when protecting the client
- fill out a full consultation card and carry out a contra-indication check prior to every treatment
- never knowingly endanger others.

It is not only the employer's responsibility to provide health and safety management, it is also the responsibility of each employee to follow the rules.

All beauty therapists work very long hours and are often on the go all day. They are in a busy salon environment with other people present all the time — their own clients, other therapists' clients, other staff, outside representatives, management, receptionists, cleaners and so on. If the therapist does not have a sense of personal safety and respect for the safety of others, accidents will occur.

You must also have a thorough understanding of the health and safety policies within your salon that affect your working day. This includes your conduct and personal presentation, which will ensure the health and safety of yourself, your clients and your working colleagues.

You should always carry out your work in relation to your level of competence, your workplace instructions and manufacturers' instructions, as well as the legal requirements. You should be capable and know your job responsibilities; this will allow you to control health and safety risks where you can. Never knowingly endanger the health of others and do pass on to your supervisor or manager any suggestions that you think might help to reduce risks to yourself or others.

To be safe the therapist should consider the following:

- Make sure personal appearance combines safety with professionalism.
- Wear shoes that are smart but comfortable. High heels are not only uncomfortable but also not particularly stable to walk on. Open-toe sandals will not protect the toes from damage from either spillage or impact injury. Most Awarding Organisations have a strict dress code for assessments which you will also need to adhere to.
- Avoid stooping and slouching. This will prevent back problems occurring.
- Have good posture and distribute body weight evenly by standing correctly with feet slightly apart. This will help prevent accidents and injury.
- Always wear the correct protective clothing to shield a uniform.
- Always wear gloves when using chemicals or if there is a possibility of coming into contact with body fluids.
- Always follow the correct disposal regulations for gloves and waste materials.
- If an establishment provides a uniform as part of a corporate image, wear it!
- Keep hair tidy and wear it short or tied back. Loose long hair may fall in the eyes and cause eye problems.

A high standard of cleanliness will ensure no cross-infection can occur. This should include the following:

- Wash hands between clients.
- Keep nails short.
- Cover cuts or open wounds.
- Do not attend work with an infectious disease.
- Do not spread cold or flu germs.
- Do not wear dangling jewellery that may be a hazard.

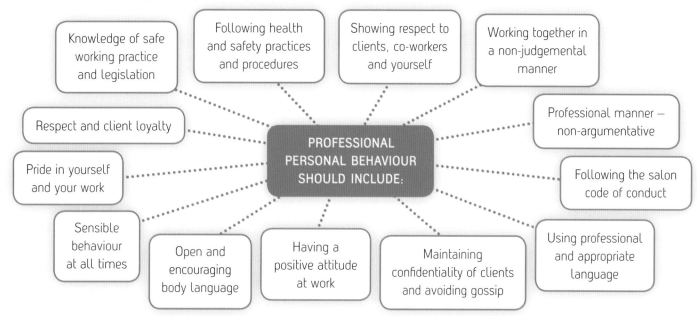

PROFESSIONAL PERSONAL BEHAVIOUR SHOULD INCLUDE:

- Knowledge of safe working practice and legislation
- Following health and safety practices and procedures
- Showing respect to clients, co-workers and yourself
- Working together in a non-judgemental manner
- Professional manner – non-argumentative
- Respect and client loyalty
- Following the salon code of conduct
- Pride in yourself and your work
- Using professional and appropriate language
- Sensible behaviour at all times
- Open and encouraging body language
- Having a positive attitude at work
- Maintaining confidentiality of clients and avoiding gossip

Good conduct cuts down any risks. This should include the following:

- Do not run in the salon or rush.
- Use equipment properly.
- Follow manufacturers' instructions at all times.
- Do not take short cuts when cleaning the salon and equipment.
- Always leave the equipment ready to be used by the next person.
- Do not block fire exits for any reason.
- Do not deliberately endanger anyone – even as a joke.
- Do not behave negligently – such as playing with fire!
- Use proper lifting procedures.
- Take responsibility for yourself, machinery and problems such as spillage that may occur – do not expect someone else to clean up after you!

Dealing with hazards

The three key areas to consider are:

- a **hazard** in the salon
- the **risk** that the hazard will be harmful
- the **control** by which you reduce the risk if possible.

> **Key terms**
>
> **Hazard** – anything that can cause harm or that has the potential to cause harm.
>
> **Risk** – the chance, however great or small, that the hazard will cause harm to someone.
>
> **Control** – the means by which risks identified are eliminated or reduced to acceptable levels.

Follow health and safety practice in the salon

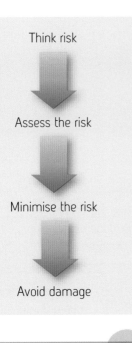

Think risk

Assess the risk

Minimise the risk

Avoid damage

Looking for a risk, and acting upon a risk assessment, is not necessarily a complicated matter, but it does need to be thought through thoroughly. Be logical. Start with the most obvious risks. Visualise making a cup of tea. What is the most hazardous part? Boiling and pouring the water is the most obvious answer, as boiling water has the potential to burn the skin quite seriously. You may get a stomach upset if the milk has gone off, or the handle on the teacup may break, or the spout on the teapot may leak, but these are secondary probabilities. Go for the main hazard, even if you think it is probably too obvious, and you cannot go far wrong. So, you have to recognise the potential of the hazard to cause injury or harm, but you also have to know what to do in order to neutralise the risk, or to make the risk as low as possible.

Promoting a safe working environment

A sensible and intelligent question to ask when attending a job interview for any salon position is what staff training is available, not just for advancement of skill areas but also for health and safety.

Think about it

Simple precautions can often be the most effective, and common sense will always help to prevent accidents. Ignorance is not an acceptable excuse, nor is it accepted as a defence against misconduct or a damage claim within a court of law. There is no justification for not being fully aware of your responsibilities and duty to yourself, your clients and your colleagues.

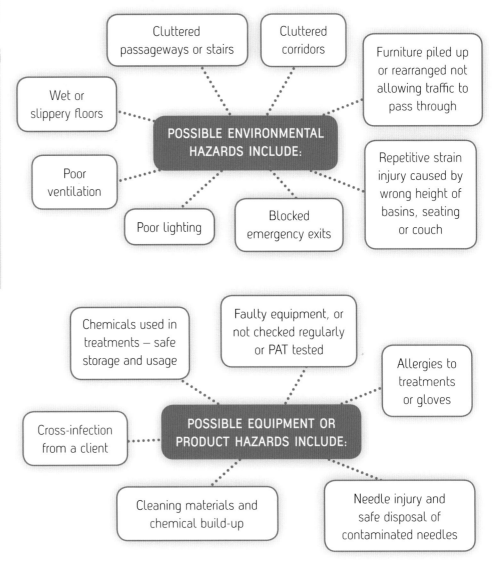

Regular guidance for all levels of staff will help to identify and minimise the hazards. All salons should have a workplace policy to include:

◉ the workplace/environmental factors

◉ safe working methods and equipment use

◉ the safe use of all hazardous substances in the workplace (not just for your particular job role)

◉ general policies for eating, smoking, drinking and drugs

◉ expected personal presentation

◉ what to do in the event of an accident, breakage or spillage

◉ all emergency procedures

◉ behaviour policies for all personnel

◉ corrective action where required.

If you are told at interview not to worry about any of the above and that it really doesn't matter, then you need to consider whether you want to work in a place that has so little regard for the safety of staff and clients, as well as health and safety legislation.

Identifying workplace instructions relevant to your job

'Employers have a general duty under section 2 of the Health and Safety at Work etc Act 1974 to ensure the health, safety and welfare of their employees at work so far as is reasonably practicable. People in control of non-domestic premises [e.g. beauty salons] have a duty (under Section 4 of the Act) towards people who are not their employees but use their premises [e.g. clients]. The Regulations expand on these duties and are intended to protect the health and safety of everyone in the workplace, and ensure that adequate welfare facilities are provided for people at work.

These Regulations aim to ensure that workplaces meet the health, safety and welfare needs of all members of a workforce, including people with disabilities. Several of the Regulations require things to be 'suitable'. Regulation 2(3) makes it clear that facilities/the workplace should be suitable for anyone. This includes people with disabilities. Where necessary, parts of the workplace, including in particular doors, passageways, stairs, showers, washbasins, lavatories and workstations, should be made accessible for people with disabilities.'

(Source: Health and Safety Executive (2007), 'Workplace health, safety and welfare: A short guide for managers')

A salon only has a legal requirement to have written risk assessments and documentation if it employs five or more people. However, the sensible salon owner will have that in place regardless of how many staff are employed. Many insurance companies insist on written risk policies before they will agree to insure the business.

The other health and safety requirements for a small business are:

◉ to inform the HSE area office or the local authority's environmental health department of the business's name and address

◉ to inform the HSE area office or the local authority's environmental health department of any new employees

Follow health and safety practice in the salon

◉ to display the health and safety law poster (available at your local Trading Standards Office) or hand out leaflets containing the equivalent information

◉ to make an assessment of the risks at the workplace — which must be acted upon and kept as a written record if the business has five or more employees (this includes fire risks)

◉ to bring the business's written statement of its health and safety policy to the attention of employees, and keep it up to date

◉ to register with the local health authority if appropriate — this will apply in particular to therapists who carry out skin piercing.

Workplace health, safety and welfare

In each of the practical units you must take into account the lighting, ventilation, heating and general comfort of the client — refer to Organisational and legal requirements in the section 'What you must know' of the National Occupational Standards. This is not only for client safety but also for yours. The client may be in the sauna for a ten-minute treatment and you will be looking after her. Not only is her body temperature rising, yours is too, but she will be able to relax and rehydrate while you will be working!

Although you may think that salon ventilation and lighting is not part of your job role, these environmental factors affect you, your colleagues and the clients, so you need to be aware of them. You will therefore need to consider all aspects of the salon, both for client comfort and safety and for all workers in the salon. These include:

◉ ventilation

◉ temperatures in indoor workplaces

◉ environmental factors, e.g. humidity and sources of heat in the workplace

◉ personal factors, e.g. the type and quantity of clothing a worker is wearing and how physically demanding their work is

◉ thermal comfort in the workplace — this applies to both workers and clients

◉ supervision — to ensure the implementation of precautions put in place to safeguard workers' health in the workplace environment

◉ lighting

◉ automatic emergency lighting, powered by an independent source, should be provided where sudden loss of light would create a risk

◉ cleanliness and waste materials

◉ room dimensions and space

◉ workstations and seating

◉ safety and training in the precautions to be taken

◉ maintenance

◉ floors and traffic routes

◉ loading bays

◉ open sides of staircases — these should be fenced with an upper rail at 900 mm or higher, and a lower rail

◉ transparent or translucent doors, gates or walls and windows

◉ windows and skylights — these should be designed so that they may be cleaned safely

◉ doors and gates — internal and external

Think about it

All aspects of the workplace are pertinent to you, and should be researched.

Think about it

Therapists who work in large salons within department stores are expected to unpack their own deliveries in loading bays, so health and safety for this area should also be researched — it is all part of your job role in a salon.

- escalators and moving walkways
- sanitary conveniences and washing facilities
- drinking water
- accommodation for clothing and facilities for changing
- facilities for rest and to eat meals — canteens or restaurants may be used as rest facilities provided there is no obligation to purchase food
- suitable rest facilities for pregnant women and nursing mothers. (Source: Health and Safety Executive (2007), 'Workplace health, safety and welfare: A short guide for managers'.)

For your portfolio

The questions below are from students who have just started work in a salon. Research each question to find out how the law can help them.

Maria: My salon is very stuffy. I often feel light-headed and sometimes think I'm going to faint. Can I complain to my employer, or will I get into trouble? What are my rights, if any?

Nicky: There is nowhere for me to eat lunch, and my boss says I am lucky to get a lunch break. I thought the salon should have a staff room? How would I find out?

Shreena: My work station is right next to a store cupboard. Staff are always going in and out, and the cupboard door keeps crashing into the back of my seat. It disrupts my treatments all the time, and I'm usually feeling a bit sore by the end of the day. What do the rules say about working areas? Surely we have to be safe?

Sam: In my salon we just put all the waxing strips (even the ones with blood spots on them) into the normal bin. I don't think that is hygienic or allowed by law. What do we have to do and how can I find out about this?

Jasmine: The lighting in the passageway to the stock cupboard is very dull and I think it is a bit of a hazard. Someone could easily fall over. What does the law state?

Identifying aspects of your workplace which could be harmful

For your portfolio

Obtain a copy of the Health and Safety Executive's booklet 'Workplace health, safety and welfare: A short guide for managers' (2007). The booklet is available online. It will help you in your research of workplace topics.

Think about it

When you inform your local Health and Safety Executive office that you are going into business, they will check out your business premises whether you work from home or in a salon. The requirements and level of inspection may vary from area to area and depend on your local authority. They will also depend upon the types of treatment your salon is going to offer; for example, face and body massage will require registration in large cities such as London, Birmingham and Manchester to show you are a legitimate massage business, but may not if you are in a small village. The same is true of treatments which involve skin piercing and the disposal of contaminated needles, ear piercing and electrolysis and milia removal.

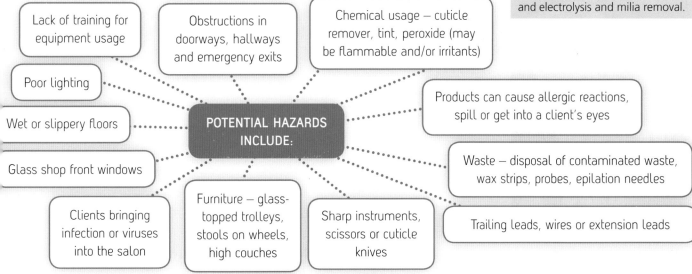

- Lack of training for equipment usage
- Obstructions in doorways, hallways and emergency exits
- Chemical usage — cuticle remover, tint, peroxide (may be flammable and/or irritants)
- Poor lighting
- Wet or slippery floors
- Glass shop front windows
- **POTENTIAL HAZARDS INCLUDE:**
- Products can cause allergic reactions, spill or get into a client's eyes
- Waste — disposal of contaminated waste, wax strips, probes, epilation needles
- Clients bringing infection or viruses into the salon
- Furniture — glass-topped trolleys, stools on wheels, high couches
- Sharp instruments, scissors or cuticle knives
- Trailing leads, wires or extension leads

Follow health and safety practice in the salon

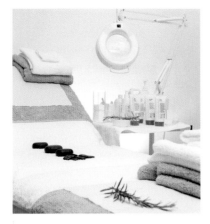

A safe work station

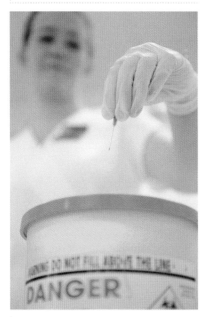

Waste must be disposed of safely

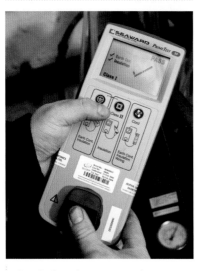

Electrical equipment must be checked by a competent person on a regular basis

Although these are identified as possible hazards, not all of them will become actual hazards, and certainly not all at the same time. For example, in all the years an experienced therapist works in a salon, there may not be a fire caused by faulty equipment overheating and bursting into flames. But the important thing is that the therapist will have recognised the possibility and will have her equipment regularly checked by a competent person. She will also keep a safety logbook with all equipment checks dated and signed, as recommended in the Electricity at Work Regulations 1989. The risk has been minimised, and should a fire start, the logbook will show that responsibility has been taken and the therapist or salon owner has not been neglecting her duty.

In this unit the Health and Safety at Work etc Act 1974 is the only piece of legislation specifically referred to, as it is the main piece of legislation under which nearly all of the other regulations fall. However, you should also refer to You, your client and the law (see Professional skills, pages 42–64) for other health and safety legislation. This includes the Electricity at Work Regulations 1989 and Environmental Protection Act 1990 for safe disposal of contaminated clinical waste.

Each practical unit has its own particular hazards which will be addressed in the unit itself. These risk factors are often out of the control of the therapist and should be the responsibility of the salon owner, for example ventilation required for nail varnish and artificial nail chemicals, or adequate ventilation in the sauna and steam suites.

However, if the sign to the salon was hanging off and about to drop onto a client or unsuspecting passer-by, you would be neglectful if you did not report it. Structural damage does happen to older buildings. If the salon is in, say, a Tudor building, which may be protected and listed, then the amenities will not be as modern as in later buildings. Oak beams and lead windows may be very attractive, but if water is dripping down a wall into an electricity socket, the building is not safe! Older buildings may be very expensive to maintain and can present many more hazards.

Identifying salon hazards in the workplace which present the highest risk

Some areas of the salon will be more high risk than others. For your own personal safety and that of others, it is up to you to know, understand and carry out workplace instructions particular to your job role, to identify those areas which are potentially harmful and control the risks, to be responsible and to be safe.

Environmental hazards

Hazard The working environment	What to check
The building A high-risk factor	Is the building safe and stable? Is there any asbestos present in the roof or walls? Is the outside of the building in good repair, with no probability of anything falling on the customer? Is the sign for the salon secure? Is the large salon window decorated with stickers to stop anyone walking into it? Is the window made of safety glass to minimise damage should an accident happen?
Floors A high-risk factor	Are they clean and dry? Has there been any spillage? Have they been over polished and become slippery? Are there any loose carpet edges or rugs to trip on? Are the floor coverings hygienic and easily cleaned?
Doorways and hallways A high-risk factor	Are they clear of obstructions? Are they full of clutter, which could cause harm? Is a fire exit being blocked? Are the doors too heavy to open safely?
Windows and curtains A medium-risk factor	Is any electrical equipment near to a curtain that could catch fire? Are the windows safe and lockable? Do the windows open to allow sufficient ventilation and airflow?
General décor and facilities A low-risk factor	Is the paint on the walls lead-free? Are the light fittings secure? Does the building have safe wiring for lighting and plug sockets? Is the boiler regularly maintained and serviced? Are gas mains and water pipes new and working properly?

Equipment hazards

Hazard Equipment	What to check
Beds A high-risk factor	Are the brakes on? Is it at the right height for the therapist to work comfortably, and not too high for the client to get on to easily? Is the bedding a danger by being too long and trailing on the floor, ready to trip someone up? Is the bedding easily cleaned, protected during the treatment and hygienic?
Chairs A high-risk factor	Are chairs secured and at a suitable height? Are hydraulic chairs regularly maintained? Are all chairs stable? Are they on castors? Are they hygienic and easy to keep clean?
Trolleys A low-risk factor	Are they glass topped and liable to shatter? Are they secure on their castors? Are they regularly maintained? Are they hygienic and easy to keep clean? Are they up to the job given to them, or is the equipment too heavy?
Electrical appliances A high-risk factor	Are they regularly maintained by a competent person? Are they PAT tested regularly? Are they used by qualified personnel only? Are they safely stored? Are they used with the correct products only? Are they bought from a reputable manufacturer to ensure safety? Are they used at the correct socket with the right plugs and fuses? Are there any trailing leads? Are they placed on a safe surface, rather than balanced on a windowsill?
Bins for disposal of waste products A high-risk factor	Are the correct bins available for different waste products? Is contaminated waste separated from other waste (e.g. body fluids, blood, etc. from waxing or eyebrow shaping)? Who is responsible for emptying the bins and how regularly will they empty them? Is infection control in place to minimise risk?

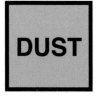 Dust  Toxic   Flammable 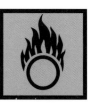 Irritant 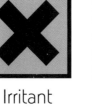 Corrosive   Oxidising agent

COSHH symbols showing the different types of hazardous substances

Products and chemical hazards

Hazard	What to check
Products A very high-risk factor	Are they clearly labelled? Are they stored safely and correctly? Has a COSHH (Control of Substances Hazardous to Health) sheet been completed for each product? Do therapists know how to use them correctly? Are they stored in the proper containers, not in other bottles? Is the shelf life taken into account? Are lids secured properly? Is a designated first-aider available in case of accidents? Do staff know what to do in cases of personal injury caused by poor product use? Are correct patch tests being carried out to prevent allergic reactions? Is regular product training being offered? Are toxic products stored correctly?
People A very high-risk factor	Should they be there? Are they going to create a hazard (e.g. workmen doing repairs and leaving tools out where clients are walking by)? Do they know where they are going? Are they aware of steps and the salon layout? Is their behaviour suitable for the salon, or are they using threatening behaviour? Are they intruders? Is there a risk they may be able to steal something?
You – the therapist	Do you lead others by giving a good example in health and safety matters? Does your behaviour endanger others? Are you fully trained to use equipment/products? Are you as hygienic as possible to avoid cross-infection? Do you follow the correct procedures for the workplace? Do you actively take part in regular training sessions for health and safety? Do you report possible hazards to the correct person? Is your uniform a health or safety hazard? Do you wear safe shoes? Do you wear a lot of jewellery? Do you walk around with sharp scissors in your pocket? Do you look out for the safety of others? Do you keep up-to-date client record cards? Do you use the correct lifting posture, i.e. keeping your back straight and bending your knees?

All of these hazards, checks for risks and tips for minimising the risks are very general, and mostly common sense. Each practical unit needs to be looked at specifically as each will have its own problems and risk potential.

By asking yourself the questions given here, you will soon start to identify and then rectify any risks.

Who is responsible for health and safety in your workplace?

Health and safety regulations apply to all businesses all the time. They should not merely be referred to when there has been a near accident at work – they should be a full-time concern.

The Health and Safety at Work etc Act 1974 is largely about employers – but since you may be an employer yourself one day, the following extracts from the Act will be very important to you.

The general duties of employers to their employees are set down in section 2(1) of the Act:

'It shall be the duty of every employer to ensure, so far as is reasonably practical, the health, safety and welfare at work of all his employees.'

In addition to responsibilities to employees, an employer has a duty to protect other persons, for example members of the public. These are stated in section 3(1) of the Act:

'It shall be the duty of every employer to conduct his undertaking in such a way as to ensure, so far as is reasonably practical, that persons not in his employment who may be affected thereby are not thereby exposed to risks to their health or safety.'

All persons who are self-employed also have responsibilities under the Act. These are dealt with under section 3(2):

'It shall be the duty of every self-employed person to conduct his undertaking in such a way as to ensure, so far as is reasonably practical, that he and other persons (not being his employees) who may be affected thereby are not thereby exposed to risks to their health or safety.'

Even if you have no intention of owning a salon, employing anyone, or becoming self-employed, you still have responsibilities as an employee. These include:

- correct use of systems and procedures
- reporting flaws or gaps within the system or procedure when in use.

Employers and employees have a shared responsibility for:

- the safety of individuals being cared for
- the safety of the working environment.

Employees also have responsibilities to take reasonable care of themselves and other people affected by their work and to cooperate with their employers in the discharge of their obligations.

The employee has a responsibility to:

- her/himself
- other employees
- the public.

Dealing with hazards in accordance with workplace instructions and legal requirements

All professional salons should have a set of rules and procedures for everyone to follow. Employees should be familiar with these rules and regulations for the safety and protection of all within the salon.

By law, the salon has to:

◉ display the health and safety rules and regulations on the wall in a prominent position (see Professional skills, page 43, for an example of this poster)

◉ display fire evacuation procedures.

Professionally, the salon will also have:

◉ codes of practice to follow from its professional body with regard to set procedures

◉ certain standards to maintain for insurance cover to be valid, which are usually linked to the codes of practice.

Legally, the employer is responsible for putting into place the rules covering the health and safety of all employees and clients and ensuring that safe practice is followed by all staff. These responsibilities may be carried out by:

◉ providing regular training, with staff meetings to update employees on safety issues

◉ giving a clear outline at the initial interview as to what is expected

◉ maintaining records of injuries or first aid treatment given

◉ monitoring and evaluating health and safety arrangements regularly

◉ providing a written health and safety booklet

◉ consulting the experts and being knowledgeable — ignorance is not an excuse.

Refer to You, your client and the law on pages 42–64 for a full breakdown of legal obligations of the employer and employee.

Reporting hazards of high risk

Hazards can and do happen and everyone should be aware of the safety implications.

As part of their personal responsibility, the therapist needs to be able to recognise when the hazard can be dealt with immediately and when help may be needed. It is very important to know who to go to when a salon problem arises that is a potential health and safety issue and there is any risk of harm. Salons will have different staff members with different areas of responsibility. One or two staff members will be trained in first aid, one person will assume responsibility for filling out the accident and report book and keeping health and safety records up to date, another will be responsible for building maintenance and the replacement of light bulbs, and so on.

Think about it

A hazard will need to be reported to a supervisor/lecturer/technician/manager/the person responsible for health and safety.

For your portfolio

Find out who is responsible for each aspect of health and safety in your salon. Make a list, so that in the event of an incident you know who to go to.

Follow health and safety practice in the salon

Follow health and safety practice in the salon

ACCIDENT/ILLNESS REPORT FORM

Beautiful Secrets

This form is to be completed by the injured party. If this is not possible, the form should be completed by the person making the report. If more than one person was injured, please complete a **separate form for each person**.

Completing and signing this form does not constitute an admission of liability of any kind, either by the person making the report or any other person.

This form should be completed immediately and forwarded to the Health and Safety Officer and Salon Manager.

If it is possible that an accident has been caused by a defect in machinery, equipment or a process, isolate/fence off the area and contact the Health and Safety Officer or Manager immediately.

SECTION 1 PERSONAL DETAILS

Surname: Lung   (Mr/**Mrs**/Ms/Miss) Forename(s): Jenny

Date of birth: 29/01/57   Address: 89, New Street, Glasgow

STAFF ☐   CONTRACTOR ☐   VISITOR ☐   GENERAL PUBLIC ☑

SECTION 2 ACCIDENT / INCIDENT / ILLNESS DETAILS

Accident (Injury) ☑   Illness ☐   Date: 19/04/12   Time: 13:07   (24-hour clock)

Location: Salon room 3

Nature of injury or condition and the part of the body affected:

Slipped on floor, twisted ankle

Account

Describe what happened and how. In the case of an accident state clearly what the injured person was doing.

Small patch of water on the floor – client got off couch and slipped on it.

Name and address of adult witness(es): Jo Benfield, Beautiful Secrets

Details of action taken

Ambulance summoned ☐   Taken to hospital ☐   Sent to hospital ☑

First aid given ☐   Taken home ☐   Sent home ☐   Returned to work ☐

SECTION 3 PREVENTATIVE ACTION

Recommended: to ensure that all spillages are mopped up straight away

Implemented: **Yes**/ No   Date: 19/04/12

Report raised by

Name: Catrina Waldron

Position: Therapist

Signature: C Waldron   Date: 19/04/12

FOR OFFICE USE ONLY

Copy sent to: Salon Manager ☐

Health and Safety Officer ☐

An accident report form

Examples of hazards which need reporting:

Hazard	Way to avoid hazard	When referral may be necessary
Breach of security	Shut windows, lock cupboards and doors	When something is found open or something is believed to be missing
Faulty or damaged products, tools, equipment, fixtures or fittings	Handle correctly, store correctly, treat with care Follow manufacturer's instructions	When something is found to be broken
Spillage	Take care when mixing, pouring and filling	When spilled material is corrosive or irritant
Slippery floors	Make others aware by blocking the area with a chair to prevent an accident Sweep up powder spills, mop up spills of liquid; refer to COSHH sheets for correct method	When acid, grease or polish is spilt
Obstruction to access and exit	Move large equipment away from doorways if able to do so Put bags and coats on a rack or shelving	When object is too heavy to be moved, it should be reported

These hazards should be reported to a manager or the health and safety officer within your workplace. There are also hazards that need to be reported to the local health officer or the Health and Safety Executive – refer to You, your client and the law, pages 42–64, for more information.

Dealing with hazards of low risk

This is largely common sense. If the risk is low and you can deal with it straight away, then do so to prevent an incident occurring. This could be something very straightforward, such as a client's handbag on the floor which could trip someone up. Pick it up off the floor, put it under the trolley out of the way and carry on with what you were doing.

This low-risk hazard does not need reporting, but it still requires prompt action to prevent it becoming a bigger problem.

Always act within the policy of your workplace. For example, if there is a policy on where clients' handbags and coats are stored to prevent congestion in the salon, then use the correct place.

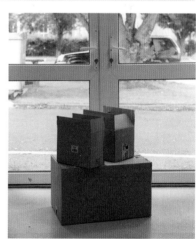

If something obstructing access is too heavy for you to move then it should be reported to the manager who will arrange to have it removed using sack trucks or similar

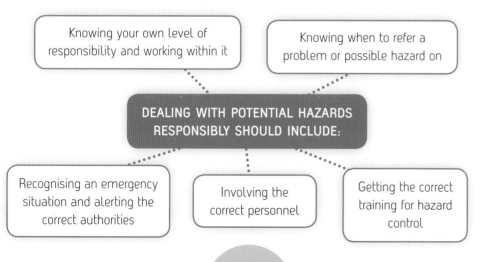

Knowing your own level of responsibility and working within it

Knowing when to refer a problem or possible hazard on

DEALING WITH POTENTIAL HAZARDS RESPONSIBLY SHOULD INCLUDE:

Recognising an emergency situation and alerting the correct authorities

Involving the correct personnel

Getting the correct training for hazard control

For your portfolio

Any low-risk hazard has potential to become a high risk – if action is not taken. What would you consider to be a low-risk hazard in your salon? Look around your place of work and have a detailed review of possibilities. What would be a high-risk hazard? Keep a risk assessment form handy and write down what you see – in many companies bonuses are paid to workers who prevent accidents from happening.

Follow health and safety practice in the salon

Salon security and reducing workplace risks

There are many areas to keep secure in a business.

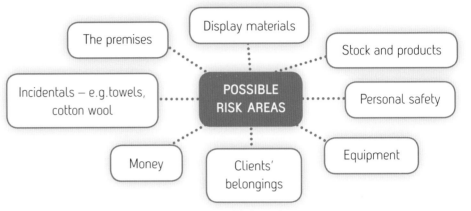

The premises · Display materials · Stock and products · Incidentals – e.g. towels, cotton wool · **POSSIBLE RISK AREAS** · Personal safety · Money · Clients' belongings · Equipment

The premises

For insurance and mortgage applications the salon owner must have adequate security measures in place for the salon. It is worth consulting the local police station for guidance. The crime prevention officer will survey the premises and give advice regarding the most vulnerable areas and the most common forms of entry by a burglar.

Externally

◎ Deadlock all doors and windows. Double-glazing is expensive but is more difficult to break into – the older the window and frame, the easier the entry.

◎ Fit a burglar alarm if possible, or even a dummy box on the wall, which will deter a burglar.

◎ Closed circuit television (CCTV) may be available if the premises are in a shopping area with other stores.

◎ Metal shop front shutters are probably the most effective deterrent. If the premises have a shutter system, use it.

Internally

◎ Internal doors can be locked to prevent an intruder moving from room to room.

◎ Fire doors and emergency exits should be locked at night, and reopened by the first person to arrive in the morning.

◎ A light left on in reception may deter would-be burglars, who may feel that well-lit premises will make them more easily seen.

◎ Stock and money should be locked away or should be in the bank so that nothing is visible to entice a burglar in the first place.

◎ Lock expensive equipment away in treatment rooms or in the stock cupboard.

◎ Very large businesses employ night security guards to patrol their premises, but as with alarmed infrared beams, these are not affordable for the average small salon owner. If, however, the salon is situated within a shopping centre or business park, night patrols may be included in the lease or purchase agreement or offered at a set fee per year. Costs would need to be considered, but it may be a worthwhile investment and save money in the long term.

◎ The local police station can be contacted.

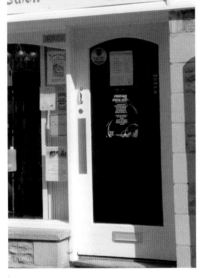

Fit a burglar alarm if possible – even a dummy one will put off a potential thief

How to minimise security breaches

Of all the temptations to the thief, smaller items may prove irresistible if they are small enough for a pocket and are very accessible. Unfortunately, this form of shoplifting costs many businesses a great deal of money, as stock can be expensive to replace and can be a big chunk of the capital outlay of a salon.

A sad fact is that the average thief may be rather closer to home than is comfortable. Staff may 'borrow' an item of stock for home use and think that their behaviour is acceptable. Also clients may like the look of a lipstick and 'forget' to pay for it!

Stealing small items is referred to as 'pilfering'; a polite word for stealing, and stealing larger items is referred to as 'shoplifting'. Either way, it means the salon has bought an item of stock from the wholesaler that has not been paid for by a customer, so it has to absorb that financial loss. If unchecked, it could eventually bankrupt the business, so tight precautions such as the following are called for:

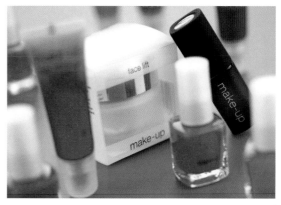

Small attractive items may prove tempting and easy pickings for a thief

- Have one person, usually the senior therapist or senior receptionist, in control of stock and limit keys and access to stock.
- Do a regular stock check, daily for loss of stock and weekly for stock ordering and rotation.
- Use empty containers for displays, or ask the suppliers if they provide dummy stock – this will also save the product deteriorating while on display.
- Keep displays in locked glass cabinets that can be seen but not touched.
- Encourage staff and customers to keep handbags away from the stock area, usually at reception, to stop products 'dropping' into open bags or supply lockers so bags can be safely locked away.
- Have one member of staff responsible for topping up the treatment products from the wholesale tubs.
- Hold regular staff training on security and let staff know what the losses are and how it may affect them – some companies offer bonus schemes for reaching targets of both sales and minimising pilfering. Heavy losses may affect potential salary increases.
- Bank money from the till at different times of the day and do not keep too much money in the till at any one time.
- Do not leave the till key in the till if the reception is to be unmanned for any length of time – it is too easy to get into.

Client security

- Where possible, don't take a client's belongings from them unless they go into a locker facility with the client holding the key – otherwise you leave yourself vulnerable to accusations. A lost purse can easily become an accusation of theft if there is an element of doubt in the client's mind.
- Encourage the client to bring as little cash or jewellery as possible so that the salon is not responsible for too many valuables. If a client is attending for a manicure, suggest they leave their rings at home so they cannot be mislaid. This minimises the risk of loss.

Think about it

Do not leave the reception area unattended for any length of time – one salon lost its till when someone unplugged and stole it – there were no keys in it but the drawer could be forced open and the money stolen. The salon had to recoup the loss of money and the cost of replacing the till. This advice is particularly pertinent to small salons.

Follow health and safety practice in the salon

● Encourage clients to empty pockets when hanging up coats. In this way valuables are not left unattended in reception and in a pocket – this is very easy to do, especially with mobile phones.

● Try not to confuse staff belongings with those of clients: staff should keep their belongings in the staff room under lock and key so that there is no confusion.

Reducing risks for staff

The salon should provide lockable storage cabinets or similar so that personal belongings can be locked away. Handbags and purses are always vulnerable to the opportunist thief, who may look like an ordinary member of the public, come in off the street and be gone in no time with someone's valuables. Large amounts of cash should not be brought into work.

Staff should be discouraged from wearing expensive jewellery to work. This will have to be removed during treatments and is therefore vulnerable to loss or theft.

Large amounts of takings should be removed from the salon daily and put into a bank or night deposit. Avoid taking the same route to the bank at the same time of day. Someone may be watching!

Be very aware of clients' jewellery – let them see that their items of jewellery are placed in a bowl on the trolley and make sure you return them after finishing the treatment. Do not risk being called a thief by slipping them into your overall pocket!

Be aware of suspicious packages left unattended – inform a supervisor and if necessary call the emergency services. The salon should have a list of telephone numbers by the phone in case of emergency, such as the local police station or security guard room. This will save time in an emergency situation.

Make sure you are protected – do not leave outside doors open when working in a treatment room, do not leave the till drawer open and do not be naive enough to think that it could not happen to you. If unsure, seek professional advice from the local crime prevention officer who will be able to advise you on both building security and personal safety hints for staff and clients.

As a professional therapist do not allow yourself to become a victim – follow your professional guidelines:

● Do not treat a male client alone in the salon late at night.

● Always work in pairs, at least on winter evenings.

● Always lock up the premises together.

● Be aware of where you have parked your car. In daylight that alley may look fine, but it may not be in the dark after work.

● Do not walk home alone in the dark – phone a taxi or friend.

● Do not put yourself at risk in any way.

Think about it

Your legal responsibilities form the first part of every practical unit – refer to Organisational and legal requirements in the section 'What you must know' of the National Occupational Standards. Reducing the risks to health and safety in the workplace is part of your legal responsibilities, so it is important to link this to your treatments.

Think about it

If a manufacturer's instructions do not comply with the practice in your salon, then always ask for clarification from your supervisor or manager, rather than endanger a client.

Think about it

You should always follow environmentally friendly practices where possible. This means being thoughtful about recycling rubbish, and separating waste such as plastic bottles for recycling. Try to be economical with product usage so waste is minimised and avoid lots of plastic packaging where possible. Many product houses now use recyclable cardboard rather than plastic packaging.

My story

Security conscious

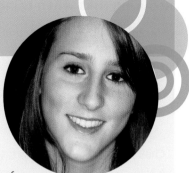

Hi, my name is Amelia and I work in a busy salon in the high street. We get a lot of walk-in customers off the street for treatments. I was just on my way out to do some shopping in my lunch hour when I realised I needed the toilet. I left my handbag on a chair in reception. I was only gone two minutes. During that time the receptionist went into the salon to see a client – and my purse was stolen from my handbag! I just couldn't believe it – it all happened so quickly. I lost my cash, my bank cards and receipts for work, which I needed to claim back, my loyalty cards, which had quite a bit on them, and a photo of my mum, who died last year. I was as upset about that as much as anything. You can always replace bank cards and I immediately stopped them with my bank – but you never get back the personal things that are irreplaceable.

Reducing risks in the working environment

Hazard The working environment	Actions to minimise risk
The building A high-risk factor	Take out property owner's liability insurance, often known as buildings insurance. This covers damage to the outside of the salon building such as roof repairs, wall repairs, etc. Internal major fittings such as toilet facilities and kitchens are also often covered. Maintain and check the outside of the property regularly and repair small damage before it becomes a major hazard.
Floors A high-risk factor	Only use the correct products for floor cleaning and allow plenty of drying time. Major stripping and recovering of the floor surface can be done outside normal salon times. Repair or avoid carpets and rugs with frayed edges and those not easily kept clean. Pay for professional cleaning companies to chemically clean carpets outside normal salon hours.
Doorways and hallways A high-risk factor	Have a regular inspection from your local fire safety officer who will advise the salon on the correct walkway exit route in case of fire. Keep corridors tidy and clutter-free. Ensure stairs and corridors are well lit, and replace blown light bulbs immediately.
Windows and curtains A medium-risk factor	Keep all electrical equipment away from the window area. Employ a handyman to ensure the windows open, are hinged properly and are safe and secure. Invest in double-glazing if possible, or make sure older style windows are properly maintained as loose windows are the ideal entry point for a potential thief. If your salon has a large window front and glass doors, remember to put lots of display stickers on them. Magnification mirrors without covers placed near to a window can become a fire risk if the sun's rays pass through the window, through the middle of the lamp and then on to a couch or curtains – the material may smoulder, then catch fire. Always cover the magnification lamp and do not leave by unshielded windows.
General décor and facilities A low-risk factor	Invest in safe decorating products bought from a reputable DIY store. Lead-based paint is hazardous to health and should not be used. Avoid positioning product displays, ornaments and plant pots where they are likely to be in the way of heavy traffic flow of people through the salon – they could be a trip hazard or knocked over. Regularly check and maintain the utility services – many companies provide a regular service agreement for a yearly overhaul of gas and electricity parts including boilers and central heating, etc.

Follow health and safety practice in the salon

Reducing risks when using equipment

Hazard Equipment	Actions to minimise risk
Beds A high-risk factor	Buy from professional suppliers only, with guarantees, and maintenance and repair agreements. Ensure the bed is the correct height to avoid back problems and buy an adjustable bed where possible. Use protective coverings that are washable, and minimise the risk of cross-infection by regularly disinfecting the bed and covering.
Chairs A high-risk factor	Buy from professional suppliers only, with guarantees, and maintenance and repair agreements. The recommended chair for use by professionals is the five-castor movable chair with adjustable height and backrest, often called the 'super secretarial chair'. Make sure the height of the chair is suitable for you – you should be able to sit squarely with your bottom at the back of the chair and your feet firmly flat on the floor. Regularly maintain the chair and lubricate the castors.
Electrical appliances A high-risk factor	Buy from professional suppliers only, with guarantees, and maintenance and repair agreements. Always buy from a reputable manufacturer who provides training, suitable products and an after-sales service, and offers repairs and servicing. Comply with the Electricity at Work Act 1989 and have the equipment tested by a competent person. Keep a logbook of testing, dated and signed, with a system of labelling and removing faulty equipment from use. Ensure regular training to update all staff as well as training in fire fighting and the use of an extinguisher. Make sure staff know who to report to in case of electrical fires.

Reducing risks with waste

Hazard Waste	Actions to minimise risk
Disposal of waste products A high-risk factor	Environmental Protection Act 1990 The Controlled Waste Regulations 1992 The Special Waste Regulations 1996 This legislation requires all clinical waste (waste which consists wholly or partly of animal or human tissue, blood or other body fluids, swabs, dressings, syringes and needles) to be kept apart from general waste and to be disposed of to a licensed incineration or landfill site by a licensed company. A contract can be arranged with a local firm who will take away yellow bins with contaminated waste and replace them on a daily or weekly basis.
Products A very high-risk factor	The Control of Substances Hazardous to Health Regulations (COSHH) 2002 require you to assess the risk of all hazardous substances used in the workplace as well as those that you may become exposed to during your work activities or which are produced at the end of any work or process. Keep manufacturers' data sheets and ensure that products are used in accordance with the manufacturers' recommendations. COSHH sheets also have a space for the recommended first aid requirements if the product is in contact with the skin, is ingested (swallowed) or enters the eye. Learn these and be prepared for any eventuality. Proper labelling and clearly identifiable bottles or tubs for caustic ingredients will help to prevent accidents. Keep thorough and up-to-date record cards for clients' treatments and products, especially if there has already been a reaction or allergy to a particular product, or if the client has a severe allergy to a specific substance, such as nuts. Go on regular commercial training to keep abreast of new products, and never guess a product use or equipment usage.

Reducing risks with people

Hazard People	Actions to minimise risk
People A very high-risk factor	There are many risks involving people – operator error with equipment, visitors to the salon, untrained people using equipment they shouldn't and even opening windows they shouldn't. With visitors, be informed about who is coming and going in the salon. Many salons employ a badge or name labelling system to identify visitors, sales reps, tradespeople, delivery drivers and so on. They may be expected to sign in using a visitor book and have suitable identification with them. Minimise the risk of client harm by asking workers to carry out repairs in the quieter part of the day, or when the salon is closed. Major repairs would necessitate the salon being closed, as the clients' safety cannot be compromised. Do not be intimidated by a person shouting or by abusive behaviour. Firmly ask the person to leave, or consult with the manager or salon owner, and if necessary call the police.

Risk assessments in the workplace

A risk assessment is simply a careful examination of what, in your workplace, could cause harm to people, so that you can weigh up whether you have taken enough precautions or should do more to prevent harm. You are legally required to assess the risks in your workplace so that you put in place a plan to control those risks. According to the Health and Safety Executive's leaflet 'Five steps to risk assessment', 'The law does not expect you to eliminate all risk, but you are required to protect people as far as "reasonably practicable".'

How to assess the risks in your workplace

When thinking about your risk assessment, remember:

- a **hazard** is anything that may cause harm, such as chemicals, electricity, working from ladders, an open drawer etc
- the **risk** is the chance, high or low, that someone could be harmed by these and other hazards, together with an indication of how serious the harm could be.

Follow the five steps:

Step 1 Identify the hazards
Step 2 Decide who might be harmed and how
Step 3 Evaluate the risks and decide on precautions
Step 4 Record your findings and implement them
Step 5 Review your assessment and update if necessary

Using the scale of probability, severity and danger ratings, you can clearly identify the potentially harmful working practices and aspects of your workplace which present the highest risks to you or to others.

> **Think about it**
>
> You cannot blame anyone else for your own actions – you need to take responsibility for everything that you do. Suing for damages if there is an accident is becoming common practice, so do not allow yourself to be vulnerable or open to a negligence claim. The law is very clear on what amounts to negligence, so be well informed and knowledgeable to minimise risk in all you do.

(Source: Health and Safety Executive (2006) 'Five steps to risk assessment') (This leaflet is available to download from the HSE's website.)

The risk rating is:	The probability rating is:	The severity rating is:
Low = 1–7	1 – Highly unlikely	1 – trivial injury (no first aid required)
Medium = 8–16	2 – Possible	2 – minor injury (first aid required)
High = 17–25	3 – Probable	3 – major injury (hospitalisation)
	4 – Likely	4 – major injury to many persons
	5 – Inevitable	5 – death (of one or more persons)

Scale of probability, severity and danger ratings

Using the ratings, a risk assessment would look like this:

RISK ASSESSMENT FORM:

NAME OF EQUIPMENT:

A magnifying lamp

STEP 1 WHAT ARE THE HAZARDS?

Accident:

- placing the lamp too close to the client's face during the consultation
- the hinges not supporting the lamp head so risk of dropping / not staying in position
- trailing wires from lamp to wall socket

Fire: if placed by window with no cover on the lens, there is a risk of the sun's rays being magnified, heat being produced and a risk of smouldering /fire

STEP 2 WHO MIGHT BE HARMED?

Client

Therapist

All in the salon if fire occurs

WHAT IS ALREADY IN PLACE?

Lamps are covered when not in use

Lamps are not stored near windows

Equipment is regularly maintained

Extension leads used where necessary if workstation is far away from wall socket

WHAT FURTHER ACTION COULD BE TAKEN?

Training in use of equipment

Health and safety notice put up

Fire precaution and evacuation procedures put in place

| The **risk rating** is: 10 | The **probability rating** is: 2 | The **severity rating** is: 2-5 |

Follow emergency procedures

Health and safety procedures

Fire procedures

The Fire Precaution (Workplace) Regulations 1997 require all premises to undertake a fire risk assessment. If five or more people work together as employees, this risk assessment must be in writing. Employers must also take into account all other persons on the premises, not just employees.

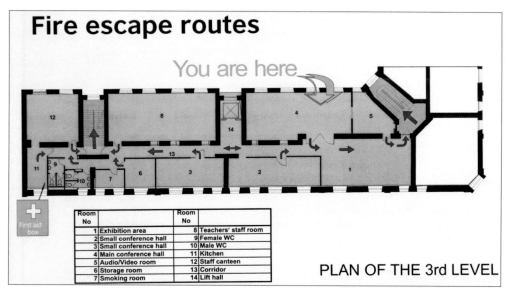

Fire escape routes

You are here

Room No		Room No	
1	Exhibition area	8	Teachers' staff room
2	Small conference hall	9	Female WC
3	Small conference hall	10	Male WC
4	Main conference hall	11	Kitchen
5	Audio/Video room	12	Staff canteen
6	Storage room	13	Corridor
7	Smoking room	14	Lift hall

PLAN OF THE 3rd LEVEL

In premises of any kind, staff must be aware of evacuation procedures and where to take their clients

There must also be a fire and evacuation procedure. In every period of one year there must be at least one fire drill, which involves everyone. Everyone must be fully informed, instructed and trained in what is expected of them. Some people will have special duties to perform.

All employees, trainees, temporary workers and others who work in any business must, by law, agree to cooperate with the employer so far as is necessary to enable them to fulfil the duties placed upon them. This means cooperating fully in training courses and fire drills, even when you know it is only a practice.

Most large training establishments will have their own policy on fire evacuation procedures and may carry out a fire drill once a term, that is three times per year. This is especially important with large groups of people or students, and any people with disabilities who will need special consideration.

Many fire-training exercises are organised with a fire safety officer from the local fire station. Often the fire engines will take part in the exercise to test their own

Think about it

Take precautions with all electrical equipment:

- Make sure there are no trailing leads to trip over.
- Carry out regular maintenance checks to ensure machines are working efficiently and safely.
- Follow manufacturers' instructions.
- Follow health and safety guidelines.

attendance time from the station to the premises. Everyone should be made aware of their own particular roles in the evacuation.

When joining any business or establishment the new person should be briefed on all health and safety issues, especially fire evacuation procedures. It is standard practice to include the information in a handbook containing all the establishment's policies.

Below is an example of an evacuation procedure.

Building evacuation procedures in the event of fire or bomb alert

The following procedure has been agreed and must be followed. Any staff member who does not comply is committing an infringement of the college disciplinary code. Whenever a fire occurs, the main consideration is to get everybody out of the building safely. Protection of personal or college property is incidental.

Raising the alarm

Anyone discovering a fire must immediately raise the alarm by operating the nearest fire alarm and report to the controller the fire location.

On hearing the alarm the receptionist will immediately contact the emergency services and then evacuate the building.

In the event of a fire being discovered when the reception is unmanned – the premises officer on duty will contact the emergency services and assume control.

On hearing the alarm

All those in senior positions proceed to the control point, normally at a main entrance to the building – where one person must take control of the proceedings.

All other staff: close windows; switch off machinery and lights, and close doors on leaving the room.

Assist less able colleagues, leave the building by the nearest marked route and proceed quickly to the appropriate assembly point. Staff must supervise their class.

Staff evacuating the building must check their locality is clear.

Assembly points

Everyone must remain at assembly points well away from buildings and clear of access roads.

Report to control in person or via two-way radios where allocated.

Everyone must remain at assembly points until further instructions.

DO NOT re-enter the building until you are told it is safe to do so.

An evacuation procedure

Emergency procedures

Fire drill relevant to the working area:

- Switch off all electrical equipment.
- Close all windows.
- Lead clients to a safe area and wrap them up warmly if necessary using blankets and towels. This is especially important when the client has been having a body treatment.

- If possible, take the client's valuable possessions with her, such as her handbag and jewellery, but not if they are safely locked away, or if it puts the client or therapist in any danger (usually clients' belongings are kept under the trolley and therefore are within easy reach).

- Be aware of the treatment being performed during the evacuation — if the client has chemicals on the skin, it may be easier to remove them immediately. This would need to be at the judgement of the person in charge of the workshop — certainly a client having an eyelash tint will need to have it removed before being able to proceed to the assembly point. Take appropriate remover and damp cotton wool or tissues to remove products on the skin such as facemasks. While it is not dangerous to the skin if left on, the client will probably be more comfortable and the skin less dry if it can be removed.

- Be aware of the client's footwear, and if possible encourage the wearing of shoes to prevent an accident occurring during the evacuation.

Bomb alert:

- Follow the procedures for a fire drill.

- Do not look inside a suspect package but do act quickly if an abandoned parcel or bag arouses suspicions.

Gas leak:

- Open all windows.

- Evacuate the building following the fire drill instructions.

- Do not turn off or on any electrical equipment as it may cause a spark which may ignite the gas.

Sensible fire precautions:

- Be informed — know what to do and where to go when the evacuation begins.

- Be sensible and do not panic — this will only make the client feel panicky too.

- Make sure that the location of the fire bell, fire extinguishers and fire exit are familiar.

- Never ignore smoke or the smell of burning — it is far better to have a false alarm.

- Do not misuse or mistreat electrical appliances that are a potential hazard — a healthy respect is needed.

- Do not ignore manufacturers' instructions for the storage and use of highly flammable products that are very common within the salon.

- Be sensible with naked flames and matches or the disposal of cigarette ends — a smouldering tip can burst into flames that will destroy the salon in minutes.

- Be able to account for clients — the appointment book can be taken outside to check which clients should be present. A college lecturer or trainer should do the same with the class register to check the correct numbers of students are present.

- Do not use a lift for the evacuation — the fire may affect the electric mechanism which then becomes another emergency.

- If you are not at the correct location for the fire evacuation, please return to the correct assembly post or you may not be accounted for. This may mean a fire-fighter taking risks to go back into a burning building to check — and all the time you are around the corner!

Fire-fighting equipment

Not every fire extinguisher is suitable to fight every fire — using the wrong one can make the situation worse. It is better to evacuate the building and call the fire service than it is to use the wrong extinguisher.

Only a person specially trained in the use of a fire extinguisher should attempt to use one. Never put yourself at risk. Personal safety is more important than saving material items that can be replaced — a human life cannot be replaced. Fire service safety leaflets recommend you never endanger life or stay in an area with a fire in an attempt to put it out — it is safer to leave it to the professionals.

In small premises, having one or two portable hand-held extinguishers of the appropriate type readily available may be all that is necessary. In bigger, more complex premises larger equipment will be needed, training should be given and the location should be indicated. This is usually in a conspicuous position on an escape route, near the exit doors.

Fires are classified by the type of material that has caught alight. The class of fire determines which fire extinguisher to use.

Class of fire	Fire extinguisher
Class A: Fires involving solid materials, e.g. wood, paper or textiles	Extinguishers with an 'A' rating, e.g. 13A Water extinguisher, foam extinguisher, dry powder extinguisher (size according to risk) Water extinguishers are the cheapest and most widely used, but are not suitable for Class B fires or fires involving electricity
Class B: Fires involving flammable liquids, e.g. petrol, diesel or oils	Extinguishers with a 'B' rating, e.g. 34B Foam extinguisher, CO_2 extinguisher, dry powder extinguisher (size according to risk) Foam extinguishers are more expensive than water, but can be used on both Class A and Class B fires
Class C: Fires involving flammable gases, e.g. propane, butane	Foam extinguisher (according to risk). Seek specialist advice Dry powder extinguishers are multi-purpose and can be used on Class A, B and C fires. However, they can obscure vision
Class D: Fires involving metals	Special powder extinguishers (size and type according to risk), dry sand (quantity according to risk). Seek specialist advice
Class E: Fires involving electrical apparatus	CO_2 extinguisher
Class F: Fires in cooking appliances, e.g. oil	Extinguishers with an 'F' rating, e.g. 15F Wet chemical extinguisher

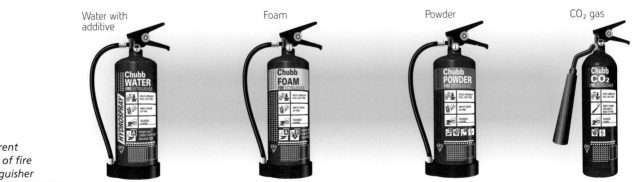

Water with additive   Foam   Powder CO_2 gas

Different types of fire extinguisher

A quick guide to selecting an extinguisher:

Type of fire	Type of extinguisher	Colour	Uses	NOT to be used
Electrical fires	Dry powder	Blue marking	For burning liquid, electrical fires and flammable liquids	On flammable metal fires
	Carbon dioxide	Black marking	Safe on all voltages, used on burning liquid and electrical fires and flammable liquids	On flammable metal fires
Non-electrical fires	Water	Red marking	For wood, paper, textiles, fabric and similar materials	On burning liquid, electrical or flammable metal fires
	Foam	Cream/yellow markings	On burning liquid fires	On electrical or flammable metal fires

Fire blankets are made of fire resistant material and are intended to extinguish cooking oil fires or to wrap around a person whose clothing is on fire. A fire blanket must be used calmly and with a firm grip. If the blanket is flapped about, it may fan the fire and make it flare up, rather than put it out. The hands should be protected by the edge of the cloth and the blanket should be placed, rather than thrown, into the desired position.

Never lean over the fire. Remember — if you cannot control the fire, leave the room, close the door and phone the emergency services.

Fire blankets conforming to British Standard BS 6575 are suitable for use in the home. These will be marked to show whether they should be thrown away after use or used again after cleaning in accordance with the manufacturer's instructions. Fire blankets are best kept in the kitchen or in the salon rest room, where there are likely to be domestic appliances such as kettles, microwaves and cookers, and where small fires can occur.

A bucket of sand can be used to soak up liquids that are the source of a minor fire. However, it is impractical to have large quantities of sand available to try to stop a major fire, so the instructions would be the same as for fire blankets — if in doubt never risk injury.

First aid

The Health and Safety (First Aid) Regulations 1981 set out the essential aspects of first aid that employers must address, because people at work can suffer injuries or fall ill. It does not matter whether the injury or illness is caused by the work they do. It is important that they receive immediate attention and that an ambulance is called in serious cases.

First aid can save lives and prevent minor injuries becoming major ones. First aid in the workplace is the initial management of any injury or illness suffered at work. It does not include giving tablets or medicines to treat illness but sufficient first aid personnel and facilities should be available to:

◉ give immediate assistance to casualties with both common injuries and illnesses and those likely to arise from specific hazards at work

◉ summon an ambulance or other professional help.

Follow health and safety practice in the salon

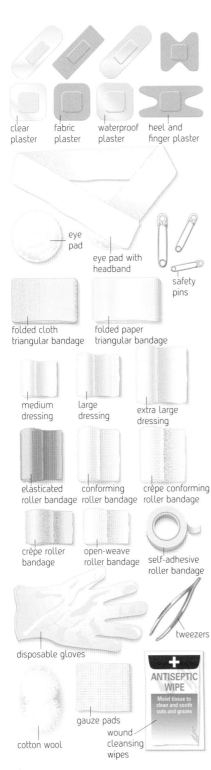

clear plaster

fabric plaster

waterproof plaster

heel and finger plaster

eye pad

eye pad with headband

safety pins

folded cloth triangular bandage

folded paper triangular bandage

medium dressing

large dressing

extra large dressing

elasticated roller bandage

conforming roller bandage

crêpe conforming roller bandage

crêpe roller bandage

open-weave roller bandage

self-adhesive roller bandage

disposable gloves

tweezers

cotton wool

gauze pads

ANTISEPTIC WIPE
Moist tissue to clean and sooth cuts and grazes

wound cleansing wipes

Items that your first aid box should contain

This will depend upon the size of the workforce, the type of workplace hazards and risks, and the history of accidents in the workplace.

Two aspects of first aid need further consideration:

⦿ Trainees — students undertaking work experience on certain training schemes are given the same status as employees and therefore are the responsibility of the employer.

⦿ The public — when dealing with the public these regulations do not oblige employers to provide first aid for anyone other than their own employees. This means the compulsory element of public liability insurance does not cover litigation resulting from first aid to non-employees. Employers should make extra provision for this themselves. Education establishments must also include the general public in their assessment of first aid requirements.

First aid kits

The minimum level of first aid equipment is a suitably stocked and properly identified first aid container.

First aid containers should be easily accessible and placed, where possible, near to hand-washing facilities. The number of containers will depend upon the size of the establishment, and the total number of employees in that area. The container should protect the items inside from dust and damp and must only be stocked with useful items. Tablets and medications should not be kept in there.

There is no compulsory list of what a first aid kit should contain, but the following would be useful:

⦿ a leaflet giving general guidance on first aid (such as the HSE leaflet 'Basic advice on first aid at work')

⦿ 20 individually wrapped sterile adhesive dressings (assorted sizes) appropriate to the type of work

⦿ two sterile eye pads

⦿ four individually wrapped triangular bandages (preferably sterile)

⦿ six safety pins

⦿ six medium-sized individually wrapped wound dressings

⦿ two large sterile individually wrapped unmedicated wound dressings

⦿ one pair of disposable gloves

⦿ antiseptic cream or liquid

⦿ eye bath

⦿ gauze

⦿ medical wipes

⦿ a pair of tweezers

⦿ cotton wool.

Do not forget that if in doubt, do not treat — phone for an ambulance immediately.

First aid training

First aid certificates are only valid for a certain period of time, which is currently three years. Employers need to arrange refresher training with retesting of competence before certificates expire. If a certificate expires, the individual will have to undertake a full course of training to be re-established as a first aider. Specialist training can also be undertaken if necessary.

Records

It is good practice for employers to provide first aiders with a book in which to record incidents which require their attendance. If there are several first aiders in one establishment, then a central book will be used. The information should include:

- date, time and place of incident
- name and job of the injured or ill person
- details of the injury or illness and what first aid was given
- what action was taken immediately afterwards (e.g. did the person go home?)
- name and signature of the first aider or person dealing with the incident.

Think about it

A first aid kit should be kept in a proper first aid container – an old biscuit tin will not do. It needs to be regularly checked to keep it fully stocked. You shouldn't be finding out that your kit is not fully stocked during an emergency!

Check your knowledge

1 Who is responsible for ensuring gloves and an apron are worn during waxing treatments?
   a) Salon manager
   b) Client
   c) Therapist
   d) Salon owner.

2 A hazard is defined as:
   a) something that will harm you
   b) something that will kill you
   c) something which has the potential to cause harm
   d) the risk you take at work.

3 The two fire extinguishers suitable for use on any electrical fire are colour coded:
   a) blue or black
   b) red and cream
   c) blue and red
   d) black and cream.

4 Which of these is just the employer's responsibility?
   a) Report faulty goods or equipment.
   b) Wear protective clothing or work wear.
   c) Provide information about health and safety and security.
   d) Take care to ensure the health and safety of others.

5 The definition of a risk is:
   a) the likelihood of a hazard's potential being realised
   b) the risk of an accident occurring
   c) the elimination of an accident occurring
   d) the potential to cause harm.

6 Your job description should have within it:
   a) your national insurance number
   b) your driving licence
   c) your health and safety responsibilities
   d) your qualifications listed.

7 The symbol for a toxic substance is:
   a) a big red cross
   b) a big black cross
   c) a skull and cross bones
   d) a flame.

8 If there are blood spots on a wax strip, you must:
   a) wrap it in newspaper and put it in the bin
   b) put it in a bin liner and put it in the dustbin
   c) put it in the contaminated yellow waste bin
   d) take it to the hospital for disposal.

9 How many steps are there in a risk assessment?
   a) Ten
   b) Six
   c) Five
   d) Eleven.

10 HSE stands for:
   a) Housing Standard Economy
   b) Health and Safety Executive
   c) Health and Safety Election
   d) Human Safety Executive.

Follow health and safety practice in the salon

Getting ready for assessment

The first part of Follow health and safety practice in the salon requires that you identify the hazards and evaluate the risks in your workplace and gather evidence to support your work such as:

- Take part in an evacuation procedure following all the guidelines safely. This will have to be a simulation as hopefully the building will not actually be on fire! Keep a log or diary of the date, time and exactly what happened, and the assessor will accept this as evidence.

- Attend a health and safety training day as part of your job role outside college. A formal letter from your part-time employer confirming that you attended the training day, dated and signed, will also provide evidence. It may be an accident procedure demonstration, a risk assessment training day or a training day covering maintenance of equipment. This will ensure your performance criteria – what you must do – will be covered.

- You should be able to show you can identify the possible risks of your own working practices. This means you should immediately report a spillage in the salon, a frayed wire, a faulty piece of equipment or a blocked fire exit. You could be in the middle of a facial assessment when you notice the wire to the steamer, which you are about to use, is a potential risk. Follow the set procedures for reporting it, and you will have an assessment for both Follow health and safety practice in the salon and Provide facial skincare.

In the second part of Follow health and safety practice in the salon you must show you have taken steps to reduce any possible health and safety risks within your own job role/responsibilities. Any of the following duties will count towards an assessment:

- If, during the course of your reception duties, your job is to decant products from large wholesale tubs into smaller ones for use by other therapists, then make sure all labelling is correct, the storage is suitable for the product and that the COSHH sheets are up to date. By volunteering to check these details you will collect a lot of valuable evidence.

- If you are designated salon manager for a day, volunteer to carry out a risk assessment on the working salon. As well as organising equipment and matching clients to therapists, look at equipment, working stations and staff with a critical eye. Are there any improvements that could be made to minimise risk? Are staff as vigilant as they could be?

- Look at the bigger picture outside the working stations. Even a light bulb blowing out could be a risk if it illuminates a stairway. Report it, minimise the risk, identify the solution. This will ensure your performance criteria will be covered.

- Be inventive. Are there risk assessment solutions that you use in your place of work that would help you at college? For example, a better design of record cards with allergy or medical conditions highlighted, better storage facilities or a particular training programme that you would recommend? Write up a proposal – the assessor can then investigate it and if it minimises risk, this will ensure your performance criteria will be covered.

Think about it

Advice is available from the Health and Safety Executive.

Client care and communication in beauty-related industries

What you will learn

- Communicate with clients
- Provide client care

Introduction

Excellent client care and communication skills are essential in the beauty industry. Clients expect more than just fantastic results – they are also paying for outstanding client care and want to have a good relationship with the beauty therapist. There are two types of clients:

◉ those who have treatments occasionally and go to a salon as a treat – perhaps they have received a gift voucher

◉ regular clients who enjoy being pampered and want their appearance maintained.

Whichever type of client, treatments can be costly, so it is important to pamper clients as well as ensuring perfect results. You can do this by performing the treatments correctly and demonstrating good communication skills. With so many salons and spas providing treatments, there is a lot of competition and clients can afford to be selective. Having outstanding client care and communication skills can give you the edge your business needs.

Top tips

To encourage clients to return, a salon may offer **incentives** such as money-off vouchers and monthly promotions.

Communicate with clients

In this outcome you will learn about:

- using effective communication techniques
- using client consultation techniques to identify treatment objectives
- providing the client with clear advice and recommendations.

Key terms

Incentives – something to entice clients to return, for example discounted treatments or 3-for-2 offers.

Different forms of communication used to deal with clients

You will need to communicate effectively with everyone you come in contact with, develop specific relationships and adapt how you communicate, depending upon the situation and the person you are with, as shown in the diagram below.

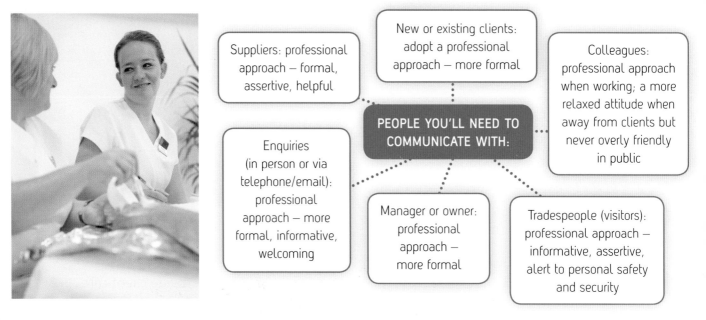

Suppliers: professional approach – formal, assertive, helpful

New or existing clients: adopt a professional approach – more formal

Colleagues: professional approach when working; a more relaxed attitude when away from clients but never overly friendly in public

Enquiries (in person or via telephone/email): professional approach – more formal, informative, welcoming

PEOPLE YOU'LL NEED TO COMMUNICATE WITH:

Manager or owner: professional approach – more formal

Tradespeople (visitors): professional approach – informative, assertive, alert to personal safety and security

The table below identifies the personality **traits** required to be a high-performing beauty therapist and how to avoid being a poorly performing one.

High-performing beauty therapist	Poor-performing beauty therapist
<ul><li>Good communication skills – an **active listener**, speaks at appropriate times, good questioning skills, good body language, can communicate with all, without discrimination</li><li>Skilled and motivated – has the qualifications, experience and drive to succeed</li><li>Efficient and **proactive** – has excellent time management skills and can allocate tasks and activities themselves</li><li>Discreet – demonstrates high level of professionalism and maintains client confidentiality in line with the **Data Protection Act 1998** (see page 59)</li><li>Pleasant and friendly approach – evidenced by the way they deal with clients, making them feel special, and demonstrating a passion for the beauty industry.</li><li>Good manners – demonstrates a level of respect for others by always being polite or generally being helpful to others</li><li>Follows **dress code and personal hygiene** rules – helps clients to feel confident in their abilities and will not create barriers.</li></ul>	<ul><li>Does not follow dress code or personal hygiene rules – creates barriers, as clients will lack confidence in their abilities and poor personal hygiene will be offensive to all</li><li>Poor communication skills – clients, employees and employers will lack confidence in their abilities and this will not generate repeat bookings or retail sales</li><li>Not following salon policies – creates risks and hazards that could result in injury, damage to a client's personal effects or salon equipment and, in serious cases, death.</li></ul>

Key terms

Traits – personality qualities, behaviour, character.

Active listener – someone who listens carefully to what the other person is saying.

Proactive – being able to self-manage, i.e. not requiring someone to tell you what you need to do.

Data Protection Act 1998 – the law that protects clients' personal information.

Dress code and personal hygiene – rules from the salon's workplace policy on what you must wear and do (see also Follow health and safety practice in the salon, pages 11–12).

Think about it

Look at the traits of a good and poor therapist, then write a list of your own personality traits. Are there areas you can improve on?

Personality traits of a good and poor beauty therapist

Types of communication

As soon as a client walks through the door, you will naturally start to communicate with them, first by making eye contact and smiling. This greeting makes the client feel welcome and important.

The diagram below summarises the main types of communication.

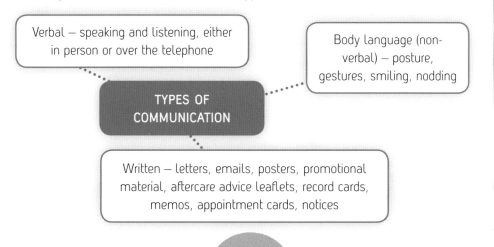

Verbal — speaking and listening, either in person or over the telephone

Body language (non-verbal) — posture, gestures, smiling, nodding

TYPES OF COMMUNICATION

Written — letters, emails, posters, promotional material, aftercare advice leaflets, record cards, memos, appointment cards, notices

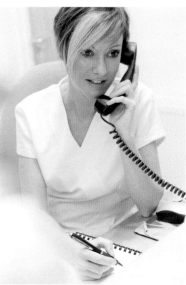

Be prepared when you communicate over the telephone

Client care and communication in beauty-related industries

Top tips

- Always make eye contact and smile when a client walks into the salon, as it makes them feel important. Imagine how you would feel if you were a client and the receptionist ignored you when you entered the salon. Never treat clients in this way.

- When the telephone rings, answer it quickly, demonstrate good verbal skills and have the information you might need, which could include business opening times, appointment availability, treatments offered and prices. An example of a telephone greeting might be: 'Good morning, The Beauty Studio, Samuel speaking. How may I help you?'

Top tips

- When you give important information to a client who speaks English as a second language, check that they have understood by asking them to repeat back what you have said or reinforce their understanding by providing a written copy.

- Clients who are visually impaired will often have a guide dog. Ensure the client is positioned safely so the dog is not obstructing walkways or doorways.

Using verbal communication

- ◉ Speak clearly.
- ◉ Avoid jargon; use plain English.
- ◉ Actively listen and do not interrupt.
- ◉ Be polite and attentive.
- ◉ Use good questioning techniques.
- ◉ Some hearing-impaired clients can lip read, so demonstrate good communication skills by keeping still when you speak and they are trying to lip read.
- ◉ Clients who are visually impaired will need you to be very descriptive, as often they cannot see the treatment results fully, or at all.
- ◉ Never use over-familiar or overly friendly words, such as 'Love' or 'Babe', as this is not professional and some clients may find it offensive.

Using non-verbal communication (body language)

- ◉ Nod when you are actively listening to a client to acknowledge them.
- ◉ Make eye contact and smile.
- ◉ Never fold your arms, keep them relaxed.
- ◉ Do not point with your fingers.
- ◉ Give clients 'personal space' — never get too close, as it may cause them to feel very uncomfortable.
- ◉ Stand up when a client approaches you.

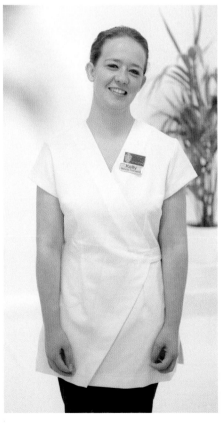 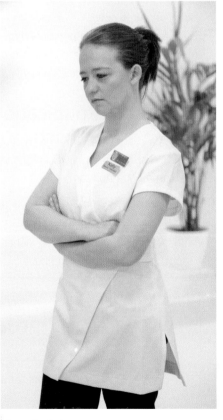

Good body language *Poor body language*

Using written communication

- Check presentation is clear.
- Use ICT skills when appropriate, for example when creating a poster or writing an email.
- Avoid jargon; use plain English.
- Use correct spelling, good grammar and punctuation.
- Provide correct information, for example when filling in an appointment card or taking a message.
- Clients who are dyslexic will have special requirements. For example, they might need promotion letters to be on yellow paper. Ask them what you can do to help, as this will demonstrate good client care.

Understanding a client's body language

When recommending a treatment or retail product to a client, you need to learn how to recognise whether they are interested or not. Their body language will give you clues, for example they:

- may look uninterested
- do not ask any questions
- provide little or no eye contact
- fiddle or play with their hair or jewellery
- look nervous or confused
- frown.

How to use consultation techniques to identify treatment objectives

The main purpose of completing a **consultation** is to:

- build a good **rapport** with the client
- gain the client's confidence
- discuss the treatment plan and the client's requirements
- establish any **contra-indications**
- discuss future treatments and retail recommendations
- complete the record card and obtain the client's signature.

Communication techniques in practice

Gathering all the information required may be difficult if the client is shy or nervous and perhaps does not feel comfortable discussing either themselves or the treatment. This is where you will need to demonstrate excellent communication and questioning skills. The following table shows the techniques you will need to be an effective communicator.

Key terms

Consultation – a discussion before a treatment begins.

Rapport – relationship between people.

Contra-indications – skin and nail diseases or disorders that would prevent or restrict a treatment.

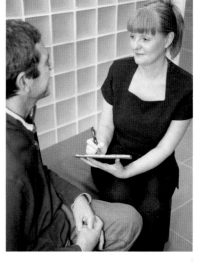

Sit facing your client during a consultation and use positive body language

Client care and communication in beauty-related industries

Key terms

Open questioning techniques – questions asked in a way to get a detailed answer.

Closed questions – questions that only obtain a yes or no answer.

Technical jargon – words used by beauty therapy industry professionals, for example 'epidermis'; when talking to clients, refer to the skin instead.

Contra-action – a bad or adverse reaction of a client to a treatment, for example redness or blistering of the skin.

For your portfolio

Look at the communication techniques shown in the table.

In pairs, use role-play to practise your communication techniques, taking it in turns to be the therapist and the client. Perform a consultation and discuss aftercare advice, then evaluate your performance. What areas do you need to perfect before you are assessed on this unit for your qualification?

Communication techniques

Key terms

Modified – a treatment can be adapted or changed to take into account a contra-indication. For example, a bruise can be worked around, or if a client has bitten nails then adding a heat treatment with massage will help to stimulate growth.

Communication technique	What is involved
Active listening	Listen carefully to what the client is saying. Do not be distracted when performing the consultation – sit down in front of the client at the same level and focus on what they are saying. Never interrupt or finish a client's sentence to avoid any misunderstandings.
Questioning techniques	Use **open questioning techniques** to obtain as much information as possible from the client, e.g. 'How do you care for your feet at home?' will give you a detailed response. Avoid **closed questions**, such as 'Do you have a routine at home to look after your feet?', which will give you a yes or no answer.
Understanding	Ask the client questions to check they have understood what you have said. You might need to rephrase and repeat a question or information. Never use **technical jargon** – use plain English so clients will understand.
Location of the consultation	Only the therapist performing the treatment should complete the consultation, which should be carried out at the workstation, in a discreet manner.
Body language	Use open, friendly gestures, e.g. smile, nod and maintain a good posture.
Written communication	The therapist must complete the record card and ask the client to check and sign it before the consultation process is complete. The client must sign the record card to document what has been discussed and for insurance purposes to protect the therapist and business. Any retail products purchased by the client, aftercare or homecare advice can be written down for the client to reinforce the information and help promote retail sales. Providing aftercare advice will also minimise or prevent possible **contra-actions** and inform clients of what to do in the event of a contra-action.

Treatment objectives

During the consultation, your aim is to:

- identify what the client's needs and expectations are
- discuss the possible treatment options and prices
- discuss the treatment effects
- discuss the benefits of regular treatments
- identify any contra-indications – if they are not contagious, then the treatment can be **modified**
- state what the realistic treatment outcomes will be.

Using consultation techniques

You will need to use your communication techniques during a consultation to aid understanding between you and the client.

- Help the client to feel relaxed by positioning them in front of you.
- Use appropriate body language, verbal and written skills.
- Complete the record card and check for any contra-indications.
- Ask the client what they want from the treatment. For example, it could be to improve a condition such as dry skin or to improve the appearance of fine lines. In this case, it could be either a facial to hydrate and moisturise the skin or an acid peel designed for mature skin.
- Establish whether the client's requirements are achievable.
- If not, explain why and offer alternatives.
- Discuss the treatment plan and ask the client questions to check that you both understand what the plan will include.

The importance of using effective communication to identify client needs and expectations

Good communication will establish the client's needs and expectations, which need to be realistic. If you do not establish what effects are achievable, at the end of the treatment the client will either be very disappointed and will never return or they will complain to you and the manager. If the client is dissatisfied, this will cause a delay with your next client and they might overhear what has happened. This could impact on your next treatment. Use the communication skills discussed above to help you prevent this type of situation from occurring.

If you believe you cannot achieve what the client wants, it is important to tell them, as you might be able to recommend something else. For example, if a client with excessively bitten nails and a small nail plate wants fibreglass nail extensions, it is better to recommend a way to improve their nails so that may be able to have nail extensions as a treatment in the future. On page 106 there is a suggested alternative treatment plan.

Top tips

Don't sit on the couch while your client sits on a chair – you will be higher than them and this can be very intimidating. It may also put you at risk of **repetitive strain injury**.

NAILS RECORD CARD

Name:		Date:	
Telephone no:		Medical history (treatment, comments):	
Address:			
		Appointments:	Weekly	
Date of birth:			Monthly	
Occupation:			Other	

Condition of nails

	Left hand:	Right hand:	Key:
Thumb			BR – broken
Index finger			BI - bitten
Middle finger			F – fungus
Ring finger			L - lifting
Little finger			N - normal

Record card used during a consultation

Top tips

For clients who are nervous, hearing impaired or where English is spoken as a second language, you could use **visual aids** to ensure you understand fully what the client requires.

Key terms

Visual aids – pictures or images to help understanding.

Client care and communication in beauty-related industries

Treatment plan and recommendations for a client with bitten nails and a very small nail plate

- Weekly manicure to speed up nail growth and improve the condition of the nails.
- Use a hand cream at home and massage skin, nails and cuticles.
- Wear gloves when using chemicals or gardening to protect the area.
- Use hand soaps that are pH balanced and moisturising.
- Buff the nails to stimulate growth.
- Use a cuticle cream.
- Gently file any rough edges to avoid the need to bite the nails.
- Do not bite the nails — use unpleasant-tasting clear enamels, wear gloves at home.

What is 'personal space'?

It is important to provide enough personal space for the client to feel comfortable when you are performing a treatment. Ensure your working space is not too small, allowing you enough room to work comfortably and safely. If you are uncomfortable when working, you may start to suffer from repetitive strain injury (RSI) — and having muscular aches and pains will affect your performance.

Some clients, especially those who are nervous or anxious, will not feel instantly relaxed when having a treatment and might find it difficult being touched — their stress levels might increase if you are too close. Be aware of your clients' feelings and do not invade their personal space — this will ensure a successful treatment and instil client confidence in your abilities.

The importance of providing the client with clear advice and recommendations

The consultation enables you to establish the client's individual requirements and then to consider their future treatment needs, appropriate aftercare advice, homecare advice and retail products to maintain the effects of the treatment and to improve any areas of concern. (For information on specific recommendations, see the Practical skills units.)

When to provide advice and recommendations

You can provide advice and recommendations at certain points during your time with the client — during the consultation, if the client asks you a question during the treatment, and at the end of the treatment. It is better not to provide advice during the treatment, as the client will want to relax and enjoy it and they might feel you are trying to pressure them into rebooking or to purchase retail products. However, if you do not provide advice and recommendations to improve a condition, your client will be unaware that they have these options.

Top tips

If a client has a contra-indication, do not name what you think it is, as you might be wrong. Beauty therapists are not medically qualified to assess a condition and you could cause unnecessary worry. The client might decide to treat it themselves, which could make the condition worse and cause discomfort. Instead, advise the client to see their GP, but remember to be tactful as the client could be very embarrassed. Perhaps offer them an incentive to return, such as a money-off voucher.

Think about it

Select a Practical skills unit and read about the different types of client needs, for example hard calluses. Think about the advice and recommendations you would give them, in preparation for your assessments.

Professional ethical conduct

It is important that beauty therapists apply a professional, ethical approach towards their chosen profession, by adopting a positive and proactive attitude. This is essential in creating the right environment to develop good client, colleague and employer relations and generate loyalty and respect. The simplest of actions, like good time management, punctuality, pride in work and personal presentation, will help to reinforce your position within the business. Professional conduct also includes confidentiality — you must not gossip or share confidential information about the business, your colleagues or the clients.

Provide client care

In this outcome you will learn about:

- maintaining client confidentiality in accordance with legislation
- gaining feedback from clients on client care
- responding to feedback in a constructive way
- referring client complaints to the relevant person
- assisting in client complaints being resolved.

Maintaining client confidentiality in line with the Data Protection Act 1998

All employees must comply with the Data Protection Act when handling clients' personal information that is stored on the premises, such as record cards, computer files and accident report forms. Clients' personal details include their name, address, contact number, medical history and GP's details.

The Information Commissioner's Office (ICO), the UK's independent authority set up to regulate businesses that handle the public's personal information, is responsible for enforcing the Data Protection Act. Businesses must register with the ICO and can participate in **audits** to ensure that they are complying with current legislation. The act sets out eight principles that businesses must follow when handling information. Data must be:

1 fairly and lawfully processed
2 processed for limited purposes
3 adequate, relevant and not excessive
4 accurate and up to date
5 not kept longer than necessary
6 processed in line with the individual's rights
7 secure
8 not transferred to other countries without adequate protection.

> **Think about it**
>
> Visit the ICO's website and research its purpose and role in the regulation of businesses.

> **Key terms**
>
> **Audits** – checks performed to ensure procedures have been followed.

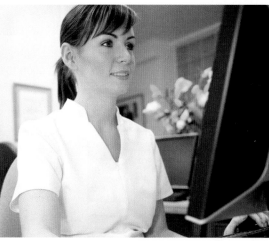

Store computer records according to the Data Protection Act

Think about it

Record cards and accident/illness report forms must be stored in a locked, secure cabinet, with access restricted to the client's personal beauty therapist(s) and manager. Any information stored on the computer must be stored securely and be password-protected. Only authorised individuals should be allowed access.

Key terms

Feature – what a product contains, for example cocoa butter.

Benefit – what the feature does, for example cocoa butter nourishes the skin.

Top tips

Appropriate timing is important to achieve retail sales and repeat bookings. Remember to use good communication skills and read your client's body language, especially if they do not appear to be interested.

Think about it

Look at the products you use in your training establishment and select three examples. List their features and benefits. In pairs, practise your selling techniques, taking it in turns to be the therapist and client.

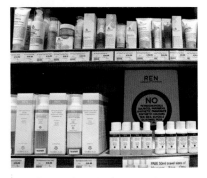

Display products in the reception area

The importance of communication techniques to support retail opportunities

Retail sales are a way for businesses to boost their profits and employees should recommend retail products to all their clients. Not only does use of the correct products maintain the effects of the treatment and generally improve the appearance of the skin and nails, it also identifies the business as one that offers the 'whole package', creating a more prestigious salon. Selling retail does not come naturally to everyone, so employers should provide staff training that covers:

- the use of role-play to demonstrate selling techniques
- practising the correct communication skills
- appropriate timing of when to discuss retail
- reading the client's body language signals
- product training including **features** and **benefits** from the suppliers
- location when promoting a product – either at the workstation or at reception.

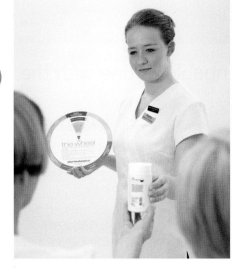

Staff training is important in areas such as communication skills and product knowledge

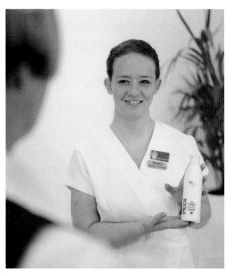

Provide accurate product information

Below are some suggested ways to generate and increase retail sales.

- Display a range of products suitable for the type of clientele. This will depend upon the location of the business. For example, city centre salons may be able to offer more expensive products than those in towns or villages.
- Offer at least a couple of brands, with one cheaper than the other – if a client is unsure, they may want to try the cheaper alternative, which might persuade them to buy the more expensive product next time.
- Offer a range that has a good selection of products for all types, such as all ages, gender, ethnic backgrounds, vegans.
- Display stock in an eye-catching way using a range of visual props (see also Display stock and promote products and services to clients in a salon, page 117).
- Maintain stock levels – if a therapist achieves a sale but the product is not in stock, this amounts to lost earnings for the salon and loss of commission for the therapist.

- Provide targets and offer bonus incentives for employees — incentives can create friendly competition between staff and inspire a stronger personal drive to sell.
- Special offers and promotions — these will entice clients to purchase and generate sales.
- Fully trained employees — employees need the knowledge to sell effectively.
- Good marketing strategy and advertising — hold regular team meetings to discuss these; use posters, website advertisements, mail shots, demonstration events, radio and newspaper advertising, leaflets/brochures, packaging and carrier bags with company logo and information to help promote the salon's services and products.

The importance of client feedback and responding constructively

Clients might comment generally on how they enjoyed a treatment, but they do not usually give feedback on client care. However, understanding if you or other employees have provided excellent client care is important, as this will affect repeat booking and retail sales. Ways to gather this information can sometimes come from managers asking clients in person, but some clients might find this uncomfortable and will not give their true opinion. Surveys can be used to find out the information; for example, you could ask 'How good was the client care you received today?' and 'How could it be improved?' The survey's findings can be used in staff training sessions to improve communication skills of the beauty therapists. The table on page 111 summarises the advantages and disadvantages of different survey methods.

Designing a survey

Here are some things that you will need to consider when designing a survey.

- Check that the survey is clear and to the point, and contains no jargon.
- Make sure the design is attractive — it needs to be eye-catching.
- Explain in a covering letter or email why it is important that the client completes the survey and include an incentive for completion.
- Put the most important questions at the beginning.
- Pitch questions at the correct level — do not use technical terminology.
- Only include a few questions — the client may get bored if you ask too many.
- Include a balance of multiple-choice questions (easier to complete) with a few questions where clients have to write a more detailed answer.
- Perform a trial run to see how effective the survey is.

Respond to feedback in a constructive way

Gaining feedback on your performance is the way you learn to become more professional and an outstanding beauty therapist. While training to become a therapist, you will need to encourage constructive feedback, especially from clients, peers and trainers. Feedback on your techniques will help you to produce better effects, and feedback on your client care and communication will make you more attentive and understanding of your clients' needs. Do not be offended or become hostile or defensive when you are told the areas that require improvement — it will help you to improve overall techniques or performance.

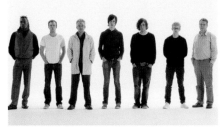

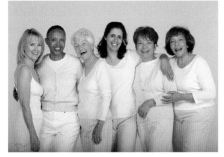

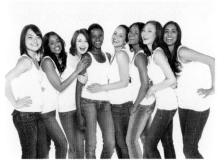

Target all types of people to increase your client base

Client care and communication in beauty-related industries

My story

Salon life

My name is Shailini. I am a newly qualified beauty therapist and recently started work in a large, prestigious city-centre salon. Everything was going well, except that I was failing to reach my retail targets. I just did not feel confident selling retail. Fortunately, I have an excellent manager, who asked to see me regarding my retail sales. I explained that I had no experience in selling and as I was new to the salon I was unaware of what retail products they stocked or what they were used for. From this, my manager organised a training session on retail products and selling techniques, which gave me more confidence. I now realise the importance of retail sales to the business and the client.

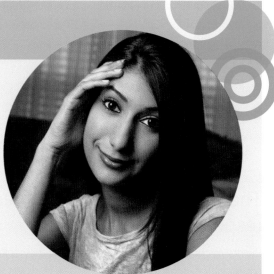

Ask the experts

Q How many products and treatments should I recommend at one time?

A You need to determine this from the type of client you have. Regular clients, for example, are likely to purchase more and book in more frequently than walk-in clients. Assess a client's initial needs. If they are having fibreglass nail extensions, they will need to rebook for their infill. If the client has a problem growing their nails, then recommend they come at minimum once a month or maximum once a week and allow them to decide. When recommending retail assess your client, then start by suggesting one or two products and offer another on their next visit. Some clients are more confident and will initiate most purchases.

Q What should I do if a client asks me a question about a product and I don't know the answer?

A Be honest, excuse yourself politely and go and find a more experienced therapist for help. Listen and observe them and use this opportunity to learn from someone with more experience.

Benefits of providing excellent client care and good communication

- Gives the client confidence in the therapist's abilities.
- Creates a good rapport between client and therapist.
- Client feels important and relaxed.
- Enhances the enjoyment of the treatment.
- Client is more open to recommendations of future services and retail sales.
- Promotes a professional beauty therapist and salon.

Top tips

When you are quiet at home, read the product manual to increase your product knowledge. Try the testers or samples to see how the products feel and what their effects are. You need to be confident, which will grow the more you practise your selling skills.

Type of survey	Advantages	Disadvantages
In person (existing or new clients)	Can target new clientele who will be more honest about client care from other businesses.	Passers-by do not often want to stop. Existing clients might not feel comfortable saying anything critical.
By telephone	Clients might explain in more detail verbally than they would in writing. Can encourage clients to make an appointment if they have not been to the salon for a while. If a client was previously unhappy and has not returned, this might encourage them to discuss the issues and rebook.	Costly and time-consuming. Can only target existing clients.
Postal	Can target the whole client base. Can be completed when clients have the time.	Costly and most people ignore this type of mail. Old clients might have moved address.
Business website	Surveys can be completed at any time during the year and are less time-consuming to complete online. Can be a cheaper option.	Clients would need to have access to the internet and know the business had a website. Clients would not necessarily want to complete a survey without being enticed with an incentive.
Emails	Can easily be sent out to client base. Cheap option.	Would need to have clients' email addresses. Clients might not regularly read emails. They might want an incentive to complete. Junk emails are often ignored.

Survey methods – their advantages and disadvantages

How to refer and assist in client complaints

When a client wants to make a complaint, take them somewhere quiet away from other clients so that it does not create an embarrassing and awkward situation for others. Often when a client complains they can become loud, distressed and hostile, which is not a good advertisement for a business. The salon manager should deal with a complaint and involve the beauty therapist if necessary. Be professional, demonstrate a calm, pleasant manner and be objective while discussing the complaint.

Reasons for complaints

When a client complains there can be a mix of emotions — they may feel angry, disappointed, in pain, confused, upset, impatient and anxious — depending on what has happened. There are various reasons why a client decides to complain, including:

- poor quality of treatment or results
- inexperienced therapist
- products or tools used incorrectly
- no pride in the beauty therapist's work — too tired or poor attitude
- poor communication regarding the desired effects
- treatment took too long or was not long enough
- parts of the treatment were not completed, for example no heat treatment in a luxury pedicure
- time restrictions or delays in starting the treatment

Top tips

- Offer an incentive to complete the survey, such as a discount or free treatment.
- By making the survey anonymous it will be more appealing to complete, as clients can be very honest in their answers.

Top tips

It is better to understand what you need to improve while you are training rather than when you enter the industry, as it will hold you back professionally and may affect your enjoyment and confidence later on. So encourage feedback, ask lots of questions and observe any demonstrations.

Client care and communication in beauty-related industries

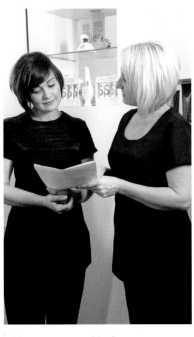

Always react positively to constructive feedback

Think about it

In pairs, create a script for a short play, in which a client makes a complaint. You choose what the complaint will be and how it should be correctly resolved.

Remember to include:

• where the complaint takes place

• procedures for dealing with complaints

• verbal communication and body language of the characters – manager, client and beauty therapist

• how it is resolved.

◉ salon too hot or too cold, which affects product's results

◉ injury or damage to client's belongings

◉ theft of client's valuables

◉ client had an allergic reaction – no skin test performed

◉ unidentified contra-indications that result in cross-infection – client in pain or the condition made worse

◉ client unhappy with a product they purchased or has had an allergic reaction

◉ unsafe environment or obstruction in the workplace leading to a client having an accident.

Resolving a complaint

If the beauty therapist or business is at fault, it is up to the manager to try to resolve the issue. If an accident or injury has occurred to the client and the business is at fault, it may be sued by the client. If a client is unhappy with their treatment results or effects, the manager may offer a refund or to correct the error. Occasionally, clients do not have a genuine complaint but do so because they do not want to pay for their treatment. If the manager cannot find fault in the therapist or treatment results, they will often challenge the client and the client does not return.

Product returns

A client may be unhappy with a product they have purchased and request a refund. For example:

◉ they may have suffered an allergic reaction

◉ the product may already be out of date when they purchased it

◉ they may have chosen the wrong product

◉ the product has not had the desired effect

◉ the product smells unpleasant and is of the wrong consistency (possibly out of date or stored incorrectly)

◉ the product is damaged.

What you must do next:

◉ Evaluate the situation for the best course of action.

◉ You could offer the client an exchange or credit note.

◉ Perform an allergy test before suggesting any further products.

◉ Contact the suppliers if the product is damaged or has caused a reaction.

◉ Seek advice from more experienced colleagues.

◉ Keep a record of refunded goods.

Complying with consumer legislation when selling and refunding products

There are several laws that protect consumers when buying and returning goods. You will need to understand these when selling and refunding products.

Sale and Supply of Goods Act 1994

Under this act, goods must be:

- of good quality with no defects
- fit for purpose
- described correctly.

If a product sold by a salon does not comply with this act, the consumer is entitled to a full refund.

The Sale and Supply of Goods to Consumers Regulations 2002

The regulations protect consumers who have purchased faulty goods within the European Union — they are entitled to a repair or replacement.

Trade Descriptions Act 1968

This act covers the false description of goods. It is illegal to mislead consumers by incorrectly describing a product or making false statements about it, so goods should have clear and accurate labelling.

Supply of Goods and Services Act 1982

This act protects consumers against bad workmanship or poor provision of services. It covers contracts for services and materials, but also applies where no contract is required, such as having your nails done at a nail bar. Services should be carried out with reasonable care and skill, within a timescale and at reasonable cost.

Consumer Credit Act 1974

This act helps to safeguard consumers who enter into a credit agreement (purchase on credit) which does not exceed £25,000. It is unlikely that a salon would provide this service. However, a salon owner might wish to purchase goods or equipment using a **hire purchase agreement**.

Businesses which allow consumers to purchase goods or services on credit agreements must be licensed by the Office of Fair Trading (OFT).

The Cosmetic Products (Safety) Regulations 2008

Products must be safe for their intended use and labels must be clear and accurate, including ingredients, weight, storage information, disposal methods, how to use.

The Consumer Protection (Distance Selling) Regulations 2000

The regulations refer to goods not purchased in person, for example on the internet or via telephone, fax, TV or mail order catalogue. Goods and services must be clearly described. The supplier must also display their delivery procedures and costs, business details and the procedure to cancel orders (consumers have seven days to cancel an order).

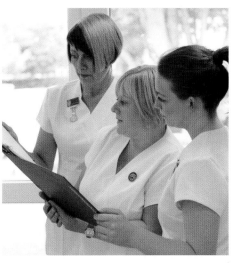

If in doubt, ask for guidance from a more experienced therapist

Top tips

Local authorities' Trading Standards departments regulate and monitor local businesses to check if they are following consumer laws and will investigate any complaints.

Key terms

Hire purchase agreement – the owner rents equipment to a purchaser and if all payments are made over a set period of time, the purchaser will then become the owner of the equipment.

Client care and communication in beauty-related industries

Top tips

- Hand-written price labels are easily damaged, so invest in a good pricing gun.
- Check the sell-by date and condition of the products before you sell them to the client.

Prices Act 1974

Prices must be clearly labelled or displayed to prevent the consumer from being misled.

Resale Prices Act 1976

This act made it unlawful for suppliers to set the retail price of goods. The recommended retail price (RRP) could be used only as a guideline.

Consumer Safety Act 1978

This act protects consumers from unsafe or defective goods/services, which do not reach safety standards. Employees must be trained fully to use such goods or services. Goods should be stored correctly, with accurate labelling and the prices must be clear and up to date.

Disability Discrimination Act 1995 and 2005

It is unlawful for businesses to discriminate against people on the grounds of disability — everyone should receive the same quality of service. Businesses must also provide easy access for disabled people.

Check your knowledge

1 What is an active listener?

2 When you ask a question and receive a detailed answer, what type of question has been asked?
   a) open
   b) closed.

3 What do the terms 'feature' and 'benefit' mean when discussing retail products?

4 What are the three types of communication?

5 Read the description of how a client reacts while they are being recommended retail products and choose the answer that reflects how the client is feeling.

   The client is not asking any questions, gives little or no eye contact, is playing with their hair, looks nervous/confused and is frowning.

   a) The client does not want to buy the product.
   b) The client is in a rush and wants to buy the product.
   c) The client does not understand what you are saying.

6 Who deals with client complaints?

7 A client comes back to the salon after buying a nail enamel and has had an allergic reaction. What do you do?
   a) Give a full refund.
   b) Call the client a liar, as she must have used enamels in the past and probably doesn't like the colour she has bought.
   c) Ask her if she has any allergies and check other products' ingredients for differences or find a range for sensitive skins as an alternative, before offering a refund or exchange.

8 How should you react to feedback that identifies areas for improvement?
   a) It's their fault if you have done something wrong, as they haven't shown you properly.
   b) By being embarrassed and annoyed.
   c) Constructively, as this identifies areas that need to be practised.

9 What law states how we are to handle a client's personal information?
   a) Consumer Safety Act
   b) Data Protection Act
   c) Consumer Protection (Distance Selling) Regulations.

10 How should we store a client's personal information?

Getting ready for assessment

There are no maximum service times that apply to this unit.

Evidence requirements

It is strongly recommended that evidence be gathered in a realistic working environment and simulation is avoided where possible. You should also ensure that you meet the required standards, i.e. that all outcomes, assessment criteria and range statements have been achieved. This unit is **internally assessed only** – but because of this it will almost certainly be internally verified, and the External Verifier may also want to view the portfolio. This is standard when there is no external paper – the Awarding Organisation just want to double check evidence is full and well rounded.

Practical outcomes are achieved two ways:

1 The practical criteria covered when doing the assessments

2 Knowledge and understanding of task through oral questioning.

Your assessor will observe your performance of practical tasks on **at least three occasions** – maybe more if the evidence is not all there within the three assessments. If practical criteria are not covered, your assessor will make a judgment through oral questioning. So, when dealing with client complaints, and giving recommendation for treatments during consultation or gaining client feedback, make your evidence trail as full as possible. Also, do not be surprised to be asked a lot of oral questions on how and why you chose this course of action as this is how you achieve competency in this unit.

Display stock and promote products and services to clients in a salon

What you will learn

- Prepare the display area
- Manage and dismantle promotional displays
- Promote products and services to the client

Introduction

When a client first comes to your salon or nail bar, you will want them to become a regular, loyal customer. This will involve much more than the standard of the treatment they receive – you will need to inform them about the different **services** the salon offers and the retail **products** that they can buy.

With so much choice and information available, clients will be very knowledgeable on the benefits of the products and services, and the price to pay for them, too. Everyone likes to feel they have bought a bargain and promotions are an excellent way to expand on the services and products a client currently uses.

For any business, the ability to sell products is vital and, as a beauty therapist, you will be expected to perform and hit sales targets. This not only increases the salon's income but it will also increase yours by means of **commission**. In an industry known for its low pay, this is an excellent way to top up your monthly earnings. You will also increase your client base, as being a confident seller will show what a knowledgeable and experienced therapist you are.

This unit looks at all areas of promotion and how to ensure they will work successfully within the business. When you begin your career in the beauty industry you will need to show your employers that you can promote and sell confidently and successfully. Many people are put off selling as they do not like the 'hard sell', but it does not have to be forced in this way. By educating clients, selling additional products and services will be a natural part of your working day.

Ensuring clients choose suitable products and services means they will be maximising the effects of the treatments at the salon and at home. The products used at home should enhance the results achieved by you and maintain them until the next appointment.

Create displays to promote products and services

In this outcome you will learn about:

- selecting the materials, equipment and stock to use
- determining the location of the display to maximise its impact
- assembling the display carefully and safely
- labelling the displayed products clearly, accurately and in a manner consistent with legal requirements.

Identifying the purpose of displays

When a client enters a salon, they are likely to see a display and/or promotional stand which aims to inform them of the types of service and products available. Displays are used to promote the business and to increase sales. They are an advertising tool designed to attract the eye and leave clients wanting to know more, and they can range from a small leaflet stand to a larger display cabinet, filled with information and visual props.

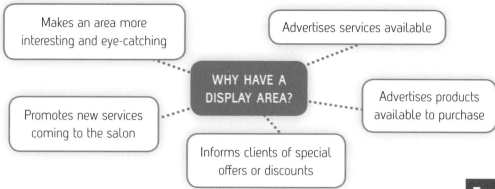

A display area may simply provide information materials for clients to read. It does not always have to be about selling – reading about the latest trends in beauty services can be enough to entice clients to try new services or at least start asking questions, which will give you the opportunity to introduce them to something new or different.

Before creating your display, make sure that you are clear about the message it is to put across. Too many different materials and visual aids can confuse a client and they will walk away. You may decide to work with a theme in mind, such as a seasonal display for summer. You will need to be sure that the theme is suitable for your salon and the time of year; for example, no one wants to see Christmas gift sets in the middle of the summer.

Selecting appropriate products and display materials

A wide range of materials can be used within a display, but they need to work together to make an eye-catching arrangement. Most of the products and equipment that you select will come from within the salon. However, it may also be appropriate to purchase materials to help enhance the display.

Products

As product companies invest time, money and effort in creating packaging that looks professional and attractive, products can work extremely well in a display. If displaying boxes, it is a good idea to remove the product and use only the empty box. You may decide to display the actual container. If so, you will need to take care where you place the product, as certain conditions can cause the product to **denature**; for example, the ultraviolet (UV) rays in strong sunlight can damage both the packaging and the product itself.

Prices should be clearly displayed with products to keep the client well informed. Ensure you have checked if any COSHH regulations apply to the displayed products, as these guidelines will need to be adhered to. To learn more about COSHH, see Essential professional knowledge, page 49.

Promotional materials

These consist of leaflets, posters, images and so on. They may be created by you; alternatively, many product companies will supply appropriate materials. The supplied materials will be of a high standard and very visual, so anything you create

> **Top tips**
>
> Empty boxes in the display area will reduce the risk of theft. Actual products can be kept in a more secure area until the sale is made.

> **Key terms**
>
> **Denature** – the chemical structures within the product may change and become more unstable, potentially leading to an ineffective product or a reaction on a client's skin.

Display stock and promote products and services to clients in a salon

should try to match that standard. Posters and leaflets should be produced using computer software to ensure they look professional. The information given needs to be basic – the aim is to attract clients' interest so they then ask you questions about what is on offer.

Stationery

Stationery materials, such as tissue paper, card and glitter pens, can be used to make the display more visually appealing and attractive. Choose colours that complement the colour scheme of your products and promotional material.

Planning and preparing the display

Preparation is an essential aspect of planning a display so that it can be assembled safely and with all the necessary components. During your planning, write a comprehensive list of everything you will need and where they will be obtained from. Be sure to highlight any health and safety issues that need to be considered. An example is given below.

Planning your display

Items	From who	Health and safety
Moisturisers	Therapist	Do not display in sunlight as it will change the colour of the varnish
Promotional posters	Product company	Display securely on unit
Gift sets	Receptionist	Check COSHH regulations and manufacturers' instructions on storage

Your display will not be effective if the standard of your materials is not consistent. You may decide to create labels yourself to give information on specific areas of your display. When creating labels and promotional material you will need to ensure that you comply with the relevant legislation (see page 57).

Locating the display to maximise its impact

Most salons have an area where promotional materials are displayed, usually in the reception area where they will be clearly visible to clients. The following spider diagram shows options for suitable display areas.

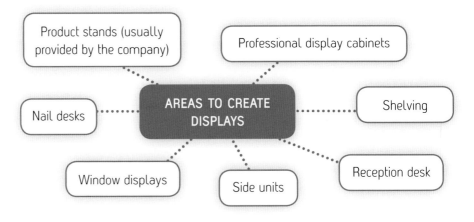

Think about it

To help you plan your display, answer the following questions:

- What is the purpose of the display?
- What features will be most suitable?
- What materials will you require?
- Who is the display aimed at?
- What will the display be placed on?

Each of these can be very effective. However, you will need to adapt your display to suit each one. For example, displays in areas of high traffic will need to be neat and sturdy to reduce the risk of items being knocked over.

Your display should have an immediate impact on clients. It should attract their attention and persuade them to enquire about the items on display. Where you choose to place the display will be affected by the purpose of it. For example, seasonal displays would be better placed in the reception area to tempt visitors, while specific treatment displays could be placed within the treatment areas. If the display is hidden away in a corner of the salon, it may go unnoticed and fail to have any impact. Placing it in a suitable area has the ability to increase sales and revenue for the business and boost commission for you as a therapist. The following table identifies the consequences of suitable and unsuitable areas for displays in the salon.

Suitable display areas	Unsuitable display areas
Attract clients' attention	Fail to stand out from other salon furniture
Cause them to ask more questions	May look old and tired as they are forgotten about
Could lead to sales of products	Products may go out of date while on display
Could lead to clients trying new beauty services	New equipment for new services will go unused
May attract new clients to business	

The consequences of selecting suitable and unsuitable display areas

If the layout of the salon prevents the movement of furniture, you may be limited to a specific area(s) when creating displays. Since the display area is static, it is important to regularly change and update it – clients will stop noticing the display if it stays the same.

Assembling the display carefully and safely

Once you have completed the planning, the display can be created. This section looks at how to assemble the display area safely and in accordance with the salon's rules.

Complying with legislation

When creating your display you will need to take account of the following legislation.

- The Control of Substances Hazardous to Health (COSHH) Regulations 2002. Due to the chemical ingredients in many products, you may be prohibited from using the actual containers in the display. You may, however, use the outer packaging such as the box to promote the product or service.

- The Personal Protective Equipment (PPE) at Work Regulations 1992. When creating the display be sure to protect yourself from injury. You may be moving boxes and furniture around, so appropriate footwear is essential.

- The Manual Handling Operations Regulations 1992. Most workplaces have posters on display to show how to lift and carry large items correctly, and you should also have been made aware of the regulations. Be sure to adhere to these guidelines to prevent any injury to yourself. It is advisable to carry out the activity with a colleague so you can support each other.

(To find out more about the above legislation, see Essential professional knowledge, pages 48–49.)

Top tips

You are creating a visual display, so use your artistic skills.

Top tips

The following issues may be specific to individual salons, but should always be considered.

- Are there any risks of cross-contamination?

- Ensure the display area is thoroughly cleaned prior to use.

- Be careful when handling equipment and stock – any breakages will cost the salon money.

- Check manufacturers' instructions when displaying products – there may be guidelines on storage and factors that may affect the shelf life of the product.

- If new display cabinets have been bought, follow instructions on assembly and work safely with any tools required.

Display stock and promote products and services to clients in a salon

Top tips

Remember, a promotional display reflects the image of a business. Old and untidy displays may mean that clients think all areas of the salon are like that.

1 Remove stationery from area – this could be reused later

2 Remove and dispose of decorative items

3 Return leaflets and educational material to storage. They can be kept in the reception area (if applicable) or somewhere that is easily accessed

4 Remove products: dispose of empty boxes; inspect products for damage – dispose of damaged items appropriately, return intact products to the appropriate storage area (following COSHH)

5 Dismantle furniture, if used. Store all parts together and be sure to pick up discarded screws and nails to prevent them becoming a hazard. If furniture is being moved, ensure this is done safely. You should not try to move anything that is too heavy or tall (follow the Manual Handling Operations Regulations)

6 Clean empty display area and the surrounding floor and surfaces, ready for the new display

7 Dispose of waste using appropriate methods. Place cards and paper in the designated area for recycling waste.

Manage and dismantle promotional displays

In this outcome you will learn about:

- maintaining the display area for the duration of the display period
- dismantling the display, restoring the area and returning stock to storage.

Managing and maintaining the display area

Promotional displays need to be changed and updated regularly so that clients know what is available. For example, your salon may decide to run monthly special offers on products and discounts on treatments that are less popular. The display itself will need care and maintenance throughout its life to make sure that it looks as good as possible and does not start to look tired and forgotten. Below are ways to help you maintain your display in first-class condition.

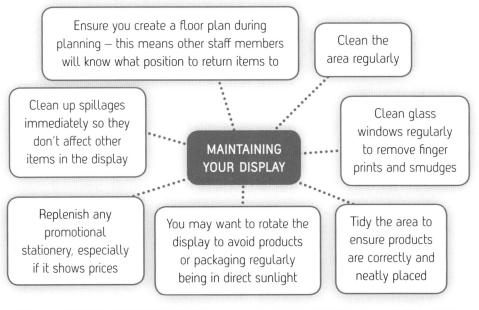

Ensure you create a floor plan during planning – this means other staff members will know what position to return items to

Clean the area regularly

Clean up spillages immediately so they don't affect other items in the display

MAINTAINING YOUR DISPLAY

Clean glass windows regularly to remove finger prints and smudges

Replenish any promotional stationery, especially if it shows prices

You may want to rotate the display to avoid products or packaging regularly being in direct sunlight

Tidy the area to ensure products are correctly and neatly placed

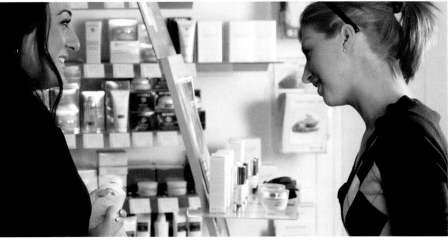

Keep your displays simple but eye-catching

Using appropriate techniques to dismantle displays

When the time for the display has ended, everything will need to be dismantled, packed away and the area cleaned and prepared for the next display. The changeover can sometimes be disruptive, and if space is already limited, you will need to keep this to a minimum. It may help to change over the display during a quieter time in the salon when fewer clients are present or, better still, when the salon has closed – in particular, this will reduce the risk of clients and staff tripping over furniture and boxes temporarily left on the floor.

Follow the seven-step process for dismantling a display as shown opposite.

As discussed earlier, all relevant legislation should be followed and adhered to during the dismantling process. There will be a high risk of injury if carelessness occurs.

> **Top tips**
>
> When dismantling your display, try to recycle as much as possible. Follow your salon's guidelines on recycling.

Key legal requirements relating to the display of stock

Prices of products and services should be clearly highlighted to clients. During a promotion, clients may be confused by the new prices. Any discounts should be clearly marked, showing the original price and the current selling price. Products need to be labelled with the price before they are put within a display. The labels can be either handwritten or computer-generated, as long as they are legible. Try to avoid using only fractions or percentages without showing the final price – leaving clients to calculate prices could cause errors and confusion and may cost the salon money.

This is the main legislation that you will need to consider when displaying stock:

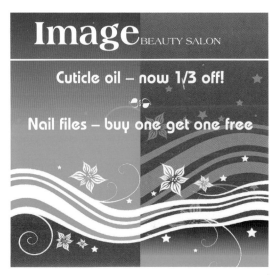

An example of a promotion

- Trade Descriptions Act 1968. Information about products and services provided by the retailer (the salon) must be accurate and not misleading. Do not exaggerate the effects of a product or service to try to increase sales.

- Consumer Protection Act 1987. The products available for clients to buy need to be safe and suitable for use. Careless storage could cause the product to deteriorate, making it unsafe to use. This is particularly important if trying to sell products near to the end of their shelf life.

- Data Protection Act 1998. Any sale made must be kept between the client and the retailer. Information on what services and products the client purchases must be kept confidential by the retailer.

- Prices Act 1974. You will need to ensure that all products and services have a price clearly attached to them so there is no confusion on the clients' behalf, particularly if running discounts.

- Sale and Supply of Goods Act 1994. The retailer forms a contract with the buyer which gives them the right to return a product if it is defective and to supply the buyer with a refund. The issue can then be taken up with the supplier.

- Consumer Safety Act 1978. The retailer must only sell reputable products to ensure they are safe for the clients to use.

Promote products and services to the client

In this outcome you will learn about:

- establishing the client's requirements
- using suitable communication techniques to promote products and services
- introducing services and/or products to the client at the appropriate time
- giving accurate and relevant information to the client
- identifying buying signals and interpreting the client's intentions correctly
- identifying services and/or products to meet requirements of the client.

Benefits to the salon of promoting services and products

When working within the industry, a salon may set the beauty therapists targets for the promotion and sale of products and services. Setting achievement targets is a commonly used method of motivation and aims to ensure you attempt to increase your sales turnover. Targets will be set according to the services a therapist can offer and how many hours they are contracted to work. A member of staff who works 16 hours a week does not have as many opportunities to sell as a full-time member of staff, for example.

Targets are set not only to help therapists increase their earnings but also to boost the income within the salon. By encouraging clients to use professional products at home, a salon will see a sharp increase in the monthly takings. Clients will also get the best results out of their treatments if they use professional products between visits.

Clients can fall into the habit of having the same treatment at each visit and never trying anything new. Promotions help to prompt clients to experience new services which they then book in for regularly. The salon will look current and up to date, keeping clients interested.

A therapist must always be aware of what their target is and identify the amount of commission they will receive. This is normally highlighted in their contract. Many establishments also offer rewards for achieving targets, such as free products or complimentary treatments. If a therapist feels their target is unachievable, they should discuss this with their salon manager, as an unachievable target is unlikely to motivate them into selling.

Each salon will have its own policies and guidelines on selling and promoting. Being an enthusiastic member of the team will be rewarding for both the therapist and the salon. If a therapist is complacent about selling, it may leave their manager with a negative opinion of them.

Although it is important to try to achieve targets, a therapist needs to be realistic about what they offer to clients. Always keep in mind how suitable the products and services are for individual clients. Sometimes therapists become so focused on hitting targets that they start recommending the most expensive items in the salon, whether they are suitable or not. This will only lead to an unhappy client who may complain or not return to the salon.

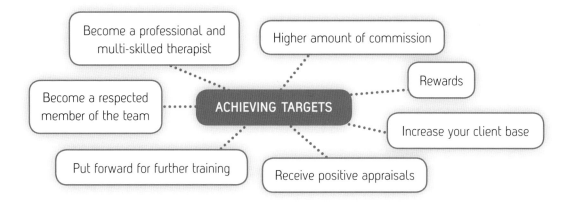

Therapists should also avoid stealing sales from other members of their team, as this will lead to tension and unhappiness in the workplace. Remember to treat everyone else in the same way you would expect to be treated. It is very common in the salon for a therapist to spend time with a client, informing them about products, without the client purchasing anything. There could be several reasons for this. If the client were to return to the salon and purchase something that was recommended to her, the sale (commission) should go to the therapist who advised the client in the first instance, as they did the work.

Listening and questioning techniques used for promotion and selling

Many newly qualified beauty therapists find the idea of selling products very daunting. They are concerned that they will feel under pressure from their manager to demonstrate that they can promote products to clients. However, advising clients on appropriate products that complement beauty services should occur naturally throughout the service they are receiving. There is no need to pressure the client into buying. Remember, a client will purchase a product or service if they feel that they will benefit from it and it is appropriate for their needs – educating clients about suitable products and services does not involve putting pressure on them.

Beauty treatments allow plenty of time to communicate with the client, so it is advisable to use this to ask them questions to help draw out their needs. Use a variety of both **open** and **closed questions** to obtain the information that you will require to make your advice specific to them. (To learn more about communication techniques, see Client care and communication in beauty-related industries, page 101.)

Having confidence will enable you to raise the subject of products and services, and clients will have faith in your knowledge. You will need to discuss the benefits to the client of purchasing the item – that is, the results they can expect to see from using it. If you lack confidence, the client will not take your advice seriously.

Clients need to understand the advice you give them, so it is important to use terminology they will recognise. Using technical terms (jargon) might prevent them from understanding why the product or service is suitable for them. Keep your explanation simple and always link the benefits of a product or service to the client's needs.

Think about it

It is important that target setting encourages a healthy amount of competition within the salon, but remember that you are part of a team.

Key terms

Open questions – allow the client to give answers in more detail and can open up the conversation.

Closed questions – usually only allow the client to answer 'yes' or 'no', which will prevent the conversation flowing.

For your portfolio

For your assessment, you will need to demonstrate that you can sell products and services to clients. Once a sale has been made, highlight it on the consultation card and use the receipt as evidence. Your assessor can then confirm the sale has taken place.

Display stock and promote products and services to clients in a salon

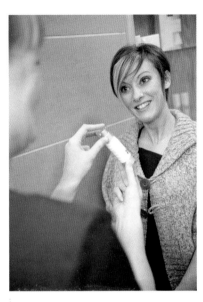

Promoting a product for sale in the salon

Top tips

Listen to the client – they will often discuss their concerns about their skin and/or nail conditions throughout the treatment.

Think about it

In pairs, discuss what signs a client would show if they were interested in a product or service. Share them with the rest of the class.

Consultation techniques used to promote products and services

During your initial consultation with the client, it is important to listen and record the information they give you accurately. This is when your client will begin to talk about their concerns and problem areas. Focusing on their needs when recommending products and services means your client will be more likely to show an interest in what you are suggesting. They will be able to see how the products and services will meet their needs.

There will be times throughout the client's service when you will be able to advise them on specific products. Choosing the right moment will ensure your client has the opportunity to listen to your advice. During a hand and arm massage, for example, the client will want to relax not discuss cuticle oil. Below are some suggestions on when might be an appropriate time to advise the client:

- while nails are soaking
- while feet are soaking in a foot spa
- when hands/feet are in mitt and booties
- when gel is curing under UV light
- as you complete the client's treatment log on their consultation card.

Remember, the client may bring up the topic themselves – do not ignore the opportunity just because you feel it is an inappropriate time.

Spotting sales opportunities

One of the most common mistakes newly qualified therapists make is to miss opportunities and signs that a client is interested in something the salon has to offer. If you spot the right opportunity, it will make the sale much easier, as the client has already expressed an interest. Below are some opportunities to look out for.

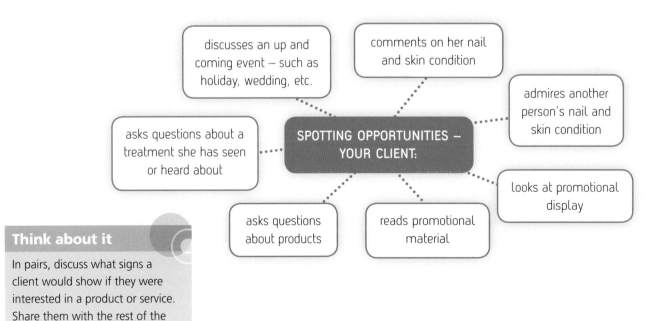

discusses an up and coming event – such as holiday, wedding, etc.

comments on her nail and skin condition

admires another person's nail and skin condition

asks questions about a treatment she has seen or heard about

SPOTTING OPPORTUNITIES – YOUR CLIENT:

looks at promotional display

asks questions about products

reads promotional material

Sometimes the client does not make it that easy for you, so it will be up to you to create the opportunities as the service takes place. This is when you will need to be confident in your approach. Generally, you can inform your clients of any new products and services and the promotions that are running in the salon at any point during the treatment – this means they will be more informed and might be tempted too. The table below suggests some links between the treatment the client is currently having and new products or services they could try.

Treatment	Links to new products and services
Eye-lash tint	eye-lash tint, eye brow shape, eye-lash extensions, tweezers, anti-septic solution
Leg wax	bikini line wax, threading, epilation, exfoliator, moisturiser
Pedicure	Deluxe pedicure treatments, waxing treatments, foot exfoliants, heel repair creams, etc.

Links between client's current treatment and new products or services

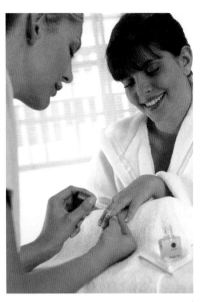

Talk to clients about new products during the treatment

Your client may not have the time after a treatment to talk about possible homecare products, but your salon should have a supply of literature and samples that you could give the client to try. At the next treatment, you can then discuss how she got on with them.

Features and benefits of services and products

The terms **features** and **benefits** should be used when informing clients about professional products and services. These are key points that should help the client to see why products and services are suitable for them. When attending product training, each product will be explained in detail, but a knowledgeable therapist should be able to identify the key features and benefits easily. To help with selling, first identify the main features, which should entice the client to find out more. The benefits should then be explained so they can see exactly how the product or service will benefit them and solve the problem areas.

The principles of effective face-to-face communication

When dealing with clients face to face, you will need to use both verbal and non-verbal communication skills. Your facial expressions will help support your selling skills; a lack of confidence will be obvious to the client, and they will doubt the information you are giving them. Positive expressions such as smiling and nodding your head will ensure the client feels you are making the right decisions for them. (To learn more about verbal and non-verbal communication, see Client care and communication in beauty-related industries, page 102.)

For your portfolio

Look at the services your local salon offers and identify which ones could be linked together for promotion.

Key terms

Feature – what will attract the client to the product; for example, cuticle cream helps keep cuticles soft and flexible.

Benefit – the advantage of using the product on the hands or feet; for example, rough skin remover helps dissolve dead skin.

Display stock and promote products and services to clients in a salon

My story

Salon life

My name is Ravneet and I have worked within the beauty industry for 10 years. At the beginning of my career I found selling very challenging and would often avoid it if at all possible. My only sales came if a client specifically asked for something.

I moved jobs and found myself working for a reputable professional beauty range. They provided me with excellent training and I began to fall in love with the products and became very impressed by the effects I saw when using them on myself. After the training I began to talk to my clients about my training and what I had learned. My clients became interested in the products and wanted to try them for themselves. My sales shot through the roof! I couldn't believe it as I wasn't trying to sell anything, I was just talking to them. I realised that my confidence in the product's ability and knowledge of the effects was capturing their attention. They trusted my opinion as a professional beauty therapist and followed my recommendation. I became the best seller at the salon and even went on to win an award from the company itself. I was completely transformed from when I first came into the industry. If you are passionate about your products, your client will be too!

Ask the experts

Q Does it matter how many products go into a display?

A No, but if you put too many different types of product on display your customers may be confused about what is on offer. Remember to keep it simple but effective.

Top tips

People like to touch displays – check glass doors regularly for fingerprints.

The importance of effective personal presentation

When assisting clients with products and services you will need to ensure your presentation reflects the standard of the salon. A client will have more faith and trust your advice if you present yourself in a professional manner. (To learn more about personal presentation requirements, see Essential professional knowledge, page 10.)

The importance of good product and service knowledge

At the beginning of your career in the beauty industry, you will be required to attend a wide range of training courses. Attending training on the services and products supplied within your salon will make you a more confident seller. The following table outlines the advantages of attending product and treatment training.

Product training	Treatment training
In-depth knowledge about effects and benefits of product	Confidence in carrying out treatment
Knowledge about use of product	Matching treatment to needs of client
Confidence in matching product to client's needs	In-depth knowledge of results achieved from treatment
Knowledge of product's key ingredients and its functions	Ability to adapt treatment to meet specific needs of client

Advantages of attending product and treatment training

By attending training, clients will notice your knowledge in the advice you give them – this will give them confidence that you have recommended correctly. You will need to use your knowledge and expertise to discuss products and services with clients. Clients tend to ask lots of questions before they will commit to a sale. As discussed earlier in the unit, displays can be used to raise clients' awareness of what the salon has to offer.

As a professional therapist, it is your duty to be well informed about the products and services on offer to your client. This should be a continual theme, as the industry changes so frequently that you will continually need to update your skills throughout your career. There are many ways to increase your knowledge:

- Attend regular training courses.
- Use the products yourself.
- Receive the treatments on offer.
- Keep up to date with new products and services on the market.
- Share information at team meetings.
- Read literature on products and services.
- Shadow a more experienced member of staff.

Product companies not only run sessions on using their range but they also often run sessions on how to increase sales. This is a valuable skill that everyone in the salon will benefit from.

Top tips

Clients will spot if you are not telling the truth – this could discourage them from purchasing the item and returning to the salon in the future.

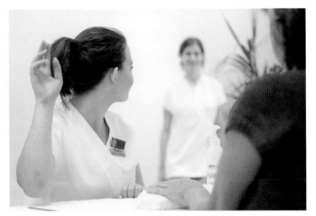

Ask a more experienced member of staff if you don't know the answer

Stages of the sale process

Ideally, all clients should use a wide range of homecare products to help maintain the service they have received, and then visit the salon regularly to receive treatments. But this can be unrealistic, so you will need to ensure you select items that can achieve the most for your client. Factors that will affect your recommendations include:

- the client's financial situation
- the client's commitment
- their nail and skin type
- how much time the client has to spend using products or visiting the salon
- how high-maintenance the service is that they receive
- the client's awareness of products and services that are available.

You might like the client to purchase five homecare products, but some clients may not wish to purchase as many as this and the quantity might put them off. Start with two key products that you know will make a visible difference and build up as necessary. Recommending products that achieve great results will win your client round and they will respect the advice you give them in the future.

The flow chart on page 130 shows the process of making a sale from the early signs of interest to closing the sale and the client making the purchase.

Display stock and promote products and services to clients in a salon

How to interpret buying signals

You will need to be able to interpret the difference between positive and negative buying signals and react to them accordingly. When a client shows positive buying signals you will need to start to close the sale. Examples of positive buying signals include:

- client nodding during conversation
- client asking more questions about the product and service
- client having a positive facial expression, such as smiling
- client identifying why they feel the product will work for them
- client describing themselves using the product or receiving the service
- client picking up products or trying out the samples.

Overcoming obstacles

Nobody likes to be pushed into making a decision, so if a client is clearly saying they are not interested, it is best to end that part of the conversation. There will be other opportunities for selling with other clients and sometimes the client just needs time to think about it before making a decision. Make sure they are aware that they can call back any time for more advice if it is needed.

Think about it

In small groups, list reasons clients may give for not making a purchase. Discuss ways of overcoming them.

1 Client shows initial interest in product or service; or therapist informs client of product or service available.

2 Client asks questions about product or service.

3 Therapist informs client about product or service and why they might be suitable for them.

4 Therapist checks client's knowledge and understanding of product or service.

5 Therapist secures client's agreement.

6 Any obstacles to the sale are handled.

7 Therapist closes the sale and client makes the purchase.

The process of making a sale

There may be times when the client is not saying no, but you are faced with objections such as 'I cannot afford to spend that much' or 'I don't have that much time to spend using products'. Here are some tips on how to turn an objection into a sale.

⊚ Finances – if a client is wavering due to the cost of the treatment, explain how long the product will last and break the cost down into how much it will cost per week. Many of the high-street brands will cost less but not last half as long. Professional products have a higher concentrate of active ingredients, so a little goes a long way. There may also be a range of sizes, so perhaps you could suggest the client takes home the smaller size hand cream this time, for example.

⊚ Lack of time – with this type of client it is important to select a product that is easy to use but has amazing results. Give suggestions to your client on efficient ways to use it, such as 'Keep your eye cream on your bedside cabinet, then apply once in bed'. This way the client will actually visualise doing it, and see that it will not take much time to do.

⊚ Already has products at home – if the client is happy with the products they have at home, they are likely to be happy with their nail and skin condition. Look back at the client's key concerns on their record card and highlight them to the client again. Perhaps you could recommend a more suitable product that will give the results that the client requires.

⊚ Out-of-stock item – this is an obstacle that may be beyond your control. As it can be very disappointing for the client, take the time to become familiar with the salon's stock. You may need to refer this to a senior member of staff for them to place the order, but you will still need to inform the client about when they can expect the item. Take responsibility to track the order, so that when it comes in you can contact the client and they can come to the salon to collect it or you can forward it via the post immediately. To keep the client happy, provide them with some samples that they could use until the product arrives.

⊚ Fully booked therapist – again, this can be disappointing for the client. Once the client has shown an initial interest in a service, it is advisable to check the diary for availability. Make the client aware that there may be time constraints. Specialised services such as 3D nail art or Minx may only be offered by a small number of therapists – explain this to the client so that you can arrange a booking which is suitable for both client and therapist.

⊚ Referring clients – unfortunately, you may come across situations where you will need to refer your client either to another stockist or to another salon for a particular service. This does not always have to be a negative experience. Clients will appreciate your honesty and trust the advice you give them. A salon, for example, may not be able to offer the full range of nail treatments, so you might need to recommend a nail bar that does. Likewise, one salon will not be able to stock every product available, so research where the client could purchase it from. It does not mean that you will lose the client to another business; if you were to turn them away without any advice you might, but by helping them you will show that you are truly professional.

Think about it

In pairs, each select one product from your beauty range. Your aim is to educate each other as if you had never seen it before. How did you get on? Were there any aspects that you found challenging?

How to secure agreement and close the sale

Securing agreement

Once the client has shown an interest in the product they would like to purchase, it is essential that they have a detailed knowledge of how to use it, including the amount, frequency and method of application. It is advisable to demonstrate the product, then ask the client to try it out too — this will also help in closing the sale, as the client can then visualise themselves using it at home.

When explaining the use of the product, keep making eye contact with your client. You need to be sure that they are still showing an interest in the product and are not getting confused with the instructions you are giving. The client needs to feel confident in using the product, as your aim is to get them to purchase it regularly. If they do not feel confident, the product will sit unused at the back of their bathroom cupboard and they will be unlikely to purchase anything again.

Most product companies offer purchasers a **guarantee** that if they are not completely satisfied with their product they may return it without any cost to the salon. It may be advisable to check your supplier's policies on this matter. You should also reassure your client that they can return to the salon if they have any queries about their purchase.

Closing the sale

The next stage is to close the sale as, at this point, there is still a risk the client may change their mind. Keep things positive and ask the client which products they would like to take home today. Give them time to make the decision. Many therapists do not feel confident enough to ask the client to make a final decision, but as you have given the client all the appropriate information they may now need a final prompt from you to make the purchase. Below are some phrases you could use to close the sale.

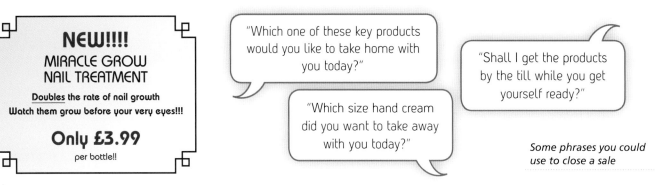

"Which one of these key products would you like to take home with you today?"

"Shall I get the products by the till while you get yourself ready?"

"Which size hand cream did you want to take away with you today?"

Some phrases you could use to close a sale

Evaluating selling techniques and their effectiveness

The way to know that a therapist has successful selling skills is to see a rise in the amount they sell. During regular team meetings, targets for sales and treatments should be discussed to identify if there are any issues. It is also an appropriate time to identify the need for further training if they are still not confident. A salon should support and help a therapist to develop strategies to increase sales and meet targets. If a therapist is continually missing targets, these may need to be negotiated, otherwise they may start to lose motivation.

Listen to your client's feedback — as a professional, you should follow up the sales you make to your clients. Check whether they are seeing results with the products they are using at home or that they enjoyed a new treatment they received. Positive

Advertisements for new products must only show the facts and not exaggerate

feedback will confirm you are matching the products and services to the client's needs; negative feedback may highlight the need to refresh your skills.

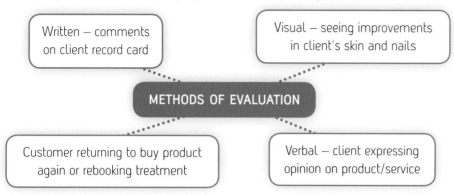

Written — comments on client record card

Visual — seeing improvements in client's skin and nails

METHODS OF EVALUATION

Customer returning to buy product again or rebooking treatment

Verbal — client expressing opinion on product/service

Legislation affecting the selling of services and products

Within this unit we have discussed how legislation affects the display of goods and services — it also affects the sales of products and services. (To learn more about relevant legislation, see Client care and communication in beauty-related industries, page 113.)

When promoting products and services to the client you must adhere to the legislation linked to the sale of goods and services. Whatever information you give to the client must be accurate and never exaggerated. Most clients will want to know what the product or service is going to do for them. The product's key features and benefits should be outlined to them. Show how it will meet their needs, but avoid getting carried away with what the product can or cannot do. Recently, some very well-known brands have been fined, as their adverts were thought to be misleading in what they claimed could be achieved with the product. Although it is important to sell products to clients, the consequences of not complying with legislation may be serious.

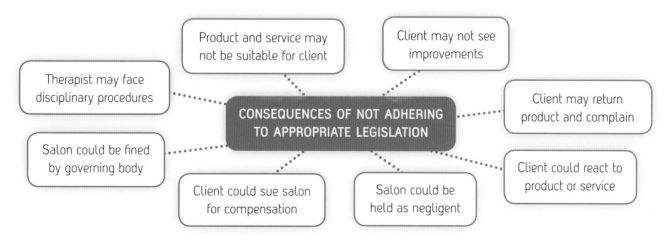

Product and service may not be suitable for client

Client may not see improvements

Therapist may face disciplinary procedures

CONSEQUENCES OF NOT ADHERING TO APPROPRIATE LEGISLATION

Client may return product and complain

Salon could be fined by governing body

Client could sue salon for compensation

Salon could be held as negligent

Client could react to product or service

Methods of payment for services and products

Taking payment for products and services will be the final stage in the sales process and shows your client's commitment. To learn more about payment methods, see Salon reception duties, page 170.

Display stock and promote products and services to clients in a salon

Check your knowledge

1   What is the purpose of a display?

2   List five items that could be used within a promotional display.

3   What is the main consequence of not placing a display in an appropriate area?

4   Why is it not always appropriate to display actual products?

5   What legislation is involved with promotional displays?

6   List five ways a client may show interest in a service or product.

7   Why is it vital to be well informed about the products and services available in a salon?

8   What are some of the obstacles clients may give?

9   What legislation covers the sale of products and services?

10 Why is it important that clients are educated on how to use a product?

Getting ready for assessment

Sources of evidence could be the following:

- On the client's record card, make a note of any products purchased, any recommendations you make for the future, and other services that would be suitable for your client's needs.

- During your consultation, or during the course of a treatment (where suitable), let the assessor hear you recommending suitable products and treatments. The client does not necessarily have to have them; rather it is your verbal recommendations that form the evidence as well as the correct knowledge that you are imparting.

- Design a questionnaire to show how little or how much the client knows about her treatment options. You could then highlight staff weaknesses in knowledge of products or services and recommend a training day. For example, of the 17 clients having a manicure this week, only five of them realised they could have a warm oil treatment to help dry cuticles.

- Design a poster to promote a particular product or service, perhaps with a seasonal theme – a free nail polish application with every Christmas makeover, or a pedicure polish carried out with every spring waxing treatment. Make the poster as informative as you can to attract new business.

- Design an aftercare and homecare leaflet for a treatment, suggesting suitable products for home use that will carry on the good work of the salon treatment.

- Organise a training seminar for other staff or students where you promote a particular treatment or product that you feel confident in, which perhaps is not selling as well as it could. Make it very 'hands on' – get others involved in using the product and demonstrate how to promote it.

- Copy and enclose in your portfolio the order form or delivery note that you may have had to complete if a product was out of stock or it was a special order.

- Include any evidence of outside selling seminars or lectures you have attended. Enclose any training certificates from commercial training you have received.

These suggestions will show you understand the requirements and mechanics of selling and linking your treatments with retail sales. It is not only important you learn how to do it but that you record it, too.

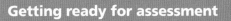

Working in beauty-related industries

Introduction

This unit is designed to help you prepare for work within the beauty industry by outlining the skills and knowledge you will need to progress. With such a diverse industry no two people's career paths will be the same and that is what makes the industry so exciting. The unit will look at the many pathways and also the skills you will need to work alongside your colleagues. Your time at college is just the start of a thrilling and challenging journey through your career.

Gone are the days when a therapist would be limited to the town's local salon, treating the same clients day in day out. There is so much choice available to you now, that every day of your career will bring you different experiences. When you become fully qualified, a whole world of further training will be open to you, taking you from being a novice to working as an expert in the beauty industry.

Whether you decide to work in a large salon or perhaps become self-employed and work by yourself, you will constantly be communicating with other people from the profession. It is important to build these relationships – they will help you to establish yourself and the business within your local beauty community. Having the skills to work with a variety of people is essential. It is not just about your relationships with clients – your colleagues and peers are equally important.

Legislation and employee rights play a vital part in creating a healthy and productive working environment. Every salon owner is responsible for ensuring that their employees are treated fairly and that correct precautions are taken to keep them safe at work. As an employee you will be responsible for adhering to the guidelines that have been set out. Even as a self-employed beauty therapist there are many laws and regulations that you will need to become familiar with to ensure your business operates legally.

Now that you have chosen a career in the beauty industry you will be surprised at the number of options that are available. This industry links with many different sectors, from sports to healthcare. Making a leap between the sectors is not as difficult as you might at first think; there is a lot of flexibility surrounding you. Your career within the industry can be as exciting and varied as you want it to be. Your determination and imagination are all that are needed. There are no rights and wrongs when it comes to your progression – so, welcome to your new career!

The key characteristics of the beauty-related industries

In this outcome you will learn about:

• accessing sources of information on organisations, services, occupational roles, education and training opportunities within the beauty-related industries.

Types of organisations within the beauty-related industries

There are many areas that make up the beauty industry, which will give you a variety of choice when looking for employment. Throughout your training you will have discovered your likes and dislikes, enabling you to focus your career in an area that particularly appeals to you.

The organisational structure of the beauty industry is rather like a family tree, with many branches you can explore. However, you will need a starting point, and the best place to gain experience of the industry will be in a busy, successful salon. This will help you to develop your professional skills and become more employable.

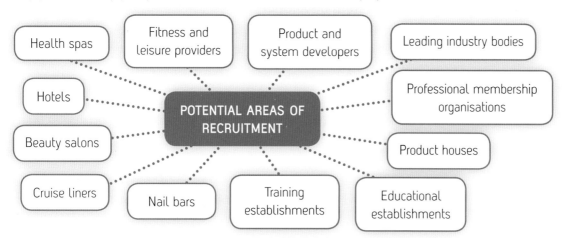

The spider diagram demonstrates the many potential areas of recruitment available to you. Nail bars, beauty salons, hotels, cruise liners, fitness and leisure providers and health spas will all give you the opportunity to apply the practical knowledge you have gained throughout your training. Working with a variety of clients who have different nail and skin types can be challenging but also rewarding. Many beauty therapists are content working within these environments, as it allows them to be creative and use the skills they have learned. Working in these types of organisations also enables you to develop your skills as a team member, as you are likely to be working with a variety of therapists and staff who may not all specialise in your area.

Training and educational establishments

These provide learners with the opportunity to complete nationally recognised qualifications within the beauty industry. The types of course on offer may differ slightly, but these establishments should be your first port of call when considering a career in beauty. Likewise, once you have gained experience within the industry you may decide to become a trainer/lecturer, which will give you the chance to help train new therapists coming into the industry and can be particularly rewarding. To progress in this area of the industry, you would be required to undertake a professional teaching qualification.

Product houses

Product houses provide training for the products that they supply. Reputable salons should ensure that you are given product training within the first few months of joining a salon. This will equip you with the knowledge that you need to use specific products effectively and safely.

For your portfolio

In pairs, make a list of all the establishments that offer beauty services in your area. Are any two the same?

Key terms

Product houses – companies or manufacturers that are responsible for the production of the professional products, packaging them ready for distribution.

Working in beauty-related industries

Professional products are developed and marketed to meet the demands of the industry and companies will support any salon that uses their range by offering training, marketing and promotional materials, and financial rewards. This may include discounts when first taking on a product range, and so on.

Awarding Organisations

The Awarding Organisations design the qualifications offered by training and educational establishments. They ensure the courses on offer meet the requirements of the industry and also set the assessment criteria — that is, what you will need to do to pass the course. This usually involves a variety of practical and written work. Some examples of Awarding Organisations are VTCT, City & Guilds and Edexcel.

Product and system developers

The developers are the brains behind the products you use on clients. It can take years to develop a product to an acceptable standard before it can go on sale. The developers continually assess and adapt products to ensure that you, as a beauty therapist, get the best results for your clients. Providing beauty services involves using complex chemicals that, if not used safely, could cause harm. Developers need to ensure that the products adhere to the relevant health and safety legislation as failing to do so could have severe consequences for the salon.

Over the years, many chemical formulae have had to be changed as the law has changed. For example, methyl methacrylate (MMA) used with acrylic systems has been banned in the USA and by many local authorities within the UK. So this ingredient has been removed from all the products and replaced with ethyl methacrylate (EMA).

Professional membership organisations

Professional bodies were established to help regulate and standardise the industry by giving guidance to therapists on appropriate conduct and behaviour. There are many different bodies and some are specific to the treatments you offer. You are not legally obliged to become a member of a professional body, but when you first start out in your career they are a good source of support in what can be a challenging industry.

Membership organisations often charge a subscription fee, so you may wish to shop around first to ensure you get the best deal with a professional body that suits the services you offer. Examples include **BABTAC**, **FHT** and **Habia**.

Key terms

BABTAC – British Association of Beauty Therapy and Cosmetology.

FHT – Federation of Holistic Therapists.

Habia – Hair and Beauty Industry Authority. The standard-setting body and creates codes of practice for the hair, beauty, nails and spa industries.

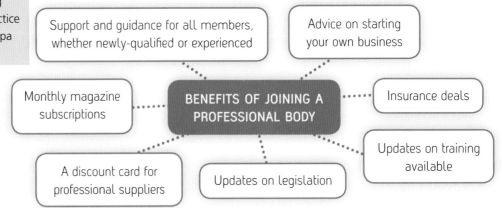

Support and guidance for all members, whether newly-qualified or experienced

Advice on starting your own business

Monthly magazine subscriptions

BENEFITS OF JOINING A PROFESSIONAL BODY

Insurance deals

A discount card for professional suppliers

Updates on legislation

Updates on training available

As a beauty therapist, you will need to keep up to date with what goes on within the industry. Similarly, a salon will not attract new clients if it continues to offer the same types of treatment that it provided ten years ago. There are many ways to access the latest information on the organisations described earlier.

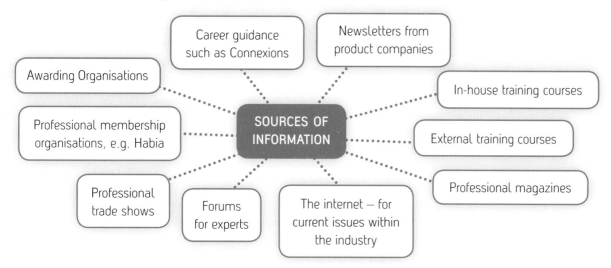

Journals

Professional journals or magazines such as *Professional Beauty* are available on subscription. They are an excellent way to keep in touch with issues within the industry and also provide information on new and upcoming treatments and products that a salon may wish to offer. Their articles can help you to overcome common problems and provide other sources of advice. Most journals have a job recruitment section, highlighting vacancies all over the UK and even Europe.

Training providers and further education colleges

Any type of training course will give you information on the industry. In-house courses such as those offered by further education colleges and training providers may help develop existing skills, but from time to time you may be required to update your qualifications. For example, therapists who trained 20 years ago may not have worked with the latest high-tech equipment and to ensure they can use it safely and effectively, they may be required to retrain. Retraining should never be seen as a negative thing – even the most qualified and experienced therapist can always learn more.

Newsletters from product companies

These are similar to magazines but may come directly from a product company. They will help to keep you informed about:

- new products available for professional or retail use
- training courses available
- hot topics and current issues within the industry
- advice and guidance that the company can offer.

Newsletters tend to be advertising tools, so will not include information on any other product range, but they can still be beneficial.

Having a good relationship with your supplier will also enhance the services you offer. Many suppliers have representatives who regularly visit salons to keep the communication and relationship positive. These visits can be very beneficial to the business, as they can motivate and inspire you.

The internet

The internet is a source of a vast amount of information and will often be a person's first port of call when seeking information about the beauty industry. Professional bodies, Awarding Organisations, training and educational establishments and so on will have websites you can access. The internet is also an excellent way to communicate with other professionals and experts in the field through **forums**.

Trade shows

Throughout the year, exhibition halls hold professional trade shows for the beauty and nail industries. New and established therapists can benefit from these exciting events, as they are an excellent way to gather information on all aspects of the industry from the different types of organisations represented there. Product and equipment suppliers and professional and Awarding Organisations will have stands at trade shows, which also run conference and training sessions giving you the chance to see the latest treatments before anyone else.

Services available in the industry

There are so many different services available within the beauty services industry that it may not be possible to offer all of them in one salon. It is also unrealistic from a business perspective for the following reasons:

- The wider the range of products and services offered, the greater the initial cost to the salon to provide them.
- Staff members may need more training, which can be an additional expense for the salon.
- Less popular treatments may lose the business money.

The range of services offered will often be decided by the salon manager, although most managers will be open to suggestions as therapists deal with clients on a day-to-day basis and might have a greater understanding of what clients want. The location of the salon may also affect the services available due to the area's **demographics**.

The role of service and training organisations

Whatever the service a salon offers or the products it uses, you will need to communicate and build relationships with service and training organisations. They play an essential role in creating well-trained, professional beauty therapists. Service organisations deal with a specific professional product range, while training organisations such as further education colleges are more general.

Key terms

Forum – discussion of questions on a professional topic, commonly taking place through the internet.

Think about it

What better way to solve a problem than to hold discussions with other professionals from your industry? Ensure you demonstrate your own professionalism when communicating with them, as they may not want to be associated with someone who is letting the industry down.

Key terms

Demographics – the age range, ethnic background, financial circumstances and so on of a range of people living within an area.

Services available:

Manicures – £18; 45 mins

Deluxe manicures – £ 22; 60 mins

Pedicures – £20; 60 mins

Deluxe pedicures – £24; 1 hr 15 mins

Nail art – prices vary; up to 30 mins

Nail enhancements – £25–£45; 1 hr 30 mins to 2 hrs

Infills/maintenance – £20; 1 hr

Rebalance – £25–£30; 1 hr 30 mins

Repairs – approx. £5 per nail; 15 mins

Removals – £20; 1 hr

Sample price list of nail services

Service organisations	Training organisations
Provide product and treatment training	Provide learners with professional qualifications for beauty services
Offer refresher courses	Provide learners with skills required for working within the industry
Provide updates on changes within companies	Ensure delivery of courses matches requirements laid down by the Awarding Organisation
Ensure products are of the highest standard and are fit for purpose	Ensure teaching staff are current and up to date with their own skills
Support salons and establishments that have invested in the products	Pass on knowledge and skills so learners achieve
Keep up to date with changes within the industry	Keep up to date with changes within the industry and qualification framework
Develop new products and treatments to reflect these changes	

Occupational roles within the beauty industry

Once you have achieved your beauty service qualifications, you may wish to research the employment options available to you. Some people have a very clear idea of where they would like to work, while others may need to try a few different roles before settling into one they are truly happy with. Remember that working within the beauty industry is demanding and also very competitive. If you want to progress it will take a lot of determination and dedication, but equally this will bring you immense job satisfaction.

When most therapists leave college they start work within a salon, to gain experience. They will be considered a junior member of staff. Junior does not mean that they are any less valued than other members of the team. It simply refers to a therapist's experience within the salon. You can quickly progress up the salon **hierarchy** by showing your professionalism and commitment and by attending training courses. As a beauty therapist you will provide a wide range of services. Due to the fast-growing nature of the industry it is possible to find employment using a specialised skill.

Experience will be needed before you can progress, so you will need to work hard to increase your **client base** and work on a wide range of people. Once the salon manager has seen your skills and you have completed further training, you will become a more senior member of the team. This may mean your responsibilities increase, something that should not be taken lightly. The business and the manager trust you to fulfil these responsibilities. At this time, you may also be asked to look after and mentor newer members of staff. This can be very rewarding, as you will remember how daunting those first few weeks can be.

Working in a salon is a good stepping stone into the industry, but there are many other roles that you may wish to explore. Spas, cruise liners, health farms and so on will all help develop your practical skills and increase your experience. Working for these types of establishment may be beneficial if you are keen to travel and seek employment outside the UK.

Experienced therapists who are thought of highly within the industry may have the opportunity to help develop products and courses by working alongside Awarding Organisations and professional membership organisations. These types of organisation rely on input from those who are working within the industry to see what changes and updates are needed.

Think about it

What beauty services would a city-centre salon offer compared to a salon in a village?

Key terms

Hierarchy – a system of people ranked one above another.

Client base – clients who come and see the salon/therapists specifically, on a regular basis.

Top tips

Shadowing a more senior member of staff will show initiative and help you learn about other roles. You will see what their responsibilities are.

Working in beauty-related industries

Becoming a salon manager or salon owner

Some beauty therapists are keen to develop their managerial skills and become a salon manager and perhaps even the salon owner. This may involve training that is not directly linked to the industry and practical skills and will include learning management techniques, relevant legislation and the principles of finance. The salon owner and manager are two completely different roles. A manager looks after the day-to-day running of the salon and supports members of the team, while the salon owner looks after the business finances and is responsible for the upkeep of the premises, equipment, staff wages and so on.

Becoming a tutor or trainer

This can be extremely rewarding and is another potential career path. Information on the qualification requirements can be found on the Internet but may vary slightly, depending on the establishment. Tutors more commonly work in a further or higher education establishment, while trainers may work in a private academy or for a specific product house, training beauty therapists who are already qualified. A sales representative would support salons with product ranges and will often have to do lots of travelling. The job involves working with a wide range of businesses as you promote a professional product range.

The diagram below demonstrates the many career paths available to you. You may decide to stick to one or experiment and gain experience in many different areas.

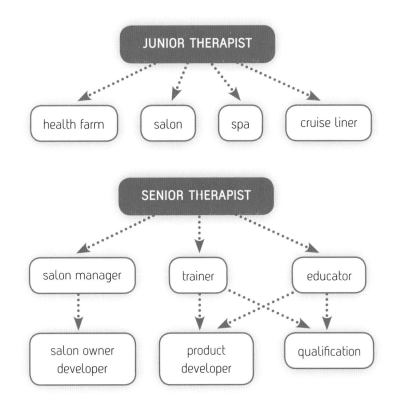

Career progression paths

Employment characteristics of working in the beauty-related industries

With all the different types of role available to you, there is also a choice of how you are employed:

- full-time
- part-time
- freelance
- on contract.

Full-time and part-time employment often depends on an individual's personal choice and circumstances. For example, mothers with young children may decide to work part-time so that they can spend time at home with the family. Some people need to work full-time for financial reasons. There is no right or wrong, and you will find the pros and cons are different for everybody. What should be clear in your contract is the number of hours you are required to work each week. The amount of holiday and sickness pay entitlement are then calculated on a **pro-rata basis**.

An employer must provide all employees with a contract, which you will need to read and check carefully before signing. Any inconsistencies should be discussed with your manager and then changed where appropriate.

A freelance therapist is usually self-employed and provides their services for a fee. For example, make-up artists are rarely directly employed by any one company. When their services are required, a company will pay the make-up artist for their time. Being a freelance beauty therapist will give you some flexibility over your working hours and your choice of work. However, the amount of work and when you work might not be consistent.

How suitable employment characteristics can open up opportunities

In order to progress in your career there are certain attributes — qualities — that you will need to have. In this section, you will look at the ones that may help you with either promotion within your existing salon or perhaps applying for a more senior role elsewhere.

Promotion does not come automatically, nor is it necessarily linked to the number of years you have worked for the company. In fact, it is common to find therapists who have never progressed within a salon, even though they have worked there for several years. Promotion must be earned and you will need to demonstrate that you are capable of taking on new challenges. For example, in the table on page 144, therapist A increases their job opportunities while therapist B decreases them. There is a big difference between therapists A and B — they are, of course, two extreme cases. However, your employer will be constantly watching and assessing your performance.

Key terms

Pro-rata basis – for employees who do not work full-time, their holiday and sick pay entitlements are calculated as a percentage of a full-time member of staff; for example if you work 70 per cent of a full-time post, your holiday entitlement will be 70 per cent of full-time.

Therapist A – increasing job opportunities	Therapist B – decreasing job opportunities
• work with a positive 'can do' attitude • attend staff training • attend and participate during staff meetings • perform treatments to the highest of standards • show enthusiasm with all tasks • shadow senior members of the team • research and gain knowledge on the requirements of the job • be knowledgeable on the industry • increase client base	• fail to update skills with new qualifications • attend staff meetings but not participate or communicate with other members of the team • lack motivation and enthusiasm when given tasks • carry out poor treatments of a low standard • receive customer complaints • show no interest in other job roles or increasing responsibility

Increasing and decreasing job opportunities

Education and training opportunities within the beauty-related industries

Developing your professional skills is a vital part of your career. To learn more, see the Importance of continual professional development, page 150.

Opportunities to transfer to other sectors or industries

The beauty industry is classified as a commercial and service industry. As the industry has developed over the years, links have been made with many other industries. This is valuable, as you can learn a lot from the way that other people work.

The beauty industry can link with:

◉ healthcare

◉ sport and leisure

◉ complementary and holistic therapies

◉ management and finance.

Therapists often work alongside healthcare professionals, and it is becoming increasingly common for recommendations to come from either side. These two industries can then work alongside complementary and holistic therapies to improve the health of a client. For example:

◉ nail services and chiropodists/podiatrists

◉ therapists and patients suffering from life-threatening illnesses

◉ therapists trained in massage have the basic knowledge and understanding to train in sports massage. Sports massage is a vital part of keeping an athlete healthy and injury-free. Many of the top football teams incorporate sports massage into their post-match cooldowns.

If you wish to own a business or become a manager, you will need specialised training. It takes a lot of hard work and business knowledge to make a success of it. There are many management and finance companies that can support you when running a business. You are likely to need the expertise of legal teams, financial advisers, accountants and so on at various times throughout your management career.

Think about it

In pairs, discuss when you might need to refer a client to another industry. Feed back your findings to the rest of the class.

Key terms

Chiropodist/podiatrist
– a member of a healthcare organisation who is trained to deal with and treat medical conditions of the feet.

Think about it

Being a beauty therapist does not qualify you to become a manager. You will need to attend further training to educate yourself and develop managerial skills.

Main legislation affecting the beauty-related industries

Information about legislation affecting the beauty-related industries can be found in other units, as shown in the table below.

Legislation	Unit name	Page number
Disability Discrimination Act	Client care and communication in beauty-related industries	114
Health and Safety at Work Act	Essential professsional knowledge	43
Data Protection Act	Essential professsional knowledge	59
Trade Descriptions Act	Client care and communication in beauty-related industries	113
Consumer Protection Act	Display stock and promote products and services to clients	123
The Performing Rights Regulations	This act protects artists and their songs. If a company wishes to play music in their premises, they will need to inform the Performing Rights Society. They will then need to pay a fee to cover the radio and/or CDs they play. This ensures that artists get financial reward for their work – royalties.	

Basic principles of finance and selling within the beauty-related industries

In order to create a successful business, the salon owner will need to have a thorough knowledge of suitable financial and marketing techniques. For information on finance and selling, see the unit Display stock and promote products and services to clients, page 117.

Main forms of marketing and publicity used by beauty-related industries

Advertising is very powerful and it is unusual to find a salon or nail bar that does not use some form of marketing to promote itself. Even relying on word of mouth is a form of marketing — you just don't need to pay for it.

There is no right or wrong marketing tool to use, but some are more suitable for different types of salons then others.

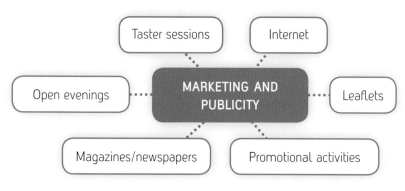

The internet

More and more people now have access to the internet, and it has become an everyday tool for organising people's lives. Having a salon website allows clients to access information about its services 24 hours a day, 7 days a week. They no longer have to wait for opening hours to find their answers. Information on a salon website should include:

- contact details
- opening hours
- services and prices
- products used and retailed
- images of the salon
- treatment information
- special offers
- customer feedback.

Some businesses shy away from websites, as they are unsure of how to set them up, but there are many specialist companies who offer this type of service. For a fee, in consultation with the salon they will design and set up the website.

Leaflets

Leaflets that provide treatment and production information and price lists should be available in a salon for clients to look at and take home. But how would people access leaflets if they never visit the salon? Leaflet drops can be used in the surrounding areas to promote the salon. Again, there are companies that can do the leaflet drop or members of staff could be involved during quiet periods. Building professional relationships with other businesses in the area could help encourage them to display your leaflets, for example GPs' surgeries, community centres and so on.

Promotional articles in magazines and newspapers

Local magazines and newspapers can be used to promote the salon to the surrounding community, through advertisements or promotional articles. This may include new promotions or services available within the salon. Advertising rates are usually quite reasonable. Professional magazines can be more expensive, so it would depend on the salon's marketing budget. However, professional magazines can help to promote the salon to other professional companies. This helps build professional relationships between companies – networking events are often advertised within magazines.

Promotional activities, taster sessions and open evenings

Promotional activities may involve setting up information stands in busy commercial areas, such as trade events or in shopping centres. They may help to increase the salon's client base by attracting potential new clients. The cost of a promotional activity will vary depending on the location, but they have proven to be very effective.

Taster sessions and open evenings are aimed at both new and existing clients, giving them a chance to perhaps try new treatments and gain advice from professional therapists and beauty therapists. They are also very effective if the salon is launching a new product, treatment or promotion.

Working practices associated with the beauty-related industries

In this outcome you will learn about:

- describing good working practices and understanding the importance of personal presentation
- describing opportunities for developing and promoting your own professional image
- the importance of **continual professional development (CPD)**
- basic employment rights and employer responsibilities.

Key terms

Continual professional development (CPD) – updating skills in your professional area throughout your career.

What are good working practices?

Everybody would like harmonious working conditions but this requires effort from the whole team. Your personal actions will contribute to the effectiveness of the salon and the effectiveness of the team. Working safely also contributes to an effective working environment – to learn more about PPE, COSHH and methods of sterilisation, see Essential professional knowledge, page 9.

As a beauty therapist, you will mainly work independently with clients, which may cause you to become detached from the rest of the team. Directly carrying out treatments on clients does not involve a lot of teamwork. However, your behaviour and actions throughout the day may affect other staff members. For example:

- Running late with a client may prevent another therapist using the products and equipment or the working area.
- Poor service will reflect badly on the whole salon, not just you, causing a decrease in the client base, which will affect everyone.
- Failing to tidy up after your treatment, leaving it for someone else to do, is not good teamwork. It could cause your colleague to run late or mean the equipment is not prepared for their client.

During a busy salon day, when you have clients back to back, it is easy to be busily occupied with your own tasks. However, take the time during gaps to check on your team members. Look to see if they need help setting up, seeing a client out, taking payments and so on. There is nothing worse for team morale than one therapist sitting down doing nothing while everyone else rushes around getting tasks done.

Each workplace will have its own set of guidelines for professional expectations. As a new member of staff, be sure to familiarise yourself with the policies and ensure you adhere to them at all times.

To learn more about professional ethical conduct, see Client care and communication in beauty-related industries, page 99.

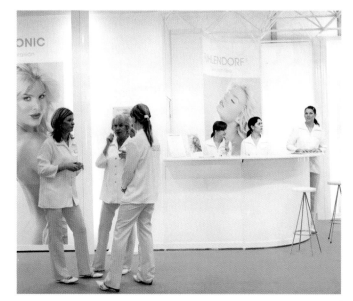

Working in a nail studio needs a lot of teamwork

Working in beauty-related industries

147

The importance of personal presentation in reflecting a professional image

To promote yourself as a professional beauty therapist, you will need to show you can present yourself appropriately. This will help to build working relationships with other companies. Other professionals will form a negative opinion of you and your establishment if you are dressed inappropriately. To learn more about personal presentation requirements, see Essential professional knowledge, page 10.

Opportunities for developing and promoting your professional image

To progress in the beauty industry, you will be required to build as many professional relationships as possible. This will involve promoting yourself to companies, organisations and other professional people in order to build an image that reflects your dedication and determination to succeed.

When progressing from job to job you will need an up-to-date **curriculum vitae (CV)** which can be used during the application process. Your CV gives you the opportunity to promote the skills you have acquired during your career. In such a competitive industry, any additional skills and qualifications that show your dedication can help you win a job opportunity.

Ways to create professional links include:

- working with professional healthcare advisers for the treatment of clients
- working with the local community
- attending regular continual professional development (CPD) events (see page 150)
- building a large and successful client base
- taking part in professional competitions, for example beauty therapist awards
- building relationships with other professionals from a wide range of organisations, for example professional membership organisations and product companies.

Key terms

Curriculum vitae (CV) – a document showing the history of education, employment and professional skills; often required when applying for jobs.

Basic employment rights and employer responsibilities

As an employee or an employer, you will need to know about the following legislation and regulations, which are designed to protect both employees and employers so that everyone is treated equally and can work in a safe environment.

The Working Time Regulations 1998

These regulations set standards for working hours and holiday entitlement. This is to ensure everyone is treated fairly and enables staff to work safely. The regulations cover:

- hours of work per week (no more than 48 hours averaged over a 17-week period)
- rest entitlement (a break of 11 hours between working days)
- short break entitlement (working over six hours entitles you to a 20-minute break)
- days off (a minimum of one day off a week)
- holiday (four weeks' paid holiday a year).

The law is slightly different for employees under the age of 17, and more information can be found on the Directgov website.

The National Minimum Wage

The National Minimum Wage is the minimum amount per hour that most workers in the UK are entitled to be paid. Employers are responsible for keeping staff informed of any updates and changes to this. Many therapists who first start out in the industry will start at the minimum wage. Following are the minimum wage rates (as of 1 October 2011):

£6.08 – the main rate for workers aged 21 and over

£4.98 – the 18–20 rate

£3.68 – the 16–17 rate (for workers above school leaving age but under 18)

£2.60 – the apprentice rate (for apprentices under 19 or 19 or over and in the first year of their apprenticeship).

Employment rights

The following table summarises the responsibilities of employers and employees.

Employer responsibilities	Employee responsibilities
provide a **contract of employment**	adhere to salon's policies and guidelines
give clear **job specifications** and responsibilities	work in a safe and responsible manner
provide appropriate amount of wage	adhere to job specifications and contract
provide a safe working environment	inform employer of any inadequate policies
provide safe and appropriate equipment	adhere to employment legislation
adhere to employment legislation	

Employment Act 1997

This act was intended to bring equality to employment and ensure people are treated fairly. It covers:

- pay
- working time and leave
- termination of employment
- variation on basic conditions.

More information can be found on the Directgov website.

Consequences of failing to act professionally

As a beauty therapist, you represent a multi-billion pound industry, which has an excellent reputation. Failing to act professionally can damage a salon's business and may affect the public's positive attitudes to the industry. The consequences of unprofessional behaviour are shown in the following diagram.

> ### Key terms
>
> **Contract of employment** – a legally binding contract that sets out the specification of your job, it will outline working hours, holiday and break entitlement, sick pay, etc.
>
> **Job specification** – this will outline your roles and responsibilities within your job role so you will know exactly what is expected of you.

> ### For your portfolio
>
> In pairs, write a job description for a beauty therapist. Remember to include their roles and responsibilities.

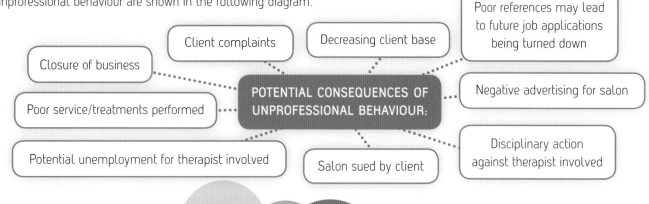

Poor references may lead to future job applications being turned down

Client complaints

Decreasing client base

Closure of business

Negative advertising for salon

Poor service/treatments performed

POTENTIAL CONSEQUENCES OF UNPROFESSIONAL BEHAVIOUR:

Potential unemployment for therapist involved

Salon sued by client

Disciplinary action against therapist involved

Working in beauty-related industries

The importance of continual professional development

Your training within the industry should never end — it should be a continual part of your career. You work in an ever-changing industry where new products and services are being developed all the time, so there will always be something new for you to learn. Continual professional development (CPD) should be a part of your contract of employment. It is an integral part of your career and should always be thought of as a positive opportunity. Unfortunately, some therapists believe CPD to be a waste of time or unnecessary — that kind of attitude will not allow you to progress in your career.

Attending regular CPD training will show you are up to date and knowledgeable about everything happening in the beauty industry, from new treatments to changes within codes of practice. The knowledge you gain will be passed on to your clients, who will be impressed by your dedication, and this can lead to an increase in your client base. It may also inspire other members of your team, as you demonstrate your knowledge and skills in the salon environment. Your enthusiasm to learn will also be reflected in the **appraisal** system.

Techniques that were developed in the early years of the beauty industry were effective and professional, and updating your skills does not mean that what you had been doing previously was wrong. However, as research is carried out and technology advances, there are even more effective techniques available to achieve incredible results on clients. Treatments are also developed to make them safer for the client and therapist and to help ensure that you comply with the latest health and safety legislation.

Organisations that can provide training

The diagram below shows the many types of organisation that can provide you with CPD training.

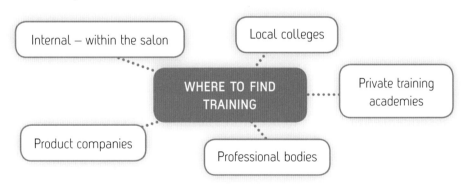

Internal training

Internal training may be provided by your employer. When you join a salon, you should be trained in its guidelines and policies. In some cases, you may also be offered treatment training by another member of staff. However, this does not always mean you are fully qualified to carry out the treatment. Where a salon uses a particular range of products, the product house may insist that every member of staff attends its training courses, without which you may invalidate your salon's insurance cover.

Product companies

Training provided by product companies varies from product knowledge (suitable for receptionists) to full-service and treatment training. Some also offer refresher training to update skills of therapists who have used their products in the past. Product companies should keep your salon notified of the training courses they are running.

The cost of training will depend on the product company. Some offer free training for all staff; others will train two members for free and the rest of the team at a cost.

Professional membership organisations

Professional bodies may not always provide practical training, but they are a good source of information for current issues within the industry. They may offer courses on changes within qualifications, legislation and so on. Attending them will ensure you have an insight into all areas of the industry.

Training establishments

These offer nationally recognised qualifications. If you have been enrolled by your employer, then they will normally cover the cost of the course. If it is something you personally are interested in, then you may be expected to pay the cost. An advantage of having a nationally recognised qualification is that all organisations within beauty therapy will recognise it, so you will be given credit for the qualification wherever you go.

Why update my skills?

You should never assume that once you become a qualified therapist your training ends. For example, if you were to compare the techniques used for manicuring 20 years ago with techniques used today, you would find they are very different.

The diagram below looks at the potential consequences of not updating your skills throughout your career.

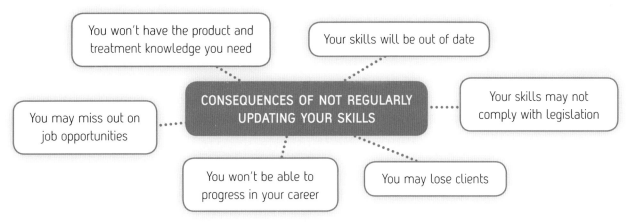

You won't have the product and treatment knowledge you need

Your skills will be out of date

CONSEQUENCES OF NOT REGULARLY UPDATING YOUR SKILLS

Your skills may not comply with legislation

You may miss out on job opportunities

You won't be able to progress in your career

You may lose clients

Building your client base is essential to a successful career. Clients nowadays are very informed about the industry – they read magazine articles, research on the internet and so on, which means they are very aware of market trends and the new treatments becoming available. If a salon fails to take an interest in new treatments, clients will eventually go elsewhere. As new products and services are being developed all the time, it would be too expensive for a salon to invest in them all, but it is important to do research and find out what is creating the most interest. Salons should also listen to clients and ask their opinion on what services they would like to see in the salon.

Working in beauty-related industries

Working in beauty-related industries

My story

Salon life

My name is Melissa and I currently teach beauty and nail services with a FE college. I fell in love with nails at college, so as soon as I was qualified I found employment within my local salon. I expected to start on clients straight away and be considered as fully qualified, due to my college certificate. This wasn't the case. I was put in as a 'rookie' and they monitored my performance very closely. After months of hard work I was told I could attend the training to become a nail technician. I had to attend the salon's own training academy, where I had to sit an exam and then perform a practical assessment. They would then decide if I was of a technician standard. Thankfully I passed, but this was not the end of my training. I then had to do the assessments to become a senior technician and then an advanced technician. At each stage I received a certificate and a pay rise.

Overall it took me three years to get to that level! It was hard work but it was very rewarding when I was told I had passed. We also had product and treatment training on top of that, whenever new systems came into the salon. When I left the salon I had a portfolio filled with evidence of my training, which helped me get the role I have today. It gave me excellent experience and taught me that you can never have too many qualifications. There is always something new to learn!

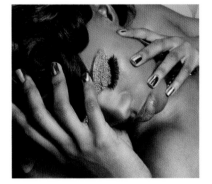

Be aware of the new products that are causing the most interest

When applying for a job, you will need to be able to sell yourself and show the new company all the skills you can offer. If your skills are too dated, it may not be interested in employing you. Potential employers will look at the cost of taking on new staff – paying for all the new training courses to update you may be too expensive for them. There will also be plenty of other candidates applying with the latest, more relevant qualifications.

Recording and evidencing continual professional development

Documenting your training is an essential part of your CPD, as this is your evidence to say you have undertaken courses to develop your skills. Depending on the type of business, there may be specific criteria for recording your CPD. It should be seen as a portfolio of evidence that could be shown to new employers, clients and so on, to promote your skills.

Within a salon environment, certificates should be on display either in the reception area or in treatment rooms. They should always be visible to the clients. This not only promotes how skilled you are as a therapist but it also rewards you for the hard work you have done by completing courses. Displaying certificates is a way of sharing the achievement with clients and other members of the team.

Within training and education establishments, there are strict policies on how much CPD a member of staff should undertake. This is usually a combination of in-house and external training courses, but should always link to the member of staff's skill area. The professional membership organisation for educators in further education, Institute for Learning (IfL), promotes professional good practice and CPD. Lecturers are required to record annually how much CPD they have undertaken and give details. Awarding bodies have also followed suit, for example VTCT. This ensures that people responsible for training and educating new beauty therapists are training them in skills that are current and relevant.

Think about it

Clients like to know how qualified their therapist is, as it gives them a sense of security that they will do a good job.

Check your knowledge

1 Where would you access information on organisations within the industry?

2 What are the advantages of being a member of a professional membership organisation?

3 State the hierarchy of staff within a salon.

4 Describe the Working Time Regulations 1998.

5 Identify ways of promoting yourself as a professional beauty therapist.

6 List five ways to market and promote a new treatment available in your establishment.

7 Why should therapists keep their skills current and up to date?

8 What does CPD stand for?

9 List four responsibilities of an employer.

10 List four consequences of not updating your skills.

Getting ready for assessment

This is a preparation for work unit, which is based on capability and knowledge. The aim of the unit is to provide learners with an understanding of our industry requirements.

Evidence requirements

You should ensure that you meet the required standards, i.e. that all outcomes, assessment criteria and range statements have been achieved. This unit is both internally assessed with assignments and/or with an online test depending upon your Awarding Organisation.

Practical outcomes are achieved by:

1 Proving you have a good understanding of the key characteristics of beauty-related industries

2 Proving knowledge of good working practice.

Patterns of delivery may vary with this unit but you will be given guidance by your assessor who will set assignments for you to complete to prove knowledge and understanding. As with other units, all underpinning knowledge must be covered, with a full range of the main services in our industry and across the various employment spectrums available. This is a big unit so expect to work on some in-depth assignments and papers. This will show you understand the full career prospects and occupational roles open to you upon completion of your course. There may also be cross references to other evidence from other units around legislation, marketing and publicity, services and specific employment law.

Working in beauty-related industries

Salon reception duties

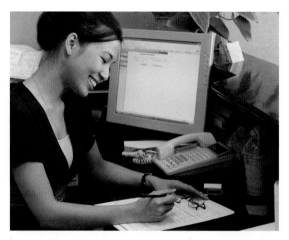

Receptionists need to be in control of paperwork and booking systems

Introduction

This unit will explore all the areas you need to learn about in order to become a successful salon receptionist. The reception area and receptionist are the first to be seen by the client on entering the salon, so a warm and inviting entrance with a confident and effective receptionist is essential.

First impressions really do count — and they become lasting impressions, so it is vital that they are positive. Reception is the heart of any salon. It needs to work properly and have the right impact on clients. It should be a place of tranquility, with order and tidiness being the key to functioning efficiently. This should be the same for a spa, beauty salon, hair salon or a salon which has combined facilities.

The way a receptionist presents themselves is vital; they should always look clean and tidy to reflect the professionalism of the salon. When sitting at the reception desk the receptionist should not slouch and when standing an upright posture should be adopted. Good posture will avoid repetitive strain and other postural problems and present a positive image to clients and other visitors to the salon.

All visitors should be made welcome and treated with equal courtesy, so that no one feels neglected or ignored. You should acknowledge clients as they appear, even if you are unable to deal with them straight away. Every client is important to the salon, no matter what the enquiry may be — they should all be given equal attention.

You will need to learn your own salon's guidelines for dealing with general enquiries and more specific problems as they occur. You will also have to gain knowledge about each treatment, how long they take and linked services offered, as well as the system for booking appointments. All of this information will enable you to offer a professional service, guarantee client satisfaction and allow maximum cost-effectiveness to your employer.

Carry out reception duties

In this outcome you will learn about:

- dealing with a variety of enquiries
- communicating and behaving in a professional manner
- presenting a positive image of yourself and the salon
- identifying the nature of the enquiry
- maintaining appropriate levels of reception stationery
- maintaining a hygienic and tidy reception area.

Reception is key to the whole functioning of the salon — it will soon grind to a halt if the receptionist is poorly organised, books appointments incorrectly and is untidy.

The therapists depend upon appointments being booked correctly, with the right time allowed for each treatment. The receptionist needs to be able to produce the correct record card, the right stock request and the correct stationery to be able to order a product for the client. That means being tidy, in control of paperwork and having a thorough knowledge of the treatments as well as good **stock control**.

Refer to Professional skills, You, your client and the law, pages 56–58, for the relevant legislation concerned with selling retail products.

Key terms

Stock control – maintaining sufficient levels of stock, such as products, consumables and stationery, for the salon's day-to-day needs.

My story

Spa receptionist

Hi, my name is Siobhan, and I'm the receptionist in a busy spa. I run the appointments for 12 therapists, who all have different areas of expertise. It is my job to ensure their days run smoothly and the clients gain the maximum benefit from their treatments. If I were to make a mistake with the bookings, it would have a huge impact on the smooth running of the salon and the therapists would get very agitated.

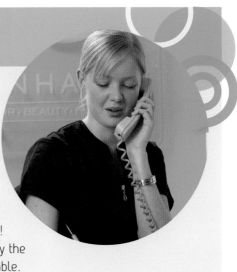

My other role is to be the 'face' of the salon. I am the first point of contact for the clients, either face to face or on the phone, so I need to be calm, smiling and polite at all times. A client can even tell over the phone if you are not smiling! I also need to keep up to date with the treatments, services and products offered by the salon to ensure clients receive the treatments and products that are the most suitable. I enjoy my job as a receptionist. It is varied and I get to meet lots of interesting people.

Dealing with a variety of enquiries

In the course of a day the receptionist will have to deal with a wide range of enquiries. It is important to understand the different types of enquiries you may be presented with so that you are fully prepared to deal with them in an efficient and professional manner.

Dealing with telephone enquiries

The telephone is now second nature to us all and mobile phones are commonplace. Not everyone can use one effectively, however. The telephone can be a very useful business tool and should be used wisely.

How to use the phone

There are key steps to a good telephone manner. These ensure that the person on the end of the phone is treated courteously, efficiently and accurately.

If a client is making an enquiry by telephone, ideally the phone should be answered within four rings. All enquiries should be dealt with in a professional manner and the same courtesy should be shown to the client as if they were in the reception area.

Email enquiries should be dealt with in the same manner as soon as practical after receiving them. Ensure that full details are given to the client to ensure that they are happy with the reply. This should always include the salon information and replies should be typed professionally with spelling and punctuation checked. It is worth remembering that you can email at any time of day, and clients who have to cancel an appointment out of hours will often use this method, so, along with the answer phone, emails should always be checked first thing in the morning. If you are unable to deal with the enquiry either forward the email to the relevant staff member or print off the email and give it to the staff member.

> **Think about it**
>
> - Always have a pen and paper handy to take messages.
> - Answer the phone promptly, even if you are busy.
> - If you do feel harassed, pause, take a deep breath in before lifting the receiver and put a smile in your voice. (It is very easy to sound abrupt on the telephone.)
> - Identify the salon quickly, after making sure you are connected properly and the caller can hear you.
> - Be cheery – no matter how pressurised you may feel, it should not show in the tone of your voice. No one wants to be greeted by a miserable-sounding receptionist.
> - Redirect the call quickly when putting it through to another extension. If the call cannot be put through, ask the caller if they wish to leave a message.

Salon reception duties

Think about it

Anyone can walk through the salon door, so it's best to be prepared!

When dealing with clients, both face to face and on the phone, it is likely that at some time you will deal with a client who may have different needs and expectations of the service they wish to receive and will challenge the receptionist. Clients may appear confused or angry, or may have a complaint. Remember to remain polite and calm at all times.

Customers with different needs and expectations

Customers with disabilities

People with disabilities may require some help negotiating doorways and assisting into the treatment area. Always offer to help, but do not assume they cannot manage — and never patronise or talk down to the client.

The hard of hearing are usually good lip readers, so the receptionist should face the client and speak clearly so the client can see the words forming. Depending upon the severity of the disability, a pad could be provided to jot down a message. A price list could be a good visual aid to help clarify what the client wants.

People who speak English as a second language might have difficulties communicating with you. Again, speak clearly, and use visual materials to help clarify and seek help if available.

Older clients may have problems with mobility or hearing. However, never assume this to be the case — never judge. Be on hand to offer assistance. If the client is very frail, then explain that some treatment adaptation might be needed.

Clients who appear angry

Never shout at clients. Be calm and precise when dealing with them. If they are in reception and appear angry and agitated, try to take them somewhere quiet, out of the public view, as an angry client, even if their anger is unfounded, does not do the reputation of the salon any good. Remember, if you cannot deal with the client's complaint, find someone in a more senior position to assist you.

Clients who appear confused

There may be a number of reasons for the client's confusion: for example, the client may speak English as a second language (see above) and have difficulty understanding; it may be related to an illness or a disability; or it could be something as simple as getting the date and time of the appointment wrong. It is important for the receptionist to remain calm and clarify things as many times as the client needs to ensure that they understand.

Wheel chair access

Deaf person

Think about it

It can be as easy to give a bad impression over the phone as in person — perhaps more so, because the caller only judges what is heard, and may not know the background to an irritable manner.

A client with a complaint

Clients with a complaint should be treated with respect and, however agitated and angry they might be, never shout or retaliate. At times, this may be difficult, but remaining calm will always give the receptionist the upper hand.

Listen carefully to the client's grievance and try to resolve the problem. If this is out of your capability, refer the complaint to someone more senior. If you are dealing with a phone complaint, you may need to say that you will ask someone more senior to phone back – if you promise this, then it's important someone does phone, as it will only annoy the client further if they do not receive the promised call.

Communicate and behave in a professional manner

Client care and hospitality are all about treating your client as you would wish to be treated yourself. No matter how good the salon treatments may be, if the client feels rushed, unwanted or is made to feel uncomfortable in any way, you will lose her business. Your salon will have a client care policy on the correct way that clients are to be greeted, both on the phone and in person. This will cover making appointments, handling payments and dealing with complaints, as well as where you store clients' coats and belongings while having a treatment and the offering of beverages in the salon.

There is a fine line between being professional, yet friendly, and being too familiar and possibly careless with your client's feelings. The old saying that 'familiarity breeds contempt' is true in business: regardless of how long you have known your clients, you must remember they are still paying for a service and deserve the best of care. The beauty therapist often learns quite personal, intimate details about her client, and there is a danger that this information could lead to a familiarity that is inappropriate.

Good client care and **hospitality** will ensure your clientele returns to the salon regularly, as they feel welcomed, pampered and cosseted.

Refer to Professional skills, pages 18–22 for treatment planning and preparation, which is all part of your client hospitality, pages 26–30 for other factors that contribute to client care, and page 18 for how to handle complaints. Good client care should be non-discriminatory and a receptionist should be non-judgmental whatever the circumstances. Above all, never argue with the client!

Presenting a positive image of yourself and the salon

The client's first impression of the salon is often formed by the way she is greeted rather than just the décor. Receiving clients into the salon is a little like greeting a guest into your home. The hospitality and friendliness should be the same. It may be the client's first or twenty-first visit; the polite and welcoming greeting should be the same. All visitors should be made welcome and treated with equal importance. This is achieved through verbal and non-verbal communication, good listening skills and questioning techniques. (These topics are fully covered in Essential professional knowledge, pages 27–30 and Client care and communication in work-related industries, pages 102–104.)

> **Key terms**
>
> **Hospitality** – being welcoming, warm and friendly, and ensuring that the clients' needs are met by offering refreshments or magazines.

Salon reception duties

It is important to maintain a balance between giving the correct amount of attention to individual clients and your responsibilities towards other clients during busy trading periods.

The approach to clients and visitors can be summed up in a simple word: PLEASE.

Posture	This should be good, both to give a good impression and to protect the spine. When standing a receptionist should not lean or slouch – this gives the impression of boredom or not caring.
Listen	Listen with your whole body, not just your ears. Look as if you are listening. Eye contact encourages the talker to continue and facing the visitor shows you are giving her your full attention. You are saying to your visitor 'you are important to me and the salon and I give you my full attention'.
Expression	This should be welcoming, open and positive. You are not there to challenge the visitor or make her feel threatened. Smile and look as if you are pleased to see her.
Appearance and attitude	These should reflect total professionalism and mirror the high standard of the salon.
Speech	Speak clearly. Your speech should not be patronising in any way, and free of any technical terms a client may not understand. If necessary use a visual aid such as a colour chart, price list or magazine to help with your explanation.
Eagerness to help others	This is a positive quality and very flattering to the client. Use it wisely to give attention without appearing insincere. A good receptionist should be patient, trusted by the clients and supportive to both the clients and staff.

How to approach clients and visitors

Think about it

Making a client angry is a sure way of losing them.

The visitor should be dealt with as soon as possible and the right action taken or the appropriate staff member informed. Eye contact and a pleasant greeting are important. Introduce yourself to the visitor as you ask about the nature of the visit, for example 'Hello, welcome to Blissed Out salon. My name is Nyesha. How can I help you this morning?'

Do not:

- ignore the client
- act as though serving the client is the last thing you want to do
- patronise the client by talking down to her.

Identifying the nature of enquiries

The receptionist should ask these questions about the visitor in order to identify the purpose of the enquiry.

- Why has the client come?
- Where has the client come from?
- Has the client come for an appointment?
- Is the client here for a price list or to purchase a product?
- What action do I take to help the client?

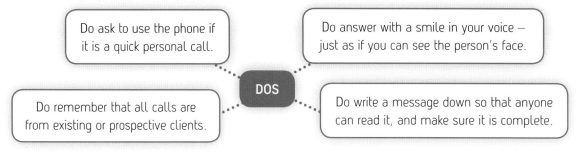

Do ask to use the phone if it is a quick personal call.

Do answer with a smile in your voice – just as if you can see the person's face.

DOS

Do remember that all calls are from existing or prospective clients.

Do write a message down so that anyone can read it, and make sure it is complete.

Don't forget that calls may come out of office hours. Most people are comfortable leaving a message on an answerphone. Enquiries can also be made electronically via the salon's website. Remember that revenue may be lost if no one follows up the message.

Don't sigh into the phone. This gives the impression that the caller is a nuisance and you are doing them a favour by answering.

Don't be curt, rude or irritated when you first pick up the phone.

DON'TS

Don't use the telephone for private calls. Itemised phone bills now show who made a call, for how long and to whom. No employer would mind the odd local call or emergency message, but do not abuse an employer's goodwill.

Don't make up an answer if you don't know. Honesty really is the best policy. If you make something up you will only get caught out and lose credibility.

Don't slam down the phone, cut someone off or talk about the caller in a rude manner.

The dos and don'ts of dealing with telephone enquiries

Eye contact and an approachable expression will encourage the visitor to give the required information so that a decision can be made as to the proper course of action. You might say:

'Please take a seat; the manager won't keep you a moment.'

'Would you like a drink or magazine while you wait?'

'I will inform your therapist you have arrived for your appointment, Mrs Smith.'

Maintaining the reception area

It is the receptionist's responsibility to ensure the smooth running of the reception at all times. Having a well organised and tidy reception area is not only crucial in creating a good first impression for clients entering the salon, it will also help the receptionist carry out her job more efficiently. This section looks at what you should consider and do in order to provide an effective reception area.

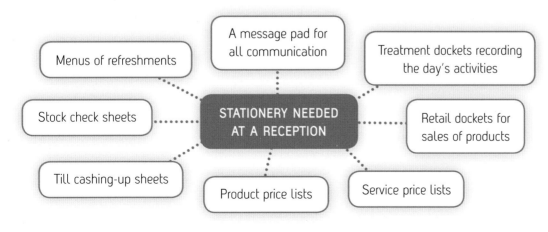

Menus of refreshments

A message pad for all communication

Treatment dockets recording the day's activities

Stock check sheets

STATIONERY NEEDED AT A RECEPTION

Retail dockets for sales of products

Till cashing-up sheets

Product price lists

Service price lists

Salon reception duties

Appropriate levels of stationery

Stationery is vital to the smooth running of reception. Running out of stationery will cause staff to use scraps of paper, or not write the information down at all, therefore forgetting vital information. Lack of the correct paperwork will affect all staff. Sales commission may be lost as the treatment and sales cannot be recorded properly. This will affect staff wages, and will not make the receptionist popular.

Vital messages may not get to the correct person, and appointments or business may be lost if there are no price lists to give out to potential clients. This is not a professional image to project. It is much better to order stationery well in advance, right down to ordering the toilet rolls! This will ensure the smooth running of all reception functions.

Maintaining a hygienic and tidy reception area

During the course of the day a reception area can become untidy just like a living room at home: the magazines and papers soon get messy, a few coffee cups may be scattered around on the table, the odd coat is thrown over a chair, and the carpet is in need of a run over with the vacuum cleaner!

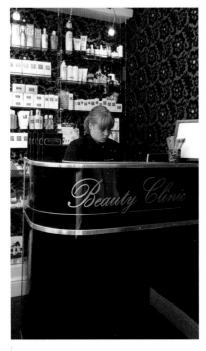

A clean and tidy reception area is inviting to clients

Think of the reception as part of your living area, with your clients as your guests, except that new ones are appearing more often than at home. At work, as at home, the living area takes regular upkeep to ensure it always looks clean and orderly.

Potential untidiness may be created by:

- clients' coats not being put away in a cupboard
- clients' umbrellas being left in a heap
- magazines and papers that are not kept in a rack or in a neat pile
- dirty coffee cups or water tumblers that are left on the table
- tables with dirty marks or stains
- delivery boxes or product trays lying around causing obstructions
- a messy floor area covered with crumbs or dust
- record cards being left out on the reception desk.

The key to being tidy is having the correct storage and being able to put things in their correct place. A salon should have a coat cupboard, an umbrella stand, a magazine rack, a table that is easy to clean and low-maintenance flooring. Suitable colours, which do not show the dirt, also help — all white, for example, would soon look grubby and would not be easy to keep clean.

Be careful though: there is a compromise to be found between being so house-proud that you hover over the client, waiting impatiently for the coffee to be drunk so that the cup can be washed up, and not tidying up until the end of the day when the mess has accumulated into a big job.

Tidying up should be carried out with minimum disruption to clients and at moments when the reception is at its quietest. This might be when there is a natural lull in client traffic flow, as they have gone into their treatment rooms. Do not attempt to vacuum around the clients when the reception is busy. Save the bigger jobs, such as floor cleaning, for morning preparation or evening tidying.

Morning preparation for the day ahead should include:

- switching on the lighting, both overhead and in the display cabinets
- putting out the day's newspapers
- getting the coffee pot ready, filling the kettle and filling up sugar and milk containers
- checking the appointments for the day and being ready to receive those clients
- putting the float money in the till
- emptying the dishwasher and putting cups away ready for the day
- collecting and sorting the post.

Ongoing duties throughout the day should include:

- keeping magazines tidy by putting them back in their rack
- removing used cups and glasses and washing them up or putting them in the dishwasher
- putting away record cards returned by the therapists
- topping up the kettle, filling the tea caddy, etc.
- wiping up spills on the table as they happen
- dusting around when quiet.

Evening tidying will include:

- leaving the reception area ready for the next morning
- putting on the dishwasher
- vacuuming the floor or other suitable cleaning for your type of flooring
- polishing all surfaces
- removing out-dated papers or magazines
- emptying the tea/coffee pots to avoid an unpleasant smell overnight or over the weekend
- filling any gaps in the display cabinets
- clearing the reception desk of all the day's paperwork
- tallying up the till and emptying the takings
- switching off all lighting.

For your portfolio

Research the display cabinets and stands that are available from various stockists. You may need to look on the internet or in salon supply magazines. Decide which would be the most suitable for your salon area and which gives you the most scope for displaying your products and displays.

Booking and recording salon appointments

In this outcome you will learn about:

- scheduling appointments to meet with salon policy and client requirements
- recording salon appointments for a variety of services
- confirming and recording client appointment details
- dealing with confidential information to meet with salon and legal requirements.

Salon reception duties

Scheduling appointments

It is usual for the appointments for each therapist to be recorded in a large book with either a column or a page for each. This allows the therapist to see at a glance the treatments booked in for the day and to make the appropriate preparation.

The golden rule is to have a system and make full use of it. Requests for appointments should be dealt with promptly and politely.

Filling in the appointments pages

Many salons now record their client appointments on computerised systems which in turn will be used to calculate takings and commission, regulate stock control both retail and for salon use and, if the program allows, many more functions. Salons can either buy the software program or they may rent software for keeping and managing their salon systems. Whether a computerised or manual appointment book is kept, the following details need to be taken:

- client's name
- client's contact details
- service or treatment required
- date and time of appointment
- therapist booked for service or treatment.

It would be advantageous to the client to know the estimated price of the treatment/service when booking and if a deposit has to be taken .

The receptionist also needs to know the length of the appointment she should book in order to ensure the most effective use of the therapist's time, thereby maximising the salon's productivity. She should also check with the client that she has enough time for the treatment/service to be carried out: for example, not booking an hour and a half treatment if the client only has an hour available. Time must also be allowed for:

- greeting the client and the consultation
- client undressing
- client preparation during the treatment
- client getting dressed, and being given homecare and aftercare advice.

The appointments page may look like the one on page 165.

Remember that if the salon has a system of coding, it should be used – it will make life easier. For example: C = cancellation, L = late arrival, A = client has arrived, and so on.

Some salons do not have columns for each therapist; instead they allot a workstation number or couch position and then fit the staff around the treatments that need to be completed. The advantage of this system is that the workload can easily be distributed between staff, and the manager can allot the jobs as fairly as possible. The disadvantage is that regular customers do not always get the same therapist.

Think about it

If time is not allowed for all aspects, the first treatment of the day will overrun, making the next appointment late. This can continue all day and the knock-on effect may be that the last client is kept waiting far too long. The therapist is put under pressure, the client may feel rushed and the benefits of the treatment will be lost.

Date: Tuesday 12th October 2012

	Lucy	Hellena	Anetta	Siobhan	
AM **9.00**	Mrs Khan	Mrs Hughes			**9.00** AM
9.15	full	full			9.15
9.30	Bodywax	B/Massage			9.30
9.45	0123445678	223335			9.45
10.00					**10.00**
10.15					10.15
10.30		Mrs Inder			10.30
10.45	Miss Jones	Pedicure			10.45
11.00	Aroma	+ ½ leg wax	Miss Westerby		**11.00**
11.15	Backmassage	01235 771540	French		11.15
11.30	357928		Manicure		11.30
11.45			+ facial		11.45
12.00			01329 815242	Mr. Vallete	**12.00**
	LUNCH	Mrs Green Eyetint 444321		Backmassage + pedicure 02271881570	
13.00	Mr. Walsh Manicure + backwax 02392815815	LUNCH	Miss Rudman Miss Allen X 2 eyebrows	Miss Binder waxing	
14.00	Mrs Suline Eyebrow tidy 413927	Miss Murphy Arm wax + u/arm wax	335215 LUNCH	e/b + lip & chin 07807577211	
15.00		223792	Miss Nair Bridal Top to toe 447812	Mrs Pattel Sugaring to X 2 leg 221335	
16.00	Mrs Wang Non-surg. facial lift 08729815111	Miss Woolford Basic facial + eyelash tint 445877			
17.00		Mrs Townsend M/up lesson 315579 ext. 222			

A page from an appointment book

When booking an appointment in an appointment book, it is important to do the following.

- Fill out the details in pencil. This allows alterations or cancellations without making the page illegible.
- Have an easy code to identify any potential problems.
- Make sure that everyone can easily understand start and finish times.
- Make sure that all names and numbers are clear and legible.
- Allow the hard-working therapist a break for lunch.
- Do not be pressurised by a persistent client into giving a lunchtime appointment to a therapist who has had no other break during the day. Good practice is to stagger the lunch breaks, so that there is always a therapist covering a busy lunchtime session.
- Give an appointment card to the client with all the details recorded on it so she has a record of when she has to come in. This cuts down the possibility of a missed appointment.

Think about it

Be aware of the new client and have a code to alert the therapist. This allows patch testing (if required) to be carried out as well as a full consultation if needed.

Date	Time	Treatment booked	Therapist
14.2.12	11:00am	Warm oil facial + manicure	Saskia

An appointment card

Confirming appointments

Appointment details always need to be confirmed. Names, times and services can sound similar, and confirming the details involves double checking, which may save confusion later on.

You will need to make sure that you confirm all the details with the client: 'So, Mrs Patel, just to confirm your appointment for Wednesday the 10th, at 4 pm, for a facial with Shauna – can I give you an appointment card with that on?' Look to the client and she will usually agree with you, 'Yes, that's correct, and yes, you had better put it on a card for me, thank you.' When making appointments over the phone, as with clients in the reception area, always confirm the service and the date and time of the treatment.

Many salons now send text messages to clients the day before their appointment to remind them. The text message acts as a prompt and allows the client to reschedule the appointment if necessary, therefore saving precious salon time through missed appointments and lost revenue.

If the client has just arrived for her appointment, acknowledge her presence and inform the therapist her client has arrived. If there is a slight delay, then keep the client informed, take her coat, make her a drink and give her a magazine.

If the client's treatment is personal, then you should not repeat it too loudly. Just confirm her arrival.

Procedures for taking messages

Enquiries cannot always be dealt with by the receptionist, and in these cases you should refer the enquiry to someone who can help. However, if the relevant person is not available you will need to take a message and pass this on at an appropriate time. During the course of your reception duties you will be asked to take messages for other staff members, the manager, or even a client having a treatment.

This valuable service also provides evidence for your portfolio. Make sure you get your message signed and dated by the person it should go to (and include the assessor number where appropriate) and it can go into your evidence portfolio.

It is very important to write down the whole message exactly as you heard it, even if you think it sounds odd, or it is difficult to understand.

You will need to include:

- the date and time of the call
- how important the message is — if necessary, write 'urgent' on it
- a brief description of the nature of the message
- whether the caller needs a reply — a return telephone number is then essential.

It is important to listen carefully and to ask the caller to repeat any part of the message you did not understand or hear properly. Always repeat the whole message back to the caller to make sure you have all the details correctly on the pad — especially the return number.

Passing on messages manually and electronically

Many large companies have computer systems that allow staff to email internally. Provided each person has access to a computer, and the system is set up centrally, anyone can receive a message on their computer. An address book is set up, you type in your message and send it, and it goes to the person's inbox.

Computer technology has the advantage of saving paper and allowing several people to be given the same information at once without having to write several messages. However, the drawback is that you cannot guarantee that the person you emailed will be able to open the email that day, or that they are in the office to do so.

Many salons use a system of a personal pigeonhole with the name above or below it. Messages can be left in the pigeonhole and can be collected throughout the day. A pin board for messages also works well — confidential messages can be sealed in an envelope and addressed as personal so that no one opens them by mistake.

Computer technology can also be used for booking appointments and taking payments. In addition, software programs can be installed to keep stock records and client record cards, and to print off price lists and gift vouchers. Many salons also have websites advertising the treatments that they offer, with price lists and the option for clients to make enquiries and book appointments. Websites can be built fairly easily today and there are a number of companies that design websites to meet any need and fit any budget, so even a mobile therapist may consider having a website to promote her business. There are also a number of companies available that work exclusively with therapists to help promote their business. Your professional body will have details of such companies. (Refer to Professional skills, Data

MESSAGE		
FOR	Deepak	
FROM	Mrs Alessi	
TEL NO.	0208 321 145	
TELEPHONED ☑	PLEASE RING ☑	
CALLED TO SEE YOU ☐	WILL CALL AGAIN ☐	
WANTS TO SEE YOU ☐	URGENT ☐	

MESSAGE: Needs to speak to you asap – you can call her on the tel. no. above up to 5.30pm

DATE: 10.05.12   TIME: 9.03am
RECEIVED BY: Amber

A message pad can be useful for recording messages

Think about it

Salons may also use email to let clients know of special offers by sending a monthly newsletter containing promotional information.

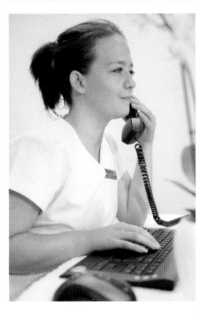

Computers can be used for booking appointments

Think about it

Urgent messages, appointment cancellations and accident or emergency messages should be given in person.

Think about it

Professionalism should be the theme running throughout your training, and integrity is a major part of professionalism. Integrity means being honest, acting with honour and being reliable and truthful in all that you do.

Think about it

If a client's health status or other sensitive or personal information is not kept private, you are breaking confidentiality. You need to be aware of, and abide by, the Data Protection Act. If you break this confidentiality, you may be subject to criminal proceedings. The Information Commissioner's office holds details of how to protect data and what is protected under the Data Protection Act and the Data Protection Registry. Clients have a right to see the information that is held by a company or organisation so care and security must be taken at all times.

Protection Act 1998, and the Data Protection Register or information on how to store and secure client data even if you do not store information on a computer database, pages 59–60.)

Regular computer training is essential so that all staff know how to access and use the information stored in a computer.

Missed appointments

Have a clear salon policy on missed appointments. Some salons make a small cancellation charge if the appointment is missed — rather like dentists or physiotherapists. This is usually in the region of £30. There is usually no cancellation fee if the appointment is cancelled with 24 hours' notice. Both staff and clients need to be clear on this policy and it could be displayed in the reception area. This is when text messages or email reminders to clients are helpful: they are less likely to forget their appointment or can rearrange if necessary.

Be flexible and be prepared to fit in the client who arrives without an appointment. The receptionist should always check first and then fit the client into a suitable slot. She should then inform the therapist, who may not be aware that another client is waiting for her.

Dealing with confidential information

It is essential to be sensitive to all confidential information. This includes the client's medical details and personal information as well as their treatment history held on record cards or electronically on the salon's computer.

A client's address, telephone number, health status/problems, medication and other personal details are all classed as confidential. You are allowed to give these details to authorised people only, such as your salon owner, manager or therapist colleagues. No persons outside the salon must have access to your clients' personal details.

Staff should also be fully trained on how to dispose of client information if a client has not attended the salon for a period of time. Different businesses may have their own rules about how long they keep client information. However, if the client details are disposed of they should be treated as confidential waste. If records are not sensitively disposed of the salon could face prosecution.

Dealing with payments

How the financial side of any business is approached is as vital as the treatment side. The client should be treated as courteously at the end of her treatment as at the beginning. Politeness is of prime importance when she is paying for her treatment.

In this outcome you will learn about:

- calculating service costs accurately
- dealing with payments for services and/or products to meet with salon policy
- following security procedures when handling payments.

Calculating costs

When it comes to totalling the costs of the services a client has received it is vital that you do this accurately. Overcharging a client could lead to a dissatisfied customer who may not choose to return and undercharging a client will lose the salon money. A client may have had multiple treatments as well as purchasing products, so it is important to check with the therapist treating them exactly what services they have had to ensure you are charging them the correct amount. You will also need to be aware of exactly what discount and special offers may be available and carry out the appropriate calculations so that this is reflected in the final amount the client is charged.

Discounts and special offers

A good way of promoting a slow-moving product, or of getting the new season off to a good start, is to offer either a discount on a service or a free service to entice clients into having the full treatment. Often supermarket promotions will be 'buy one – get one free', or you get a free small conditioner when you purchase shampoo. A salon can offer the same type of discounts: for example, at the start of summer, when everyone wants leg waxing and pedicures, a salon could offer a free bikini wax with every half-leg wax. The wax is already on, the therapist can perform the service in a short time while doing the leg wax, and the client is very happy to be receiving a free treatment! A pedicure could include a free polish – very little outlay for the salon, but again a good gift to pass on to the customer.

All these variations of costs need to be carefully put through the till, so that the stock and money add up at the end of the day. If the client has been given a free nail polish by the therapist and the receptionist tries to charge it to the client, she is not going to be very happy! The receptionist needs to know what is going on, and how to work the till to show discounts and free products.

A course of treatments often includes a free one, or payment in full for a course might offer a 10 per cent discount, so the receptionist will need to know how to work out a percentage.

How to calculate a discount

Fractions, decimals and percentages are just different ways of saying the same thing: $\frac{1}{2}$ is the same as 0.5 and 50 per cent.

These three you should know straight off without any problem:

Diagram	Fraction	Decimal	Percentage
	$\frac{1}{4}$	0.25	25%
	$\frac{1}{2}$	0.50	50%
	$\frac{3}{4}$	0.75	75%

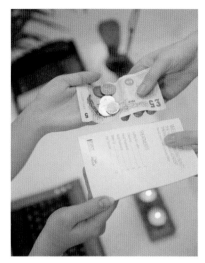

Always provide a receipt of payment

Salon reception duties

Converting fractions to decimals to percentages

For the ones you don't know, you must be able to convert them like this:

| **Fraction** e.g. $\frac{1}{5}$ | Divide using the calculator $1 \div 5$ → | **Decimal** = 0.2 | x 100 (0.2 x 100) → | **Percentage** = 20 per cent (%) |

Fraction	Decimal	Percentage:
$\frac{1}{4}$	0.25	25%

Diagram	Fraction	Decimal	Percentage
1/4	$\frac{1}{4}$	0.25	25%
1/2	$\frac{1}{2}$	0.50	50%
3/4	$\frac{3}{4}$	0.75	75%

| **Fraction** e.g. $\frac{1}{5}$ | Divide using the calculator (1/5) → | **Decimal** = 0.2 | x by 100 (0.2 x 100) → | **Percentage** 20% |

| **Fraction** e.g. $\frac{1}{8}$ | (1/8) → | **Decimal** = 0.125 | (0.125 x 100) → | **Percentage** = 12.5% |

Dealing with payments for services and/or products to meet with salon policy

Several methods of payment are available. How the client pays is very much her choice and the receptionist must be prepared and able to cope with any payment method. The client should always be told the amount politely and asked which payment method is going to be offered.

All payment methods are equally acceptable and should be handled with care. However, it will be up to the individual salon to state which payment methods it wishes to accept. Salons often have a sign in the reception area and on their price lists stating the payment methods that are accepted. Clients who phone with an enquiry or to make an appointment should be told of the methods of payment that are available to them. Many salons now require their staff to have a pin number or log in that needs to be entered each time they complete a transaction. This is not only for security but can be a valuable tool for a salon manager when working out commission for the therapist.

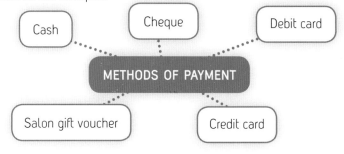

Cash

When a customer is paying cash (a rarity these days), there are several aspects to be aware of. A large denomination bank note, that is £20 or £50, should be checked to ensure it is genuine and not counterfeit.

- Look for the watermark — every note has a watermark that can be seen when the note is held up to the light.
- Look for the metallic strip which is woven into the paper — it should be unbroken.
- Compare the feel of the bank note paper — often a forged note is not printed on the same quality paper and may have a thin feel.
- Often the police circulate a list of forged note numbers to be on the lookout for. The numbers are on a stop list and this list should be kept near the till, so that numbers can be compared.

At the end of the day's business the till must be totalled and the takings matched against the recorded amount taken, either through the till roll or a docket system. If a float has been used to provide small change at the beginning of the day, then it needs to be deducted from the total takings. This can then be used for the next day's trading. The balance of the takings should be paid into the salon bank account. Most large banks offer a night safe facility, where the takings can be deposited. It is not ideal to keep large amounts of money and cheques on the premises overnight — there is always the risk of a burglary.

If there is a problem with a bank note, it will normally be because the client has accepted this money from another source, and the authorities should be notified. It is important that the note is removed from circulation and the police are informed. Ask the client quietly to step into the office away from reception to avoid embarrassment. Ask the supervisor, manager or owner to deal with the situation. The receptionist can then return to her duties at the front desk.

Even when accepting money from very regular customers, you should still check it thoroughly. Dealing with cash involves a lot of responsibility, and care must be taken to avoid errors.

Procedure for handling cash payments

Place the client's money on the till ledge to ensure you remember the amount given to you. Do not place the money straight in the till drawer as this may lead to confusion — was it a £10 or a £20 note? Count the change required from the note, and then re-count it into the client's hand. Place the client's money in the till drawer and close it. Give the client the receipt to confirm the cost of the treatment, how much was given to you, and the change you gave.

Cheques

A cheque is no more than an instruction to the bank telling it to pay a specific sum to a specified person. Most banks and building societies offer a cheque service, although a debit card service is also available (see page 173). Many stores and salons now refuse to take cheques as a form of payment and it is up to the discretion of each individual whether or not these are accepted as a form of payment. If a salon decides it does not take cheques as a form of payment a notice should be prominently placed on reception and the receptionist should tell all clients who book over the telephone. This will save embarrassment

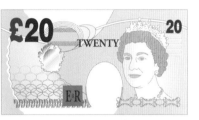

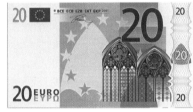

Large denomination bank notes should be checked carefully

Think about it

It is important not to feel embarrassed when checking money; it will protect the salon and the customer.

Is the name of the salon correct?

Is the amount of money in words and figures correct?

NEW BANK
TOWN BRANCH
WEST COUNTRY GROUP
P O BOX 64, ANYTOWN OS5 2GD

30 – 27 –54
46055239

Date 11th April '12

Pay **Village Gossip**   Only

Twenty pounds only ———— £20 ——

A. N. OTHER

" 203064" 30··96823·" 402229521·03

Is the date correct?

Does the signature on the cheque match the signature on the guarantee card?

Look carefully at all these items on a cheque

Think about it

Payments for all treatments need to be acknowledged by a handwritten or a till receipt, regardless of the method of payment.

Think about it

If a cheque is faulty in any way, the bank will reject it and return it to the salon. It is up to the salon to contact the customer and inform her of the fault. The customer will then need to call into the salon and alter and initial any necessary changes. It may be wise to rewrite the cheque altogether. So it is much easier to get it right first time.

A number of businesses have recently stopped accepting cheques as a form of payment, favouring the use of debit cards. If your salon has decided not to accept cheques as a form of payment, you should advertise the fact in the salon and on price lists. This will prevent potential embarrassment if the client does not have another method of payment.

A cheque payment is acceptable to a salon, providing certain checks and precautions are carried out. Always check that:

- the date is correct (day, month and year), especially important around New Year
- the name of the salon is spelt correctly – the client could be offered a stamp with the full name pre-printed on it
- the amount of money is correct, and is in words as well as numbers
- the signature is completed correctly and matches the signature on the cheque guarantee card.

Most banks do not now issue cheque guarantee cards but the signature strip on the debit card can be used to clarify the signature with that written on the cheque. With the demise of the cheque guarantee card a salon will not be able to claim money back from the bank as they used to if there is insufficient funds in the bank account.

If your salon still accepts cheques as a form of payment always check the expiry date on the card, written as 03/12 for example, for the month and year the card needs to be reissued. Also check that the signatures match and the card type is the same as the cheque; that is, both are issued by the same bank. The cheque is then treated exactly like cash and put into the till. A receipt is given and the till is closed.

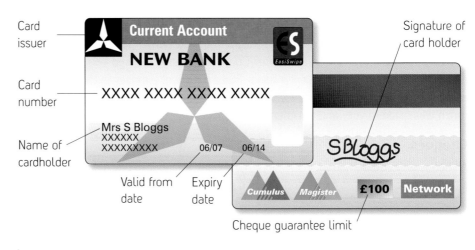

Card issuer

Card number

Name of cardholder

Signature of card holder

Current Account

NEW BANK

XXXX XXXX XXXX XXXX

Mrs S Bloggs
XXXXXX
XXXXXXXXX

06/07   06/14

Valid from date

Expiry date

S Bloggs

Cumulus   Magister   £100   Network

Cheque guarantee limit

A cheque guarantee card

Credit cards

Credit cards are often referred to as 'plastic money'. Credit card companies offer credit cards to those customers they consider creditworthy.

How credit cards work

If your salon has a contract with a credit card company, it will usually display a sign stating that credit cards are accepted. Most salons use the chip and pin linked to their computerised till for credit or debit card transactions (see below). If the amount is large, the chip and pin facility will check to see if the client has enough credit before the payment is authorised.

Debit cards

All banks now offer the convenience of a debit card. In a number of businesses these have taken the place of both cheques and cash transactions. The payment is made electronically by transferring money straight from the customer's bank account to the salon's account.

Debit cards are usually the same as the cheque guarantee card, should the customer wish to write a cheque.

The card is inserted into a chip and pin machine and the amount is entered by the receptionist taking the payment. The customer then enters their unique pin number and electronic authorisation is given by the bank. The customer is given a copy of the receipt and the business has a duplicate, which is used when calculating the takings at the end of the day. When using a credit or debit card where the client inserts a pin number the receptionist should always avert their eyes and give the customer privacy when they enter their pin number. In the same instance other customers should leave a polite distance when payment is being taken.

The salon may impose a minimum spend on debit or credit cards as the business has to pay for every transaction by this method of payment either to the bank or credit card company. This is usually 1.5–2 per cent of the transaction. In some cases, this is passed on to the customer by the business, but salons do not normally charge the client for using a debit card.

Cash equivalents and pre-paid cards

Salon gift vouchers

Bliss Salon

This voucher is for the value of £20

Redeemable against any treatment

Valid until September 2012

> **Think about it**
>
> Be careful with credit and debit cards. All the information is stored in the chip and this can sometimes become damaged and the information destroyed.

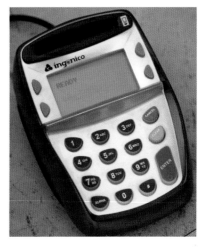

A chip and pin machine

A salon gift voucher

A gift voucher is a good alternative to giving someone cash as a present. As the name suggests, it is a voucher to the value of a set sum of money. The voucher usually includes a card with the salon details on it. The amount of money to be exchanged will also be prominently displayed. When the lucky person who has received a gift voucher presents it to the salon, the receptionist will treat it exactly the same as a cash transaction. For security, the vouchers have serial numbers to avoid duplication or reuse. This makes them easier to track.

When the voucher goes into the till, it should be kept in a separate compartment from the notes. The receptionist or therapist should put a line through it and give her initials to state that it has been used.

Pre-paid cards

There are new advances in technology that could make plastic cards obsolete within the next few years. Manufacturers in phone technology have designed a phone that thinks it's a credit card! It works by sending bank details – which are now contained in the chip on your credit or debit card – in an infrared beam from the phone to the till. After purchases are scanned at the checkout as normal, the customer selects the 'banking' menu on his or her phone, chooses the payment function and enters a personal four-digit pin code into the keypad. Pushing the 'send' key beams the information into a receiving unit in the till. This passes the information to the account to be debited, in much the same way as completing a normal chip and pin transaction. As with the chip and pin debit/credit card, no signature is required. Some salons have now adopted this increasingly popular payment method. It is hoped that fraud and stolen cards will be a thing of the past, as the process is so easy to manage.

Loyalty cards

Many salons now offer their clients a loyalty card that is stamped at each visit. This offers the clients an incentive to return to the salon. The reward is at the discretion of the salon but is usually given when the client has collected the allocated stamps on a card. Reduced price treatments or products are often given which encourages the clients to return to the salon.

Invalid payments

Unfortunately, there may be times when payment discrepancies and disputes arise. They should be dealt with calmly, without causing embarrassment to the client. If you are unable to resolve the dispute refer to a senior staff member, salon manager or owner.

Possible problems may include the following.

- Invalid currency is presented – perhaps a foreign note or even a forged note. Many salons check large denomination notes with a special pen to detect if the note is a forgery.
- An invalid card is presented – it may be out of date, or not match the cheque details.
- A cheque is filled out incorrectly, or does not have a current cheque guarantee card.
- The client has entered the incorrect pin for their card.
- Fraudulent use of a payment card is suspected – perhaps it has been put on to the stop list.

How the till works

Tills come in all shapes and sizes and vary in their functions, depending upon their age and what they are required to do. Scanning tills are automated to pick up a bar code on goods and products. The bar code includes the price and the stock levels, making reordering and analysis of sales easy. The operator has little work to do except for clearing the till when mistakes occur and loading the till roll.

Supermarket tills have a discount system built into the software. The scanner picks up the price and then automatically takes off the appropriate discount. Any till receipt will show the deductions at the end. Some larger salon chains now offer a discount or loyalty service that is often used during promotions to entice clientele.

Smaller salon tills do not often have a scanner facility. Discounts should be done manually and clearly marked on the receipt with the therapist's or receptionist's initials to verify the date and amount.

Manual tills have an adding-on button, usually a + sign, so that items that are listed separately can be added up for a final total. The whole front button panel looks a little like a calculator and includes a percentage button and a subtotal button. Staff till training should be available for all, with regular updates as the technology changes. It is important to ensure the bill is accurately totalled, before confirming the price with the client and accepting the payment.

Dealing with damaged goods

When finalising a transaction with a client, it is good practice to check products for faults, damage or leaks. It is both disappointing and inconvenient if a product has to be returned. (Refer also to the Sale and Supply of Goods Act in Professional skills, page 58.)

Often clients do not mind if a box is slightly damaged as long as the quality of the goods inside is still perfect. Do not try to sneak the purchase into the bag without telling the client – it looks as though you have something to hide. Point out the damage and explain to the client that it will not affect the goods. Providing it is within your authority to offer a discount, offer to reduce the item if the client is unhappy. If you cannot give deductions, you must ask the manager and obtain a signature on the till receipt.

If the goods themselves are damaged or leaking, they should be replaced. It can be frustrating if the product is the last one in stock and the client really wishes to purchase it. Again, some form of discount could be suggested, but details must be written on the till receipt to avoid the goods being brought back for a full refund.

All stock should be checked when unpacking the bulk purchase from the salon supplier, as the damage may have been caused in transit and not be the salon's fault. If you sign for a parcel and do not check it before the delivery person leaves, then it is unlikely your supplier will accept responsibility for the damage. If the stock arrives damaged and you have checked it and discovered the damage, you can send it back.

If stock has been around a long time and the packaging is not as good as new, then the solution is often to have a bargain basket. Prices are reduced and the goods put in a basket on display. Do be careful, though, that the basket is not left unattended as items are liable to be stolen. Damaged stock that is reduced in price will have to be written off against profits, so try to keep accidental damage to a minimum.

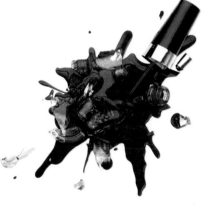

Accidents can happen and goods can be damaged or broken

Salon reception duties

Money matters – a float

At the end of the day's business, the takings in the till must be totalled and matched up with the recorded sales and treatment dockets. A set amount of money is put into the till every morning, called a float, to provide change for clients paying in cash. It is usual to count out the float and replace it in the till for the next day's trading.

A typical float would consist of a mixture of change (for example):

- 2 × £10 notes
- 4 × £5 notes
- £30 in £1 coins
- £10 in 50p coins
- £5 in 20p coins
- £5 in 10p coins
- £1 in 5p coins
- £1 in 2p and 1p coins.

This will, of course, depend upon the size of the salon, how busy it is, and how many people pay in cash. Most transactions are carried out by debit or credit cards – very few small businesses handle a lot of cash unless the cost of goods is small, such as in a greengrocer's shop.

Following security procedures

Security in the reception area is important, both for stock and for the till itself. Never leave the till drawer open when leaving the area, or leave it with the key in for easy access – unfortunately not everyone is honest. Presenting a thief with an open till will invalidate an insurance claim, as adequate measures were not in place. When cashing up two members of staff should be present to ensure staff safety.

Some salons have a wall or floor safe to keep the takings in and store the daily float money. The takings need to be banked frequently, but avoid taking them to the bank at the same time every day. This may make you a target for a thief, who may be watching your movements. Most banks offer a night safe facility, where takings can be deposited. Again, be safe, do not go on your own, and do not go at the same time every day.

Larger salons employ security firms to collect the moneyboxes from the salon and deliver them to the bank. Security guards have special headwear, eye goggles and often body suits to protect them against attack.

For your portfolio

1 Check the amount of float your salon keeps.

2 Count your takings at the end of the day. How much money have you taken? Remember to deduct the float.

3 How much have you taken in debit and credit card payments?

4 How many gift vouchers or pre-paid cards have you taken?

5 How many products have you sold?

6 Does the salon have a loyalty card scheme?

Check your knowledge

1 List five things you could do to help keep the reception area tidy.

2 Why would it be important to check emails first thing in the morning?

3 Name two benefits of text reminders for the salon?

4 List six items of stationery that are essential for the receptionist.

5 What are the two types of displays of products most commonly used?

6 What does client hospitality mean?

7 Which Act of Parliament do you need to uphold when storing clients' details on a computer?

8 What would you do if you knew the client was going to be kept waiting?

9 What do you need in order to use email?

10 What will happen if you do not know how long a treatment takes and you are booking a client in?

11 List four other functions that a computer can provide to the receptionist other than storing appointments.

12 What is your salon policy on missed appointments?

13 What is the gift voucher or pre-paid card the same as?

14 How does a credit card work?

15 Your salon usually charges £17.50 for a facial. It is currently running a seasonal promotion offering a 10 per cent discount on facial treatments. How much is the discount and what is the new price of the treatment?

16 What is the purpose of a loyalty card?

17 How many people should cash up at the end of the day?

18 Which organisation gives recommendations for salon service timings?

Salon reception duties

Getting ready for assessment

There are no service times for completion of this unit and how much time you spend in the reception role will depend on the size of your establishment. However, the role must be undertaken on at least three occasions. You will be required to show that you can:

- carry out reception duties
- book appointments
- deal with payments.

You will also be required to sit an exam and if some evidence does not naturally occur the assessor may ask oral questions or require written work to be completed so all outcomes and ranges are covered.

The evidence for this unit is quite straightforward. The best way of covering all the ranges is to spend a set time at the reception desk at your place of training. Ideally, a rota of students with no experience can be drawn up and matched with experienced students, who will pass on the skills needed to greet clients, make appointments and tend to all reception duties. An assessor can then observe your activities, and very quickly a portfolio of ranges start to develop.

Even though a new student will have little experience of booking appointments and handling payments, a day spent observing others and being guided through the process is the only way to learn these new skills.

An assessor will expect you to be professionally presented, polite and courteous, with open body language and good interpersonal skills. Those qualities are far more important than getting the till operation correct at the first attempt. Think of it like taking a driving test – stalling the engine is not the end of the world as long as the correct procedures are followed. Seeking clarification from a more senior staff member, or asking for help if you think the problem is outside your own authority, will not mean you are considered incompetent – rather it shows you are mature enough to seek help and you have an understanding of your own personal limitations (which is actually a range you need to cover).

- Keep a diary of events, problems sorted, and how you dealt with situations such as an angry customer or a disabled client. Get it signed by the senior reception staff or your assessor at the end of the day.

- Be as helpful as you can and volunteer for any extra duties – they may cover a range you are unable to cover in the normal course of the day. For example, escorting a client on a conducted tour of the facilities may be classed as handling a confused client if she is unsure of prices, what the treatment consists of, or even how to find her way to the toilet!

- If you help on the reception desk in your place of work, then an employer's letter can be invaluable as evidence. It may not be in a beauty salon, but could be anywhere where you deal with members of the public, take payments and use a till, book clients in for hair appointments or doctor's appointments, or deal with telephone enquiries. The employer's letter should clearly outline your duties in as much detail as possible and be dated and signed.

Section

3

Anatomy, physiology and the skin

You and the skin

What you will learn

- How skin type and colour is determined
- Impact of environment and lifestyle on the skin
- The pH of skin and desquamation
- How to recognise skin types and conditions
- Skin characteristics and skin types of different ethnic groups
- The photosensitivity of skin
- Tools for diagnosing skin types and conditions
- Face shapes and contours
- Contra-indications to facial treatments
- Other skin conditions – pigmentation disorders
- Allergic reactions and sensitivity testing
- Male skin
- Factors affecting the skin-ageing process
- The skin and the sun

You and the skin

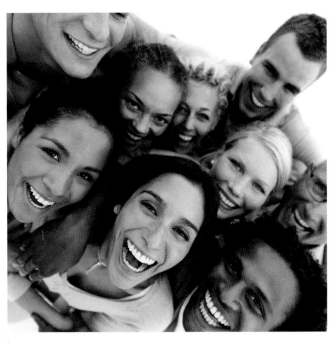

Everyone's skin is different – all clients have individual needs

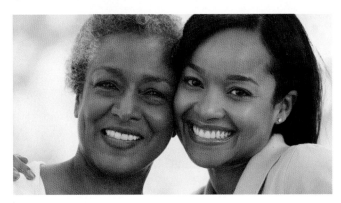

We inherit our skin and colouring characteristics from our parents

Introduction

This section looks at all aspects of the skin, which is a continuing theme throughout each unit you are assessed upon. For information on the anatomy of the skin, refer to Related anatomy and physiology on pages 235–41.

The skin is a core subject for *all* beauty therapists to understand regardless of the qualifications you are taking – and not just for completing your assessments but so that you have the knowledge to offer your clients the most suitable treatment programme for their individual needs.

Knowing how to treat the skin (and hair and nails) is essential for all the practical units, both for Level 2 and when you progress on to further treatments within Level 3. These include face and body treatments using mechanical or electrical equipment along with manual massage techniques.

A full knowledge of how the skin behaves, how it grows and what its problems or reactions may be will enable you to make sound judgements when diagnosing skin types, planning treatments and product use, and recognising any potential skin problems that would prevent the treatment from taking place at all (this is called a contra-indication to treatment).

Try this quick quiz:

- What is the largest organ of the body?
- What is the waterproof covering for the body, stopping water getting in or out?
- What makes vitamin D in the presence of sunlight?
- What protects the body from harmful ultraviolet (UV) rays?
- What makes up the majority of the contents of a vacuum cleaner?
- What helps regulate body temperature?
- What is dead and yet grows continuously?
- What is found on the body that is thin, thick and has lots of layers?
- What has a surface area of up to 6 square metres?
- What do you lose up to 20 kilograms of in a lifetime?
- What stops poisonous chemicals and germs from entering your body?
- What contains sense organs that help us detect changes in our environment?

The answer to all these questions is the skin. This illustrates how amazing, hard working and versatile the skin is – and yet most of us take it for granted until it goes wrong!

How skin type and colour is determined

The type, condition and **ethnicity** of your skin are determined both genetically and environmentally. While the ethnicity of your skin is clearly inherited, your skin type may also be inherited to some extent. However, both skin type and condition can be hugely influenced by how the skin is treated, the products that are used, external conditions and lifestyle choices.

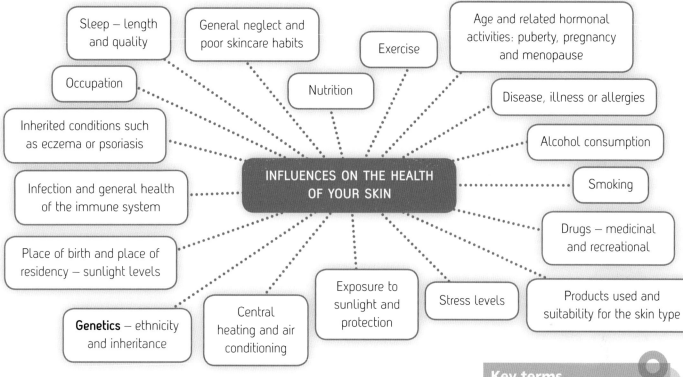

Sleep – length and quality

General neglect and poor skincare habits

Exercise

Age and related hormonal activities: puberty, pregnancy and menopause

Occupation

Nutrition

Disease, illness or allergies

Inherited conditions such as eczema or psoriasis

Alcohol consumption

Infection and general health of the immune system

INFLUENCES ON THE HEALTH OF YOUR SKIN

Smoking

Drugs – medicinal and recreational

Place of birth and place of residency – sunlight levels

Exposure to sunlight and protection

Stress levels

Products used and suitability for the skin type

Genetics – ethnicity and inheritance

Central heating and air conditioning

Influences on the health of your skin

Genetics

We are all a product of our parents and we inherit all our characteristics from our families, either directly through our mother and father, or indirectly from our grandparents and sometimes further back in the family.

Every newborn baby's cells contain an inbuilt programme for its future development and growth, a set of instructions that are predetermined. In normal, healthy babies, the instructions will be the same and will make up a basic recipe for a human being. All the organs will be in the right place and working well, and, depending upon the sex of the baby, the outer appearance will be the same for us all, and reflect our family background and ethnic origins.

You and the skin

Key terms

Ethnicity – relating to a group of people who have a number of factors in common, e.g. race, culture, religion, language.

Genetics – the study of genes, the hereditary units that we receive from our parents, e.g. blood group, eye colour, height, skin colour.

DNA – deoxyribonucleic acid; a very important molecule that contains our genes. DNA is present in the nucleus of all living cells.

Variation within humans is the result of two major influences:

- the genes you inherit from your parents
- the environment in which you live.

For your portfolio

Look at your family tree and ask your parents or grandparents about eye and hair colouring within the family. Are there any surprises that you were not aware of, such as ginger hair or taller relatives? How has your family background influenced your colouring? Where does your colouring come from? Write a short overview on your skin type and genetic influences.

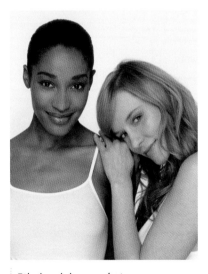

Ethnic origins vary between the Northern and Southern hemispheres

These instructions are found within an individual's **DNA**: an arrangement of codes that will produce an individual set of features. These are often called units of inheritance. They determine hair colour, eye colour, skin colouring and so on. It is so individual to each human being that forensic scientists are able to match DNA from tissue or hair found at a crime scene with the criminal. It is therefore a powerful tool to help fight crime. A DNA sample can be taken from the inside of the cheek lining using a sterile swab, its contents determined and the results stored on a computer.

How are the instructions in genes used? A simple way to visualise this is to think of a gene as carrying a set of instructions for the manufacture of an enzyme. This enzyme can be the difference between a characteristic being present or not: for example, if you have brown eyes, it is because you have the enzyme that helps in the production of the brown pigment. This enzyme can only be made if you have this gene.

Genes contain a mixture of influences from both parents. For example, a child may inherit the curly hair and dark colouring of its mother, and grow to be tall like its father. There may also be an inherited gene from a grandparent, perhaps if both the parents are blond but have a child with ginger or red hair. The genes of the grandparents may have influenced the colouring, as neither parent had a predominant red hair colour.

You can change your hair colour, or darken your skin through tanning or artificial colouring, but to begin with, like it or not, you are made up of your parents' genes! You cannot pass on something that is not natural, such as a bottled hair colour, to your children.

The environment and genetics

There are more than seven billion people on earth; we are all different, with different height, weight, shape, skin colour, eye colour and so on. To ensure survival of the human race, we have adapted as we have evolved, depending upon where on the earth we were born.

This shows within different ethnic origins. The darker the skin and eye colour, the more protection is given against the sun's rays. Those living nearest to the equator (the middle band around the earth, which is closest to the sun) have a darker skin and eye colour as the sun's rays are at their most intense.

Throughout history, nations have invaded one another. This has influenced the gene pool and therefore the skin types of people on the different continents. Immigration has also had an effect. Immigrants who settle in foreign countries and marry the people of their adopted country produce children of mixed race. If you were to look at your own family history, you may find your ancestors came from another country and your genetic inheritance comes from many different countries.

Impact of environment and lifestyle on the skin

Both the environment in which you live and your lifestyle contribute to the health of your skin.

Nutrition

Good health and therefore a healthy skin begin with good nutrition – the fuel that our bodies need to replace cells, maintain growth and repair and hydrate the skin. A variety of foods will provide the essential vitamins and minerals required to keep the body working at its optimum level. Getting vitamins from a variety of foods, rather than in pill form, means our bodies also receive fibre which helps the bowel to process waste products, and antioxidants, which are essential in the fight against **free radicals**. The body cannot overdose on vitamins and minerals found in food no matter how much we have, whereas too many vitamin pills can cause dangerously high levels of minerals that the liver then has to try to break down.

Growth and repair

In order to maintain healthy growth and repair of tissues, to keep hair and skin healthy and muscles working, to renew blood cells and improve brain function, doctors recommend a minimum of one gram of protein per day for every two pounds of a person's body weight. So, if a person weighs ten stone and is fairly healthy and active, they should be consuming about 70 grams of protein a day to keep cells healthy and able to repair themselves. This can be a problem for anyone on a very restrictive diet, e.g. a vegetarian or who doesn't eat very nutritious meals. Constant skin infections or poor repair of skin is a sign of general ill health and may indicate that a client is not getting enough protein in the diet.

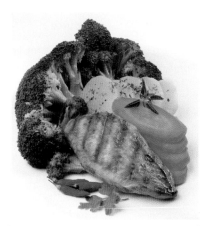

A variety of foods will ensure a healthy vitamin intake and a balanced diet

Key terms

Free radicals – highly reactive chemicals that attack molecules by capturing electrons and thereby change a cell's chemical structure. Environmental factors such as pollution, UVA rays, smoking and pesticides may cause free radical damage if production becomes excessive. Damage occurs and accumulates with age.

Nutrient	Source	Why needed
Protein	Red and white meat, dairy products, pulses and lentils, seeds and nuts	Maintains and supports body growth Essential for respiration of skin cells
Iron	Red meat, liver, egg yolk, pulses, dried fruits, e.g. apricots, raisins	With protein, forms haemoglobin to carry oxygen through the body With vitamin C taken at the same time, helps absorption Tannin and antacid medication limit absorption Deficiency causes anaemia resulting in fatigue Essential for oxygen levels in the skin
Calcium	Dairy products, whole fish (sardines), sunflower and sesame seeds	With other minerals and vitamin D, helps strengthen teeth and bones
Vitamin A (retinol)	Carrots, margarine, fortified dairy products, liver, green vegetables	Important to health of mucous membranes and resistance to infection Antioxidant essential for renewal and growth of new skin cells If applied in cream form on the skin, it can help stimulate collagen production

You and the skin

Nutrient	Source	Why needed
Vitamin B1 (thiamine)	Wheat germ, liver, whole grains, nuts, offal	Aids digestion and utilisation of energy Increases fatty acids in the skin – providing firmness to the skin and aids natural exfoliation
Vitamin B2 (riboflavin)	Milk, yoghurt, cottage cheese, liver, whole grains, green vegetables	Promotes healthy skin and eyes
Vitamin B3 (niacin)	Oily fish, whole grains, liver, fortified breakfast cereals, peanuts	Aids digestion and normal appetite needs Promotes fatty acid production
Vitamin B6 (pyridoxine)	Meat, bananas, dried vegetables, molasses, brewer's yeast, whole grains	Helps to regulate the use of fatty acids to fight infection
Vitamin B12 (cyanocobalamin)	Milk, eggs, meat, dairy products	Essential for the maintenance of red blood cells and nervous system (No vegetable source sufficient for daily needs. Vegans should see their doctor about synthetic forms)
Folic acid (folacin)	Green leafy vegetables, nuts, dried vegetables, whole grains	Essential for blood formation, therefore bringing oxygen and nutrients to the skin Vital during pregnancy to prevent possible defects in babies
Vitamin C (ascorbic acid)	Most citrus fruits (including oranges), red, green and yellow vegetables, e.g. tomatoes, peppers and broccoli	Increases resistance to infection, blood coagulation and iron absorption More required during illness Building block for collagen – the protein which provides the skin with structure, tone and elasticity
Vitamin D	Fortified milk and other dairy products, oily fish, liver, eggs, butter, salmon Sunshine on skin	Helps body to absorb calcium Calcium and phosphorus strengthen bones Essential for development of skin cells
Vitamin E	Vegetable oil, green leafy vegetables, wheat germ, egg yolk, whole grains	Protects fatty acids from being destroyed Antioxidant which helps to build and maintain good skin cells
Phosphorus	Milk products, meat, fish, whole grains, beans	Combines with calcium to strengthen bones and teeth
Iodine	Seafood, fortified salt	Regulates energy use in the body
Zinc	Lean meat, seafood, whole grains and dried beans	Makes up some enzymes and releases vitamin A from liver
Fat – unsaturated (often classed as 'good' fats)	Unsaturated fat found in olive oil, avocadoes, fish oils with omega-3 and seeds, brazil nuts	Provides supple skin, shiny hair and softness to all the tissues

Water

Our bodies are made up of 80 per cent water, and each cell needs water to function. Water also helps blood to flow around the body. Blood should flow through the veins and arteries like skimmed milk, but with low water content it becomes thick like clotted cream, which doesn't flow well at all. Besides drinking eight to ten glasses, approximately two litres a day, water can also be found in food with high water content such as melons, fruit and soups. Drinks that include alcohol and caffeine act as a diuretic, which means they remove water and really make a big difference to the hydration levels of the skin.

Skin dehydration is associated with clients who:

- do not drink enough water to replenish natural loss
- do not use the correct products to maintain the skin's acid mantle, so water is evaporated through the skin
- follow a completely fat-free diet, so are deficient in essential fatty acids
- work in a dry atmosphere, which also encourages water loss
- have a high alcohol intake, which is a factor in dehydration.

Think about it

You are what you eat – how true! Nutrition is the body's fuel, so feed it well for best performance. You would not put low grade fuel into a Ferrari and expect it to work really well, and the same applies to the body.

Sleep

Sleep is essential to the body for repair of tissue and for growth – even though adults have stopped growing in height, cells and tissues need to repair and regenerate. Lack of sleep causes all the body functions to slow down, and both mental and physical function is impaired. You are also more likely to become run down, pick up infections and generally feel low, all of which is reflected in the skin. The very young need regular bouts of sleep to help the body grow and the brain to function. Learning to walk, talk and process all of life's knowledge is very tiring on the body; children can get very irritable if they do not get enough sleep. As we age, we may need less sleep. This varies for each individual but six or seven hours per night is still essential.

Exercise

The body needs regular exercise, which increases the heart rate and gives the lungs a good workout (cardiovascular exercise). This is good for the whole body and stimulates the blood flow, which shows up in the skin. The immune system is strengthened, stress levels are reduced, and the heart functions better. General well-being is evident in a healthy, glowing skin. Walking, running and swimming are all good energy-boosting activities. Encourage your client to fit exercise into their lifestyle two or three times a week – and do some yourself and see how well you feel, with higher energy levels and the ability to cope better with your studies.

Smoking

The health risks associated with smoking are well publicised. Smoking is banned, by law, in public places, which means that the risk of passive smoking – inhaling other people's cigarette smoke – has been reduced (refer to legislation in Professional skills, pages 50–51).

Exercise will increase blood flow and give the body a boost of feel-good hormones, too, as endorphins are released

You and the skin

Smoking not only diminishes the lungs' capacity to function well, it also affects the oxygen levels in the blood stream, showing up as a sallow, dull complexion. Smokers are depriving the skin of oxygen and their skin may be prone to line more easily and age prematurely.

Nicotine, the principal alkaloid in tobacco, impairs the circulation, slowing down the progress of nutrients and oxygen in the blood stream and the removal of waste products from the cells. Skin may look pale yellow and grey, lose its elasticity and become wrinkled, over time. Smokers also find that fingers and eyebrows become stained with a build-up of nicotine if the cigarettes are untipped and rolled without a filter. Not a good look for the skin!

Alcohol

Sustained alcohol intake can have an adverse effect on the skin as alcohol stops the absorption of essential vitamins by the body, as well as providing 'empty' calories with no nutritional goodness. This may lead to weight gain, which puts extra pressure on the skin. Alcohol can act as an appetite suppressant, and a poor diet can cause malnutrition in the long term.

There is also an allergic potential to alcohol, as it contains both salicylates and yeast, which can cause the skin to break out in hives and rashes. Yeast also feeds conditions such as thrush, irritable bowel syndrome and general irritability in the nerve endings in the skin.

Stress

We all need a little stress in our lives to function fully and get our adrenalin flowing. However, long-term and sustained stress on the body can cause ill health, mental function impairment and hormonal fluctuations, which show up in the skin. Adult acne and poor skin maintenance can be the result of long-term stress.

It is important for your client to deal with the underlying causes of anxiety and stress and manage it – and take care of the body to allow it to function properly. Exercise is a good stress buster and good nutrition is essential when the body is under stress. Regular beauty treatments are very therapeutic and regular massage will help with relaxation and improve skin function, as well as encouraging the client to maintain the skin with good product advice.

Hormones

Hormones are slow-acting chemical messengers which control many of the body's functions including growth, metabolism, sexual development and coordination.

The human body is very much dictated by its hormones. Hormones are released into the bloodstream and act on the organs of the body to produce the correct level of hormones for a given situation, for example the hormone adrenaline is released when we feel under attack. It also dictates our gender: testosterone makes males predominantly masculine and oestrogen makes women feminine. Hormone production happens throughout our life but the key changes as we increase in age are outlined below.

◉ Puberty begins in the teenage years when the body is starting to prepare for adulthood. This causes significant changes in body shape, skin condition and aids the development of sexual characteristics. The skin reacts to this surge of hormonal activity and acne can develop in both boys and girls during this phase. Skin that was generally blemish free and well behaved suddenly develops spots, comedones and sometimes infections, with a tendency to flush easily. Male teenage skin is particularly prone to acne as testosterone plays a part in regulating sebum production. Male voices drop in tone, hair develops on the body and emotions can be erratic. Females develop breasts and begin their periods. In addition they may experience changes to skin and hair. Teenagers need more sleep than in previous years and can expect an increase in the speed at which they grow.

◉ Reproduction – in females monthly hormone cycles and resulting periods can have an effect on the condition of the skin, with alterations in hydration and sensitivity to blemishes and breakouts. In addition the body tends to retain more fluid around the peak of ovulation. In pregnancy, hormonal changes may affect the pigmentation of the skin and darker patches, called chloasma, may appear. These are commonly found along the hairline and on the neck or hands. However, not all pregnant women have skin problems – some gain a glow when skin is at its peak, and problems suffered before pregnancy may disappear.

◉ Menopause – this is when the reproductive cycle comes to an end, generally over a three or four year span in a female's fifties, or earlier if the woman has an early menopause caused by a hormonal disturbance of some kind (often through illness). Periods cease and oestrogen levels drop as the body is no longer trying to become pregnant. This may often bring skin problems and dryness and it can also affect the development of new healthy bone cells – density is diminished and osteoporosis is possible. Hot flushes, a rise in body temperature and mental faculties are often affected: some women may lose things, become accident prone, forget things and claim to feel 'woolly headed'. This is all due to hormonal fluctuation. The production of collagen, an elastic which supports the skin's structure, also slows down and lines and fine wrinkles appear at this time. Hormone replacement therapy (HRT) may be prescribed by a doctor to help alleviate the symptoms and good nutrition is essential. Soya proteins and plants containing natural oestrogens may help. Weight gain is probable at this time of life, too.

◉ Although men don't have a menopause, their bodies also change later in life. Hair loss and classic male pattern baldness may occur – with hair diminishing on the crown and hairline but hairs sprouting in the ears and nose. Exercise can drop off and weight gain is probable giving the male paunch or 'beer belly' appearance. Again good nutrition is vital at this stage of life to ensure growth and repair takes place.

In conclusion, therapists who treat mainly female clients will need to think about their client's age and their stage of hormone production – namely puberty, pregnancy and the menopause. All fluctuation of hormone production during these key times will affect the skin. However, this may be in a positive, not necessarily negative, way. It is important to remember, however, that it is not just the female sex hormones which affect the skin, or that just female clients are affected by hormonal changes. The pancreas, the pituitary gland and the adrenal glands all produce hormones – as do our fat deposits – and any imbalance of hormone production can cause disease or disturbance to the body.

Free radicals

Free radicals or oxidants are a big factor in the ageing of the skin. They are harmful chemicals which can accumulate in the tissues. They are generated in the body as a reaction to aggressive environmental influences such as sunlight, petrol fumes, chemicals, smoking, wind and pollution, and to internal factors such as stress and tiredness. A consequence of this attack on the skin is an acceleration of the skin's ageing process, with the loss of radiance, elasticity and tone. Free radicals are controlled by enzymes, but should the production of the enzymes slow down, due to a poor lifestyle, lack of sufficient nutrition and so on, then there is a build-up of chemicals and toxins within the tissues.

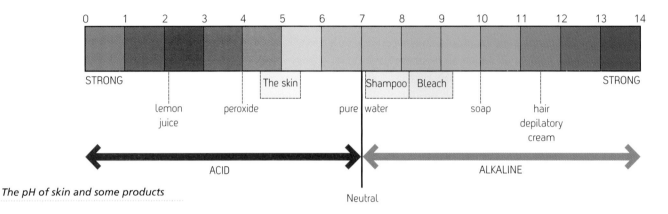

The pH of skin and some products

The pH of skin and desquamation

The pH of skin

pH stands for potential hydrogen or – if it is easier to remember – parts hydrogen, of any product. It is a number that describes whether a substance or solution is acid, neutral or alkaline. A pH of 7 is neutral, 0–7 indicates acidity and 7+ indicates alkalinity. Chemicals applied to the skin should have a pH that is neither too high nor too low to avoid skin irritation.

The acid mantle

The skin acts as a barrier against infection; this is known as the **acid mantle** because normal, healthy skin has an acidic pH between 4.5 and 5.5. The acid mantle is made up of a delicate mixture of sebum and moisture content on the skin – dermatologists refer to it as the hydrolipidic balance (hydro = water; lipid = fat). It helps to inhibit the growth of bacteria.

Fungi are controlled by sebum, which inhibits their growth. So it makes sense to maintain a steady pH balance in the skin to help fight off infection. Using products that are too harsh will strip the skin of its protective pH acid mantle and this will allow infections in and cause damage.

Key terms

pH – potential hydrogen. This is the degree of alkalinity and acidity measured on the pH scale of 1–14, where 1 is a strong acid, 7 is neutral and 14 is a strong alkali. The pH of the skin is 4.5–5.5.

Acid mantle – often termed the hydrolipid film. It is the thin coating of the skin made up of sebum and sweat. Its job is to help prevent bacterial growth. It has a pH value of 4.5–5.5.

Think about it

An impaired acid mantle is often caused by lack of essential fatty acids (EFA) in the diet – ask your client about crash dieting, fat-free diets and restricted eating – it could be the cause of her skin problems.

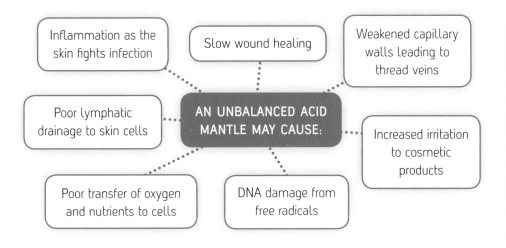

Inflammation as the skin fights infection

Slow wound healing

Weakened capillary walls leading to thread veins

Poor lymphatic drainage to skin cells

AN UNBALANCED ACID MANTLE MAY CAUSE:

Increased irritation to cosmetic products

Poor transfer of oxygen and nutrients to cells

DNA damage from free radicals

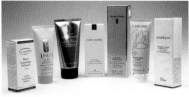

Exfoliating products

Desquamation

The epidermis is continually renewing itself – the lower layers are continually growing and dividing, pushing cells upward until they reach the surface, and then they are rubbed away. Friction within everyday movements, such as using a towel, getting dressed and scratching the skin will be enough to shed thousands of dead skin cells. This process is called desquamation or **exfoliation**. Getting rid of the old cells allows the new ones to come up to the surface, keeping the skin healthy and able to fight infection. This goes on daily and is not normally visible to the naked eye. Desquamation can only really be seen when a suntan is fading and the skin becomes dry and peels off in visible sheets.

The life cycle of a cell from the germinative layer to the top horny layer takes about 28 days and the cells go through a process called keratinisation. Keratin is a form of protein, and the cells get harder, flatter and eventually die. As the dead cells have no nucleus and no nerve endings, you don't feel your skin shedding itself.

Key terms

Exfoliation – the manual or mechanical method of removing dead skin cells from the epidermis using techniques that may include loofah scrub, dry brushing, salt glow, enzyme masks or abrasive scrubs.

Think about it

Some skin conditions and disorders are linked to skin shedding.

Psoriasis – a common skin condition where the life cycle of the cells drops to only five days from the germinative layer to the top horny layer. This happens so fast in the cells that only the nuclei are retained. This results in itchy, red, scaly patches, most common on the elbows, knees, legs and scalp. The cause is not known, but it is thought to be stress-related. Sunlight or UV exposure from a sunbed often helps the condition and there are creams available to help, too.

Ichthyosis – a chronic condition, usually present from birth, where the skin becomes rough, dry, itchy and scaly because of the over formation of keratin and a lack of natural exfoliation. In severe forms the scales can appear all over the body.

You and the skin

You and the skin

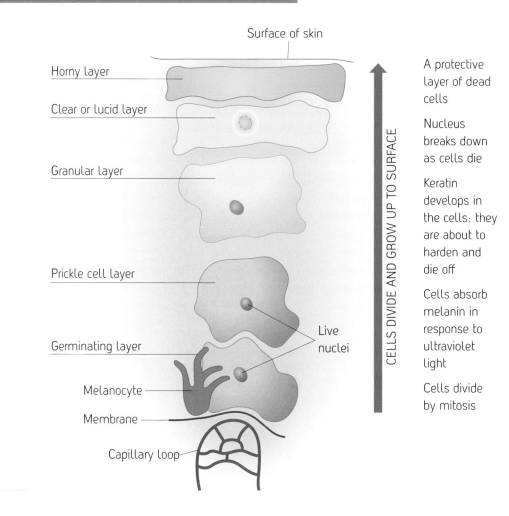

Surface of skin

Horny layer

Clear or lucid layer

Granular layer

Prickle cell layer

Germinating layer

Melanocyte

Membrane

Capillary loop

Live nuclei

CELLS DIVIDE AND GROW UP TO SURFACE

A protective layer of dead cells

Nucleus breaks down as cells die

Keratin develops in the cells: they are about to harden and die off

Cells absorb melanin in response to ultraviolet light

Cells divide by mitosis

The cells of the epidermis

How to recognise skin types and conditions

Skin types are usually described as one of four categories:

1 Normal

2 Dry

3 Oily

4 Combination.

As well as these four basic types, skin can also be mature, sensitive, dehydrated, and may have other problems. These may include: broken capillaries, blemishes, acne, comedones, milia and other minor imperfections.

The true skin type or condition may not be very easy to diagnose at first, as all skins react to the environment, to products used, and to different lifestyles.

Think about it

Everyone aspires to balanced skin in maximum condition and optimum health – that is the foundation of all the treatments that therapists carry out.

Skin types

Normal skin

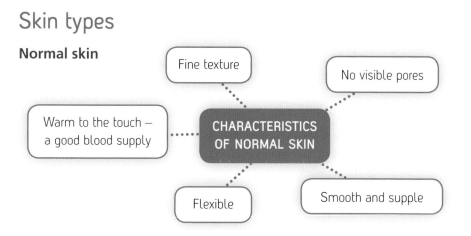

This exists when the oil and sweat glands are working in harmony, with a working acid balance to protect the skin. This skin has a good balance of moisture content and oil to keep the skin soft, supple and flexible. It is an ideal skin type, but rare. The skin is fine textured with no visible pores and smooth to the touch.

Some experienced therapists would argue that normal skin only exists in the very young, prior to the hormonal influences brought on by puberty. However, some people are lucky enough to enjoy a balanced skin, and those who look after their skin very well and enjoy a healthy life style are more likely to experience a balanced skin type.

Normal skin can occasionally become slightly dryer or slightly greasier — it should never be assumed that it is always normal. The skin should feel warm to the touch, and it heals well if damaged.

Questions to ask your client:

1 Is your skin generally in this condition?
2 Do you feel you have any problem areas?
3 Have you had problems in the past?
4 What skincare routine and products are you currently using?

Dry skin

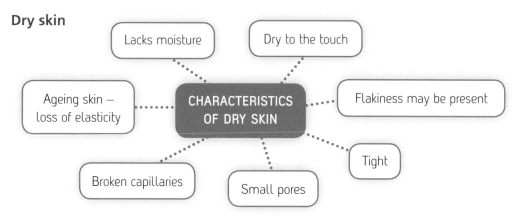

This type of skin is oil- and moisture-deficient, leaving the skin dry to the touch. There may be some loss of elasticity depending upon the client's age, and in extreme cases it can be rough or flaky. The texture of the skin is fine; dry skin can often be thin and small red veins (dilated capillaries) may be present on the cheek areas. Pores and follicles are often closed and inactive. The skin chaps easily and can be inclined to be sensitive. Lines and wrinkles may form early on with dry skin, especially around the eyes. The appearance of the skin is likely to be slightly dull, with a matt finish and it lacks suppleness.

Dry skin can be deceiving. It may not be the client's natural state but rather the effects of internal or external influences. Factors such as ill health, poor or incorrect product use, extreme weather conditions, over exposure to UV light or a poor diet (lack of essential fatty acids) all contribute to making the skin dry. It can therefore be easy to misdiagnose this skin type.

Questions to ask your client:

1 Does your skin feel tight and drawn?

2 Does your skin sometimes flake?

3 Does exposure to cold and wind make your skin sore?

4 Do you burn easily?

5 What products are you using?

Oily skin

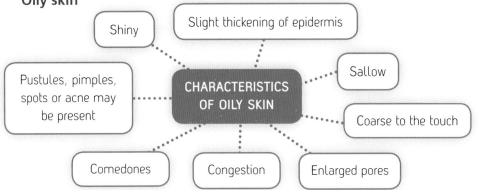

Oily skin is caused by overproduction of sebum from the sebaceous glands. This disturbs the acid mantle and the ratio of water to sebum on the skin. It looks shiny; it can be slightly thicker in consistency than normal skin, sallow, coarse and have problems associated with it. This skin is often referred to as **seborrhoeic**.

An oily skin often develops during puberty, when there is a surge of glandular activity under the influence of hormones. It often corrects itself when the hormone levels settle, and the use of the correct skin preparations can certainly help. Enlarged pores, congested pores, comedones and infection may occur on oily skins if the skin is not thoroughly cleansed and maintained, so care must be taken. It may also show signs of scarring, if there has been acne present.

Skin of this type is often over treated with quite harsh products, which can dry it out — it is possible to have an oily skin with dry flaky patches as a result of poor product use. This can be confusing for both client and therapist, so do check product use and previous treatments. The only advantage to having an overproduction of sebum is that in later life, as the skin sebum production slows down, the oily skin still has a good supply of sebum to moisturise and lubricate the skin — an oily skin is less prone to fine lines than a dry one.

Key terms

Seborrhoea or **seborrhoeic** – the name given to excessively oily skin caused by overactive sebaceous glands producing large amounts of sebum, making the skin look shiny; in some cases, may result in acne.

Questions to ask your client:

1 Is your skin prone to pimples and blackheads?
2 Does the skin shine?
3 Is it difficult to keep make-up on?
4 What products are you using?

Combination skin

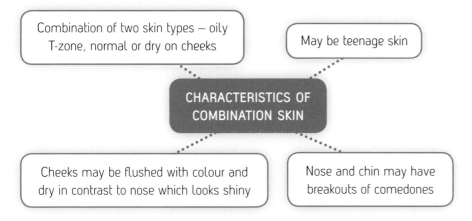

Combination of two skin types — oily T-zone, normal or dry on cheeks

May be teenage skin

CHARACTERISTICS OF COMBINATION SKIN

Cheeks may be flushed with colour and dry in contrast to nose which looks shiny

Nose and chin may have breakouts of comedones

Some skins are a combination of two or more skin types, and the most common one is an oily T-zone along the forehead and nose, with normal or dry skin on the cheek area. This is because there are more sebaceous glands along the T-zone which may therefore show all the characteristics of greasy skin. This skin type really needs to be treated as two types.

Questions to ask your client:

1 Is your nose shiny?
2 Are you prone to blackheads in the T-zone area?
3 Does the skin on your cheeks ever feel tight or dry?

Skin conditions

Sensitive skin

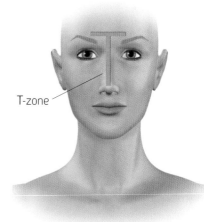

T-zone

The T-zone is commonly found in combination skin

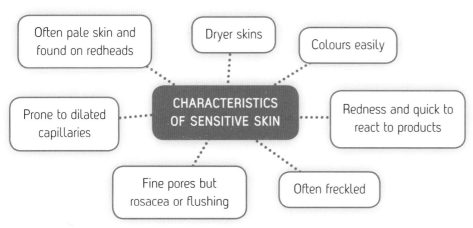

Often pale skin and found on redheads

Dryer skins

Colours easily

Prone to dilated capillaries

CHARACTERISTICS OF SENSITIVE SKIN

Redness and quick to react to products

Fine pores but rosacea or flushing

Often freckled

You and the skin

All skin needs to be sensitive for good health, but in beauty therapy a sensitive skin is really one that is super sensitive, that is it reacts to even mild stimulus. This condition is often associated with pale skins or a dry skin that lacks the protection of enough sebum. Sensitive skins have a highly flushed look, with a tendency to colour easily, and can react to beauty products or chemicals used within the salon.

More and more clients are developing allergies and sensitivity to chemicals and products – not just those found in cosmetic preparations but also cleaning products and perfumes – food intolerances and nickel found in jewellery.

Questions to ask your client:

1 Is your skin prone to allergic reactions?

2 Do you often have a high cheek colour?

3 Does your skin show signs of being dry but slightly red?

Dehydrated skin

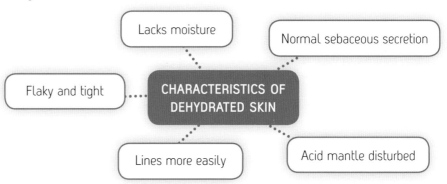

Skin may have the normal sebaceous secretions and still suffer from flaking and tightness due to loss of surface moisture – a condition of dehydration. Any skin can suffer temporary dehydration, which may be caused through using products that are too harsh on the skin or through exposure to extreme temperatures, central heating or over-stringent dieting.

The most common cause of dehydrated skin is a combination of not drinking enough water and drinking too many alcoholic or caffeinated drinks (such as cola and coffee), which are also dehydrating. When the thirst mechanism kicks in and the body needs water, it very often gets a cup of coffee instead, which makes it more dehydrated.

Questions to ask your client:

1 What skincare products are you using on the skin?

2 Have you altered your diet recently?

3 How much water do you drink a day?

Mature skin

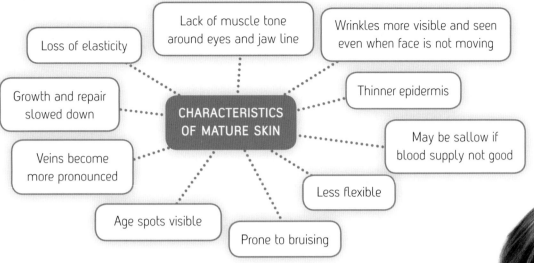

Loss of elasticity

Lack of muscle tone around eyes and jaw line

Wrinkles more visible and seen even when face is not moving

Growth and repair slowed down

CHARACTERISTICS OF MATURE SKIN

Thinner epidermis

May be sallow if blood supply not good

Veins become more pronounced

Less flexible

Age spots visible

Prone to bruising

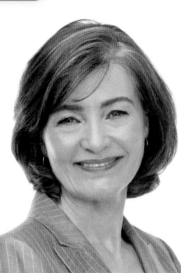

Mature skin type

All skins will age. The general rule of thumb is that a person's cell renewal rate is relative to their age – so a 16-year-old replaces skin cells every 16 days and an 80-year-old replaces skin cells every 80 days. This is only a guide, but it gives you an idea of how an older skin behaves and why.

There are two types of ageing.

1 **Intrinsic** – this describes natural ageing that occurs in the body. Your genetic programming not only dictates your colouring and height, it also dictates how fast you age. Generally, cell division stops after about 80 divisions and this cellular clock is fixed, despite our best efforts to stop or slow it down.

2 **Extrinsic** – this relates to the external factors that contribute to the ageing of the skin, e.g. exposure to UV light, free radicals, extreme weather and the chemicals found in cigarette smoke.

In a fine-textured, older skin the slower rate of the sebaceous secretions, accompanied by loss of elasticity, are contributory factors in the ageing process, leading to a mature skin type. Wrinkles begin to form. The epidermis may become thinner with a lack of springiness and loss of support from underlying muscles and collagen and elastin fibres, causing the skin to sag.

However, lots of mature clients maintain their health, use the right products and have a good lifestyle, which means that you cannot always diagnose a mature skin just by looking at the client. You may find that a younger person who is a heavy smoker (thus starving the skin of vital oxygen), with a poor diet and unhealthy lifestyle, may have skin that looks and behaves considerably older than their biological age.

You can read more about the effects of ageing of the skin on pages 216–23.

You and the skin

Congested skin

All skin types can become congested under the right conditions. Congestion occurs because the pores become blocked and sweat and sebum cannot escape on to the skin's surface, which can be seen and felt as lumpy and coarse. Whiteheads and blackheads can build up and the epidermis may harden. Poor removal of make-up, using the wrong products and excess sweat building up all contribute to this skin condition.

Comedones

Comedones or blackheads are formed when the mouth of the hair follicle on the skin's surface becomes blocked with excess sebum and hard keratinised cells. The comedone mixes with oxygen (oxidises) and turns black, and can be quite hard and embedded, or impacted. They are not infectious and do not spread but can be numerous, especially on the forehead, nose and chin, if the client has an oily T-zone. Comedones are more common in oily skins and during puberty when hormone fluctuations affect sebum production.

Infected skin

Any bacteria, fungi or viruses can penetrate broken skin and cause infection. This is usually a sign of poor health and can occur when a person is run down or ill. The acid mantle stops offering protection and the delicate balance is disrupted. This is easily recognised as swelling or irritation, with pain and tenderness. The presence of pus is also a sign of infection.

Bacteria entering the follicle, causing pore blockage to occur, causes acne vulgaris (see page 211).

Damaged skin

Think about it

Pigmentation is the production of colour in the body, caused by the deposit of a pigment called melanin, which protects the skin from UV radiation.

Reasons for damage	Signs and symptoms to look for when assessing skin type or condition
Excessive exposure to the sun, artificial sunlight (e.g. sunbeds), alcohol intake and smoking	The skin ages prematurely, causing a breakdown in collagen and elastin which supports the skin; uneven pigmentation; excessive lines and wrinkles relative to the client's age.
Pollution from chemicals, traffic and thinning of the protective ozone layer	Contamination of the skin leads to clogged and blocked pores, irritations occur and there is a tendency to comedones and allergic reactions. This causes dehydration and overactivity of the sebaceous glands; loss of oxygen causes skin to look sallow and tired.
Heat and steam	Overstretching of the skin; pores enlarge and become congested; damage to capillaries seen as thread veins on the cheeks and chin.
Incorrect use of skincare products	Inappropriate products can cause comedones to form or lead to an oversensitive, dry or flaky skin.
Excessive heat	Chapped and dehydrated skin; damaged capillaries and vascular flushness on the skin; spider naevus present on cheeks.
Poor diet containing insufficient nutrients or a lack of fatty acids; crash dieting	Sluggish and yellow or sallow-looking skin; lack of oxygen results in slow healing and repair of skin.
Impaired acid mantle due to poor product use or ill health	Increased inflammation and sensitisation; poor healing and infection.

The best way of caring for the skin is to:

- avoid skin damage — picking, bruising or scratching it
- take care of the skin internally with good nutritional habits/a balanced diet
- drink plenty of water
- avoid smoking
- limit alcohol and caffeine intake
- avoid crash diets or excluding fats from the diet
- use the correct skincare products
- have regular facials from an expert
- always use sun protection on the skin when in the sun
- maintain a good work/life balance — avoid unnecessary stress
- take regular exercise
- limit medication or drug use where possible
- try to regulate hormone levels.

Skin characteristics and skin types of different ethnic groups

Refer to the structure of the skin in Related anatomy and physiology, pages 235–40.

The skin owes its colouring to the red **haemoglobin** found within the blood vessels, yellow **carotenoids**, subcutaneous fat and the dark brown pigment **melanin**. Various degrees of pigmentation are present in different ethnic groups. The differences are in the amount of melanin produced and are not dependent upon the number of **melanocytes** present (see below).

Pigment

Certain areas of skin are very rich in pigment, such as the genital area and the nipples, while practically no pigment is present in the palms of the hands and the soles of the feet (often referred to as 'glabrous' skin, this lacks hair follicles and sebaceous glands, and has a thicker epidermis).

Pigment is stored as fine granules within the cells of the germinative layer, although some granules may also be deposited between the cells. In white/Caucasian skin the granules occur only in the deepest cell layers and mainly in the cylinder-shaped cells of the basal row. In non-white skin pigment is found throughout the entire layer and even in the granular layer (stratum granulosum).

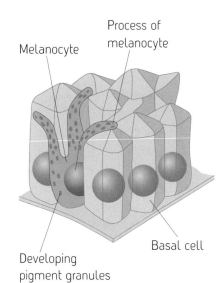

Melanocyte

Process of melanocyte

Basal cell

Developing pigment granules

Melanocytes in the skin

You and the skin

Key terms

Epithelial cells or epithelial tissue – specialised tissue that covers all external and internal surfaces of the body, made up of cells closely packed together in one or more layers. Epithelial tissue is separated from underlying tissue by a thin sheet of connective tissue called the basement membrane, which provides structural support and binds it to neighbouring structures. Simple epithelium is one cell thick and stratified epithelium is two or more cells thick.

Congenital condition – a condition that is recognised at birth or that is believed to have been present since birth. These include all disorders present at birth, whether they are inherited or caused by an environmental factor.

Melanin

All melanin is made in special cells called melanocytes and then distributed to the **epithelial cells**. The melanocytes are scattered in the basal layers of the epidermis and mature as the embryo is developing in the womb. They are influenced by the units of inheritance gene code which determines race and colouring.

Some people are born without the ability to produce melanin within their skins and with no hair pigment – a **congenital condition** called albinoism. People with this condition have pure white hair, pale skin and pink eyes.

Think about it

Not all white Caucasian skin is very light and fragile. Some skin tones are darker if the parents have brown or black hair, in which case the skin may tan more easily and be less prone to damage. Some white Caucasian skins, noticeably the Irish and Scottish, may have striking dark hair colouring with paler skin tone.

Skin ethnicity

The skin's ethnicity can be grouped into five basic categories. These are generalised only for the purposes of identification. Always remember that there are many variations within these categories.

1   White/Caucasian
2   Black
3   Asian
4   Oriental
5   Mixed
6   Mediterranean/Latino

White Caucasian skin

How to recognise it	Most likely origin	Features	Possible problems
White Caucasian skin is the most delicate or fragile of all the skin types, and is light in colour, often with blue or green eye colouring. It has blue and pink tones from the blood capillaries, which can be seen through the pale epidermis, and its melanin content is not as high as in other skin types.	Britain Northern and western Europe North America* New Zealand* Australia*	The skin of blonde or red-haired people tends to have a fine hair growth, and as the hair colour is light or fair, it is not usually noticeable. It tends to be fine in texture and thinner than in other skin types.	Light skins do not tan easily and are at risk of skin damage, especially if there are large amounts of freckles present. Light skins burn quickly and are less tolerant of UV light, so care should be taken in hotter climates. It is prone to early signs of ageing and wrinkles, and may bruise easily. It can be more prone to broken capillaries, especially if the skin is very light.

Think about it

All these basic skin categories provide only a general overview and should never be used to replace a thorough consultation with the client – and remember: there are always exceptions to the rule.

Treat each client as an individual, not just a type of skin colour. Different factors apply with each client: different lifestyles, dietary intake and use of products will determine how the skin behaves and reacts.

* People native to these countries have naturally much darker skin than those who have immigrated over the years from northern Europe. The indigenous people of Canada and Greenland are the Inuit. The indigenous people of New Zealand are the Maori and the indigenous people of Australia are the Aboriginals. They have dark skin for protection against the sunlight.

My story

My name is Sara-Jane.

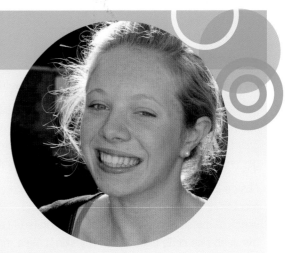

As you can see from my picture I am a white Caucasian skin type. Being very fair, I do not tan easily. When I went to Barbados on holiday, I had to be very careful not to burn my skin. I just go a bright red and then the skin peels!

I find I am quite sensitive to some products, so I tend to stick with the products I know won't irritate me – I get a strong itchy feeling and redness over my cheeks if I use anything too highly perfumed. I am prone to patches of eczema on my body if I use anything highly perfumed or change my washing powder.

Being blonde does have some advantages. Lots of people pay their hairdresser to put highlights in their hair, but mine are natural, with no regrowth showing through!

Black skin

How to recognise it	Most likely origin	Features	Possible problems
Black skins have more evenly distributed melanocytes, which are larger and more active than in a white/Caucasian skin. Black skin tends to be more robust: it has greater elasticity and strength of collagen fibres, giving support to the skin, so there is less possibility of dropped contours of the face. Black skin tends to be darker across the forehead and perimeter of the face but lighter in the middle on the cheeks.	Africa West Indies/ Caribbean North America	Sebaceous glands are larger and denser, giving good lubrication and moisture, making it less prone to premature wrinkles. This also means the ageing process is usually slower in black skin, with less cell deterioration. Because black skin flakes and is shed more quickly than other skins, cell renewal also tends to be faster.	Some black skins may be quite sensitive to products and care should be taken to avoid harsh, abrasive products, or strong alcohol-based toners. These types of product are often used to treat an 'oily' skin, but black skin is not usually oily at all – the reflection of light against black skin often gives the skin a glow or sheen. As the epidermis is thicker black skin may scar more easily, which can turn into **keloid** tissue. This is seen as an overthickening of the skin, in a pink or beige colour, which is more noticeable against a darker background.

Think about it

Skin cancer is not as common in people with black skin as they are protected from the harmful UV rays of the sun. Also, the epidermis is considerably thicker than in its white Caucasian counterpart, and it is therefore less reactive and not prone to allergies or infection: warts are rarely found on a black skin.

A condition called dermatosis papulosa nigra occurs almost exclusively in black skin, usually on the cheeks. It consists of brown or raised dark spots. Do not treat if infected – recommend that the client seeks medical advice.

Key terms

Keloid – a raised formation of scar tissue caused by excessive tissue repair in response to trauma or surgery when fibroblast cells continue to multiply and form large mounds of scar tissue. Black skins are more susceptible to keloid formation and they may appear on any part of the body.

You and the skin

My story

My name is Ogo.

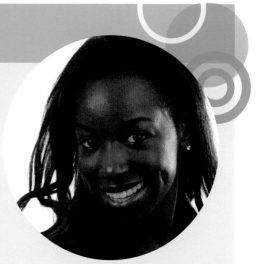

My skin is black, as my parents originally came from Nigeria in Africa.

I think I have good skin, with no real problems, although I don't wear foundation as I have trouble finding a colour that suits my skin – lots of foundations go grey on my skin tone. I can end up with darker circles under my eyes if I don't get enough sleep and my cheeks are a shade lighter than my forehead.

I use a lot of moisturiser to keep my skin from drying out – which can be a problem if I sunbathe. I do actually tan – and have a strap mark from my watch in the summer! Also if I get dehydrated I can go a grey colour because the dead skin cells build up on my skin. I need to drink water regularly and use an exfoliator to stop me looking ashen.

My only skin problem is stretch marks as I was slightly larger in my teens than I am now. They look like pink lines on my hips and tummy. I think they are fading slightly, but I am quite conscious of them, as they show up against my darker skin. I hope I have inherited my mum's great bone structure and skin condition – her skin is great even in her fifties!

Asian skin

Asian skin can be divided into two types: dark and light/oriental.

Dark Asian skin

How to recognise it	Most likely origin	Features	Possible problems
Dark Asian skin tends to be more sallow with a darker tone than light Asian/oriental skin as there is a higher proportion of melanin present.	Pakistan India Sri Lanka Malaysia	This type of skin has more sweat glands, which are also larger, to keep the body temperature at a manageable level in the heat. It has fewer problems with oil-related conditions such as acne. The skin is often smooth and line-free, strong and adaptable, with the underlying fibres being supportive well into middle age.	Wrinkling tends to be minimal, but the skin may be prone to loss of pigmentation if care is not taken. It can have a tendency towards uneven colouring and pigmentation can cause dark circles under the eyes.

My story

My name is Poonam.

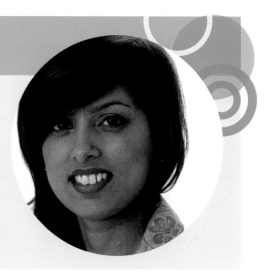

I come from a small Indian village outside New Delhi.

All of my family have very dark skin and hair. My grandmother is now greying, but both Nanna and my mum still have a thick head of hair. My skin is quite strong and healthy. I am not very sensitive to anything and I can use most products on it with no problems, but I do have quite a lot of facial hair. I also need to have my eyebrows threaded regularly. As my mum has grown older she has become prone to dark pigmentation patches on her face and neck.

Light Asian/oriental skin

How to recognise it	Most likely origin	Features	Possible problems
Light Asian/oriental skin has yellow undertones, and can develop an olive tone. The base colour is cream and this type of skin is often clear and fine in complexion.	Japan China Middle East Thailand Hong Kong	The skin is often smooth and fine, with minimal blemishes. This skin type rarely shows degeneration due to ageing. There is likely to be little or no facial and body hair. The skin has good tolerance of UV and tends not to wrinkle early.	This skin tends to scar easily and there may be irregularities in the skin's surface seen as pitting or unevenness. Hyperpigmentation may also occur; clients may be concerned about these age spots developing. As the skin can be fairly oily, especially around the T-zone, this skin type may develop a problem with open pores and comedones along the nose.

My story

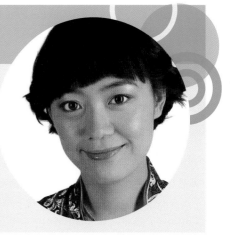

My name is Masico.

I come from Japan. Although I have an oily skin I look after it with good skincare products and I am sure my diet, which is full of fruit and vegetables, helps maintain its condition. In Japan we eat very healthily with a diet low in carbohydrates and fats/butter, so we have fewer problems with obesity or heart disease than western countries — I am sure that is also reflected in my skin's condition. I do worry about getting sun spots so I make sure I use good sun protection of SPF 30. As I have a lot of yellow surface tones if I use the wrong concealers I tend to look a bit grey — so I use a peach corrector to even my skin tone out. Still, I am lucky as I don't need to wear a lot of make-up as my skin is clear.

Mixed race (multi-ethnic) skin

How to recognise it	Most likely origin	Features	Possible problems
A client with mixed race skin will need a very thorough consultation to ensure that the skin analysis is correct, as those with this skin type are likely to have a combination of influencing factors.	Mixed parentage from any ethnic background.	These will vary considerably.	The skin will be more of a product of the mixture of parents and the environment. The correct product use will also dictate how clear the skin is, and whether the acid mantle is intact and doing its job correctly. This skin type is the easiest one to misdiagnose.

Think about it

A student with one Chinese parent and one white/Caucasian parent has skin which looks quite oily, with blocked pores and comedones present. There are dry patches on the cheek area — but is this really dry skin?

The problem might be down to product use — the top layer of the epidermis is perhaps being dried out with alcohol-based toners (for an oily skin), which are too strong. They would cause the dry patches but would not address the oil production still taking place in the sebaceous glands underneath. The horny layer would not shed properly, so a build-up of cells forms the dry patches. In a case like this, good exfoliation will help, along with gentle steaming to aid extraction and then application of the correct water-based product. Avoid any oil-based products on an already oily skin.

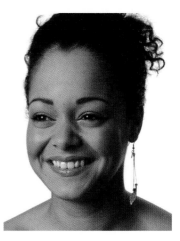

You and the skin

Additional knowledge

Mediterranean/Latino skin

There is one other skin type you may come across which, although it is not a range for VRQ Level 2, is still a recognisable skin type. That is Mediterranean/Latino skin.

How to recognise it	Most likely origin	Features	Possible problems
A golden skin with olive undertones.	Spain Italy Southern France Portugal Greece South and Central America	This skin type tends to be oilier, due to the sebaceous glands producing more sebum to keep the skin lubricated in the heat. It therefore tends not to dry out too much, and is slow to form wrinkles. As the hair colour is also darker, facial and body hair is more noticeable and often grows thicker and is coarse in texture. This skin type is robust and less prone to damage; it can withstand higher levels of UV without burning, and tends to tan more easily.	There is a tendency for excessive facial and body hair. The skin may be fairly tough and tends to thicken as it ages.

My story

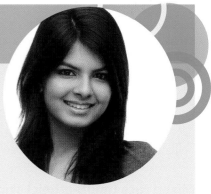

My name is Christiana.

I come from Cyprus and both my parents are originally from Greece. I have a typical Mediterranean skin – dark and tanned. I don't have to worry too much about burning and I tan really easily – we all do in my family. That is the good side about my skin – my only problem is that I tend to get blackheads around my nose and on my chin, so I am very careful to cleanse my skin thoroughly to prevent them. I have quite a lot of facial hair and have very strong hair on my head – which grows very fast, but the down side is that my leg and under-arm hair do the same. I spend a fortune on waxing!

For your portfolio

Of the skin types mentioned here, which colouring or skin type do you recognise as similar to your own? How does your skin react in sunlight? Look up which sun protection factor (SPF) creams would be most suitable for your skin. See pages 224–25 for more detail on SPFs. Fill out a consultation card as if you were your own client. What would you be noting about your skin type?

Think about it

You are not medically trained and must not recommend treatment of a medical nature. Do not pass comment on any skin irregularity you may observe; instead refer the client to her GP.

The photosensitivity of skin

This is the term used to describe how the skin reacts to sunlight and UV rays, real or artificial. The skin may break out in a heat rash; this condition is called photodermatosis. It may be caused by exposure to UV, or a reaction from a topical application of a product that reacts with UV, a metabolic defect within the body, a genetic disorder, which has been inherited, or a pre-existing skin disease.

The Fitzpatrick classification system for skin types

We have seen how skin can be classified by type, condition and ethnic origin. Some cosmetic houses base their product ranges – especially sun protection creams – around the Fitzpatrick classification system.

The system was developed in the US by a dermatologist, Dr Thomas Fitzpatrick of Harvard University, in 1975. It is based upon melanin content in the skin and how quickly the skin burns. The system classifies the skin into six different types, ranging from extremely light-skinned people, who are highly likely to burn, to extremely dark-skinned people, who may suffer serious discoloration from laser or light treatment or other pigment-altering therapies or conditions.

The Fitzpatrick classification is often used by dermatologists using laser and light therapy as it can help highlight the risks of poor reactions to treatment.

A variety of questions are asked about genetic history, physical attributes such as eye colour, hair colour and freckling, and personal observations of the skin's reaction to sunlight. Depending on the answers to the questions, most people fit into one of the six skin categories, usually labelled with roman numerals I–VI.

Think about it

The Fitzpatrick classification system should be used as a guideline rather than a definitive system for determining skincare. You must always conduct a full consultation, a manual and visual examination and employ all diagnostic tools available to you as a therapist.

Skin type	Typical features	Ability to tan
I Celtic, English, Northern European	Pale white, fair skin, blue/hazel eyes, blonde/red hair	Always burns, freckles, does not tan
II Nordic, North American	White, fair skin, sandy to brown hair, green, brown or blue eyes	Burns easily, tans poorly and with difficulty, freckles
III Central/Eastern European, Mediterranean, Maori (New Zealand)	Darker or olive white skin, brown hair, green or brown eyes	Tans after initial burn
IV Chinese, Korean, Japanese, Thai, South American, Indian, Filipino	Olive to light brown skin, brown hair, brown eyes	Burns minimally, tans easily
V East African, Ethiopian, Northern African, Middle-Eastern Arabic	Dark brown skin, black hair, dark brown eyes	Rarely burns, tans darkly easily
VI African type, American-African	Dark brown, black eyes, dark brown or black skin	Never burns, always tans darkly

The Fitzpatrick skin type categories

Tools for diagnosing skin types and conditions

The magi lamp

A good magnification lamp with a surrounding light is the ideal tool for examining the skin's surface; the magnification glass allows you to get a clear picture of blemishes and problems. Always check the lamp is working prior to putting it over the client's face: check the light bulb and the screws and joints so that it is safe, and not likely to drop suddenly.

For your portfolio

To determine your own skin type there are many websites offering complete questionnaires for the Fitzpatrick skin classification. Why not have a go to see your own skin type!

Skin scanners and black light equipment

There are some very effective diagnostic tools for use in salons which give an in-depth analysis of black skins and which measure the acid mantle, pH of the skin, melanin and water content, as well as the density and strength of the dermis. These machines have been used by dermatologists for years and salons are finding them very useful to support the other diagnostic and consultation techniques used.

Wood's lamp or black light

The Wood's lamp (often called a black light) was invented by Robert William Wood in 1903. It was designed to produce a source of UV light and was used in hospitals to detect fungal and bacterial infections and parasites. Its clinical use in salons is to detect skin conditions.

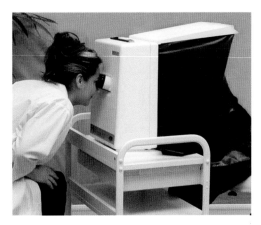

A skin scanner

Think about it

The colours produced by the Wood's lamp will vary depending upon the make of lamp. Always follow the manufacturer's instructions.

Identifying skin conditions using a Wood's lamp

Colour of fluorescence	Skin type or problem
Blue	Normal balanced skin
Weak violet/light purple	Dry skin or patches of dehydration
Dark purple	Sensitive, thin, fragile areas
Coral pink	Dehydrated skin
Strong white	Thickened stratum corneum and the presence of dead skin cells
Orange	Oily skin or patches of overproductive sebaceous glands
Brown spots	Overpigmentation/sun damage
Light yellow	Acne, comedones
Green	Presence of pathogen Pseudomonas – a bacterial infection

A Wood's lamp produces deep UV rays. It makes the skin glow, signifying different conditions and problems. There are both hand-held and box versions. The hand-held type is difficult to get a true reading from because the face needs to be in darkness. Ideally, the salon needs to be blacked out to operate the machine correctly, but this is rarely possible. With a box machine the client is seated, and the face is placed on a chin rest, rather like having an eye examination at the optician, and the curtain is pulled around the head so that the face is in darkness. The UV light can then be turned on to the skin. Certain colours will appear in patches which will indicate the skin's condition.

These areas can be noted down on the consultation card and the appropriate treatment and products recommended to the client.

Skin scanners

Hydration levels

The Corneometer® measures the skin's moisture content. It indicates whether the acid mantle is still intact and whether the skin's defence barrier is adequate. It also shows the enzyme action of the epidermis. The scanner looks rather like a pen, with a flat end, which is placed on the skin's surface; the reading appears on the attached machine. It is used in hospitals to measure a patient's intake of fluid.

Skin lipid levels

The Sebumeter® determines the amount of sebum being excreted by the sebaceous glands on to the skin's surface to check if the acid mantle protection is in good condition. The sebum of the skin or hair is taken by a film on the cassette's measuring head. Its transparency changes according to the sebum content on the film and is then analysed. If the skin's lipid or fat content is low, the acid mantle is unable to defend the skin properly. This could be because the client's diet is deficient in essential fatty acids. This is a good tool to use but is only one of the diagnostic procedures — your consultation will also reveal a lot about the skin's condition.

Melanin and erythema

There are also machines which measure melanin and blood flow in the skin. This can help determine which skincare and sunscreen products will be most useful to recommend to the client. This is used with the Fitzpatrick classification system of skin-burning capacity.

Face shapes and contours

It is not only skin colour that characterises each ethnic identity; the shape of the skull and the bones form the contours of the face.

The position of the bones of the skull gives the face its shape, as the bones provide the attachment for all the muscles. The underlying bones dictate how high the cheeks are, how far apart the eyes are and so on. The jawbone dictates the shape of the face, along with the frontal bone, making the face square, round, oblong or heart-shaped. Apart from weight loss or gain, which will alter facial contours, nothing will alter your face shape unless you have corrective surgery to alter the bones themselves or have implants put under the skin or muscles to alter the contours.

For your portfolio

Identifying face shapes correctly takes some practice. You can practise by identifying your own face shape. Pull your hair back off your face. Using a mirror, look at your own face shape. Try to analyse and match the shape of your face to one of the diagrams. If your forehead and jaw line are the same, you probably have a square face shape. If you have quite a pointed chin, you probably have a heart face shape. Draw your face outline on the mirror (using a pen that will rub off!) and see what shape you really are.

Face shape	How to recognise it		
Oval face shape 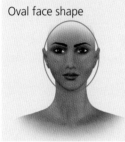	This face shape and bone structure is considered to be the ideal face shape. The chin tapers slenderly from a slightly wider forehead. The aim of make-up is to accentuate the natural shape.	Heart face shape 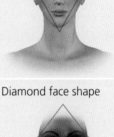	This shape usually has a wide forehead with the face tapering to a long jawline, rather like an inverted triangle. The aim of the make-up is to reduce the width across the forehead, emphasising the jawline.
Round face shape 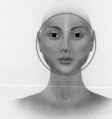	The face is usually short and broad with full cheeks and round contours. Width at the top of the head should be provided, with height from the hair, which should be worn close at the sides. The aim of make-up is to slim the appearance.	Diamond face shape	The forehead in this bone structure is narrow with the cheekbones extremely wide tapering to a narrow chin. The make-up aims to minimise the width across the cheekbones. A central fringe should be worn with hair full below the cheeks but flat at the cheekbone line.
Square face shape 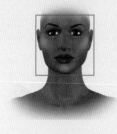	The forehead is broad, corresponding with an angular jawline. This shaped face should have a little height without width and the hair should taper well towards the jawline. The aim of the make-up is to narrow the forehead and the jawline, reducing the squareness of this bone structure.	Pear face shape	The forehead is narrow and the face gradually widens to the angle of the jaw which is broad and prominent. The make-up should aim to create the impression of width across the forehead and to narrow the jaw line. The hair should be swept off the forehead to create an illusion of width with a reverse flicking fringe.
Oblong face shape 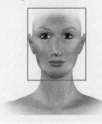	This face shape has a narrow frame. The make-up aim is to create the impression of width and to shorten the face length. A fringe with short hair would be suitable.	Triangular face shape 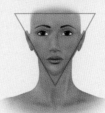	This is similar to the heart-shaped face, but not as soft. The aim of the make-up is to reduce the width of the forehead, by emphasising the jawline.

Contra-indications to facial treatments

Skin treatments must not be carried out if the client has a potential skin problem that would prevent the treatment from taking place. This is described as a contra-indication to treatment.

Contra-indications include:

- infections — bacterial, viral and fungal infections of eyes, lips or face
- open cuts and abrasions
- broken bones or bruising
- acute acne
- severe eczema or psoriasis
- recent invasive procedures such as chemical or medical peels (glycolic or AHA), Botox® injections, collagen or other filler injections in the face
- recent waxing
- certain types of medication, including Retin-A and Accutane used to treat topical acne
- recent cancer treatment
- recent dental work.

Refer to Professional skills (pages 34–36) for details of micro-organisms and the diseases they cause and also how to minimise the risk of infection.

Infections — viral

The common cold	Cold sores (Herpes simplex)	Warts
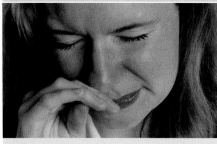	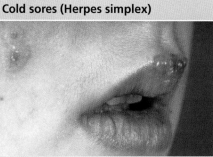	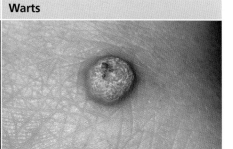
Freely recognised. Streaming eyes and nose, coughing and sneezing, easily spread.	Found on the lips, cheeks and nose. Blisters form, the skin is broken and painful; the blisters are especially likely to spread when open and weepy and then crusts form.	Small compact raised growths of skin — can be light or brown in colour, present on the face and neck.

Infections – bacterial

Impetigo	Boil (furnuncle)	Conjunctivitis	Stye
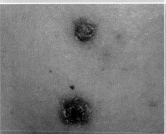	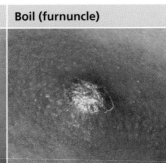	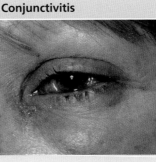	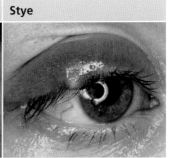
Highly infectious, this starts as small red spots, which then break open and form blisters. Most common around the corner of the mouth and, if picked, will spread. (Some strains are particularly resistant to antibiotics.) Can be spread through use of dirty equipment.	This infection forms at the base of a hair follicle. Bacteria can spread through an open scratch in the skin. The area is raised, red, and painful. Pus may be present.	This is a nasty eye condition. The eyelids are red and sore, with itching. Mainly caused by bacteria present, it can be irritated by a virus or an allergy.	This is a small boil at the base of the eyelash follicle. It is raised, sore and red; there may be considerable swelling in the area.

Infections – fungal

Ringworm (tinea corporis)	Blepharitis
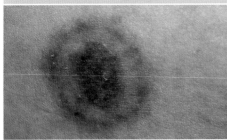	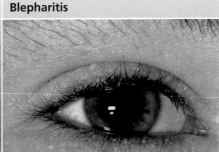
Red pimples appear and then form a circle, with clear skin in the middle. It is highly contagious and scales and pustules follow. It can be spread on to the face from any other area of the body. Can be passed on to humans by contact with domestic animals.	An infection of the lid causing inflammation, the eye will look red and sore. Depending on the severity of the condition, you could avoid eye make-up application, and focus attention on the mouth, with a pretty lipstick shade.

Think about it

All of the conditions mentioned would be a contra-indication to a facial treatment of make-up application to the face. The beauty therapist is responsible for protecting everyone in the salon from contamination via these micro-organisms.

Conditions restricting the effectiveness of treatment

The following conditions are contra-indications that will not necessarily stop the treatment from taking place, but they may mean that a facial or make-up application has to be restricted and/or adapted. Most of these situations call for common sense and professional judgement can be used. If the problem is not directly on the face or neck, where the facial or make-up application takes place, then just avoid the area.

You and the skin

Each one will depend upon the individual case, the client granting permission, and then giving written permission on the record card. (Refer to Professional skills, pages 24–26 for further information on the client record card; see also practical units on individual treatments and services.)

Cuts/abrasions/broken skin	Bruises or swelling	Recent scar tissue
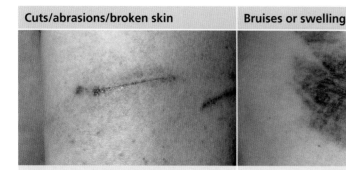	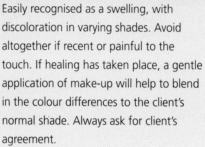	
If recent, a scab will be forming, the skin may be tender and swollen in the area, and bruising may be seen. If cuts and abrasions are recent, then avoid the area altogether. If the area has healed over, and is not too recent, get the client's agreement that gentle application can take place, with careful consideration to hygiene.	Easily recognised as a swelling, with discoloration in varying shades. Avoid altogether if recent or painful to the touch. If healing has taken place, a gentle application of make-up will help to blend in the colour differences to the client's normal shade. Always ask for client's agreement.	Usually a different colour from the rest of the skin, following the line of injury. If the scar is recent, raised or angry looking, then avoid the area altogether. If the area is healing and not very large, gentle application with client's permission. Scar tissue less than six months old, or over a large area, should not be touched with make-up.

Eczema	Dermatitis	Psoriasis
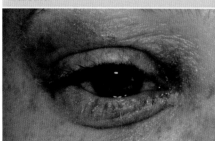	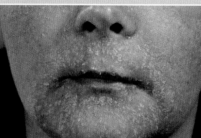	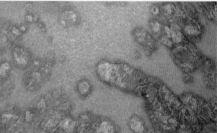
Very dry skin, often scaly and flaky, can be red and often very itchy. If the eczema covers a large area, and is inflamed with broken skin, then leave alone, and suggest a visit to the GP. You may make it worse. If the eczema has irritated the eye area, it is unlikely the client would want make-up application. If it is only a small patch of eczema, and not angry, just exclude the area from treatment. The use of hypoallergenic products is recommended and patch test if the client is very sensitive.	This is similar to eczema in appearance, but the cause is not the same. A reaction or allergy to something in contact with the skin usually causes dermatitis. See Eczema (left). Skin allergies may result in a contra-action, so if the client's skin tends to react, do a skin patch test 24 hours prior to the make-up application. It may be advisable to use hypoallergenic make-up; ask the client to bring in her own make-up if she knows she is safe using it.	Seen as scaly patches of red and/or silvery skin. This can break open and become sore. The cause is unknown but is thought to relate to the nervous system. A contra-indication would be if the psoriasis is open or bleeding. One of the common sites for psoriasis is the scalp, so the client may have a little patch visible along the hairline. If the client agrees to make-up application, and it is not directly over the area, then continue. A patch test 24 hours prior to the application of make-up is advisable to ensure that the condition is not aggravated.

You and the skin

Acne vulgaris	Acne rosacea	Skin tags

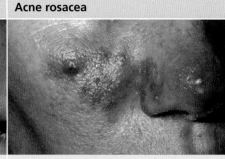

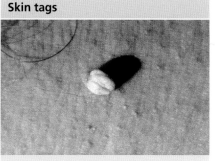

| Inflamed whiteheads, blackheads and pustules in various degrees of congestion. Mostly associated with hormones – and the presence of bacteria can make the condition infected.

Infected inflamed acne is a contra-indication. However, a client with mild acne can be treated in the salon, and a light water-based foundation applied. There may be a tendency to greasy skin, and therefore a light application of powder keeps the skin looking matt. | Seen as a flush of red over the nose and cheeks with a raised feel to the skin. Often those who have suffered acne vulgaris in youth are prone to acne rosacea in later life. If the skin is not tender and the client agrees, application of make-up can tone down the redness and therefore lessen the angry look of the skin. | Usually found on the eye area or lids and/or on the side of the neck. They resemble little 'mushrooms' of skin on a stalk which move when touched. This skin tag is under the arm.

As these are not painful or dangerous, make-up application can take place. If they become enlarged and irritating to the client they can be removed under local anaesthetic, usually at the GP's surgery. |

Milia	

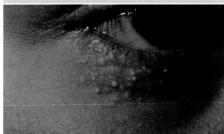

These are small white pearls under the skin, often around the eyes or on the side of the cheek, caused by a build-up of sebum. Make-up application can take place over milia, as they are not infectious.

Other skin conditions – pigmentation disorders

These disorders are caused by irregularities in the skin's melanin production. They are not infectious and are not a contra-indication to facial or make-up treatments. However, pigmentation disorders do affect the client's appearance and may make the client feel embarrassed and self-conscious; as a therapist, you therefore need to treat them sensitively. The use of remedial camouflage cosmetics may help more effectively with the matching of the pigmentation than ordinary foundations and concealers. Permanent make-up techniques can also help with pigmentation loss – it is a form of tattooing the skin but with the right colour of skin tone rather than coloured ink as in a tattoo. This is carried out by specially trained therapists as it is permanent and therefore there is no margin for error.

You and the skin

There are two main types of pigmentation disorders:

- hypopigmentation (hypo = less than normal)
- hyperpigmentation (hyper = more than normal).

Melanoderma

This is a general term used to describe patchy pigmentation. This is usually an increase in melanin caused by applying cosmetics or perfume which contain light-sensitive ingredients (e.g. bergamot oil used in the perfume industry) — the skin becomes extra sensitive to UV light. Some drugs have a similar effect. This can also follow inflammation and is sometimes the cause of brown patches following sunburn.

Hormones can often cause over pigmentation too. For example, there is a condition which occurs during pregnancy, called 'the mask of pregnancy', where the skin darkens in the shape of a mask or butterfly over the upper face, often into a deep brown colour, up to the hair line. It fades slightly after giving birth but will be extra sensitive to light for many years afterwards — sun creams should always be applied to the area as it will darken considerably more than the rest of the face.

Vitiligo	Chloasma	Freckles (ephilidies)
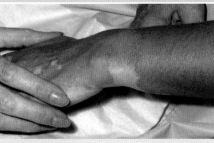	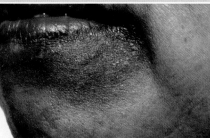	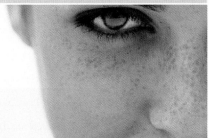
This is hypopigmentation; a condition in which small patches of skin have lost their pigmentation and appear a lighter colour than the rest of the skin. These lighter areas burn easily in the sun and need protection. They are not raised or painful to the touch. If the discolouration is in large patches a specialist camouflage make-up should be applied to conceal and match the skin tone. This may mean referral to a specialist. If the patch is small, clever choice of foundation and careful application is acceptable.	This is hyperpigmentation. It consists of irregular patches of brown pigment caused by the overproduction of melanocytes. This often appears on the face during pregnancy and is sometimes linked to the contraceptive pill. The discolouration usually disappears when the hormone balance is restored.	These are tiny, flat irregular patches of pigment on fair-skinned people, particularly blonde/redheads. They are due to the uneven distribution of melanin, and this becomes more noticeable on exposure to strong sunlight. The freckles often increase in size and join together. The skin between the freckles contains little or no melanin, so burns easily. As a therapist you should recommend a good sunscreen to the client.

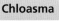

Lentigo	**Haemangioma**	**Dilated capillaries**
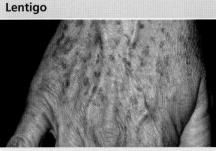	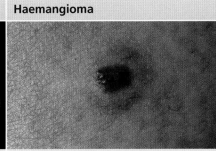	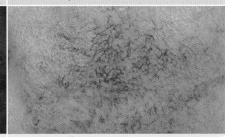
Also known as 'age spots', these are larger and more distinctive than a freckle, and may be slightly raised. This pigmentation does not increase in number or darken on exposure to UV light.	This consists of various conditions caused by the permanent dilation of superficial blood vessels. Stimulating treatments will therefore be a contra-indication to treatment, but camouflage cosmetics can be used.	This is the result of loss of elasticity in the walls of the blood capillaries – the cheeks and the nose are often most affected. Exposure to weather, harsh handling and lack of protection, along with spicy foods and alcohol, can be contributing factors. Clients with dry/sensitive skin types are most likely to be affected.

Split capillaries

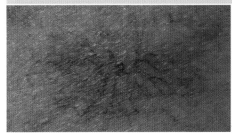 Weakening and rupturing of capillary walls – clients should avoid stimulating treatments. This condition can be treated by diathermy.

Other skin conditions – naevus

This describes a variety of birthmarks and developmental abnormalities. It is the most common disorder involving melanocytes.

Strawberry naevus	**Spider naevus**	**Port wine stain**
This is a raised and distorted area, often on the face, bright pink/red. It appears a few days or weeks after birth and usually clears up completely by the age of eight.	A central dilated vessel with leg-like projections of capillaries. The face and cheeks tend to be most affected and this often occurs during pregnancy due to the increase in oestrogen levels.	This is a bright purple, irregular-shaped, flat birthmark that can vary in size. It is thought to be due to damage by pressure during foetal development. These marks grow with the body and can be quite disfiguring. You should treat such marks sensitively with good cosmetic camouflage make-up.

Allergic reactions and sensitivity testing

Both in the European Union and the USA the law requires that cosmetic companies conduct very strict safety tests on materials they use to formulate products. Nevertheless, there will always be some people who are allergic to a substance that other people can tolerate without a problem.

An allergic reaction is a method of defence. The skin produces histamine – a compound derived from the amino acid histidine – found in mast cells in nearly all tissues of the body. Histamine causes dilation of blood vessels and contraction of smooth muscle: it is an important moderator of inflammation and is released in large amounts after skin damage.

A reaction could include:

- redness (erythema)
- swelling
- irritation to the area
- pain or itching in the area.

This is not a common reaction but may occur if clients have an allergy to any active ingredients within a product, or other common substances such as nickel, food or nuts. Some allergic reactions are life-threatening as the throat closes up and swells so that breathing is inhibited. Adrenalin needs to be administered in the form of an EpiPen® injection, and clients who suffer with this normally carry emergency medication to literally save their lives. This type of reaction can happen with strawberries, shellfish or even with a bee or wasp sting. It is therefore essential that you complete a sensitivity test if you are concerned that the client may react to a product. This can be done by testing a small sample of the product behind the client's ear or in the crook of the elbow. If a reaction occurs within 24 hours the product should not be used.

If a client does develop a reaction, stop the treatment and treat with calamine lotion and a cold compress as necessary. Always make a note on the record card so that the product is not used again on the client. (Refer to Professional skills, page 33, for information on contra-actions.)

Think about it

Lots of products used within facials are nut-based – almond oil in massage, for example. Always check with the client at the consultation stage, before starting treatment, for potential allergic reactions.

Choosing suitable products

Product labelling

By law, ingredients which are known to be irritants (or sensitisers) must be listed on the packaging, together with the precautions for use. Some facial and make-up products contain substances which cause allergic reactions in people who are hypersensitive. For example:

- lanolin – a fatty substance used as a softening agent in skin creams and lipsticks
- eosin – a red dye found in some lipsticks
- perfumes – particularly those containing bergamot, lavender and cedarwood
- alcohol – a grease solvent and astringent used in cosmetics and skincare products

- cobalt blue – a pigment used to produce eye make-up colours
- pearlising agents – ingredients which give products a shimmering effect
- gums – adhesives and binding agents in cosmetics.

Eye irritation

Although products used around the eye area are very strictly tested, and only safe pigments are used, some can still cause irritation to some clients.

Hypoallergenic products

If your client has sensitive or allergic skin you should use this type of product, which contains no perfume as well as fewer pigments and preservatives. Organic facial products are also freely available now, and are preferred by many clients; the only drawback may be that they lack preservatives and have a limited shelf life. Most large cosmetic and product companies recognise the need to produce quality products that are neither comedogenic nor allergy causing and so use food grade preservatives.

Ethical products

Consumers are very well informed about the use of chemicals and their effects on the skin and many would prefer not to have certain ingredients in a skincare range, e.g. parabens, lanolin or synthetic bases. They will look for largely botanical or aromatherapy based ingredients. They also want products which are more environmentally friendly, with packaging that is recyclable and biodegradable, with many companies refusing to test products on animals. These products are labelled as 'green' and judged to be kind to the planet. Organic skin care ranges are widely available and are very compatible with the skin. They tend not to have stabilisers in them so do not have a long shelf life.

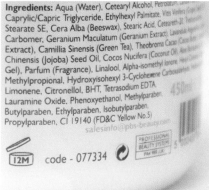

Always check ingredient labels if you know your client is allergic to particular additives

Male skin

When looking at skin types and conditions, it is important to include the male skin, as males have become big spenders in the skincare market. In 2007 a survey in the *Guardian* found that men in the USA spent approximately $10 billion on personal grooming products. Even though this includes the large number of deodorant and shaving products that most men use, it is still a lot of money. One of the fastest-growing areas within beauty is the demand for specific men's salon treatments and related care products.

Characteristics of male skin

Male skin is thicker than female skin due to the influence of the male hormones testosterone and androgen. It is therefore more resistant but can become thinner more quickly when ageing. Because of the testosterone influences, men's skin tends to be oilier than women's, so men like lighter moisturising products and products which solve their particular problems. Men also prefer less fragrance in their products or for it to have a masculine smell of cedarwood or pine.

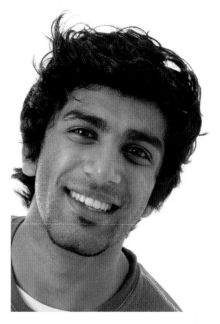

Men have become big spenders in the skincare market

Products for male skin

Previous generations of men would be happy to use their wife's moisturiser if their skin felt a little dry, but few would venture out into the salon or department store for a full consultation before purchasing their own products. Not any longer. The salon or company that caters for male skins is on to a winning formula – it is no longer seen as effeminate to use facial products, especially with high-profile sports personalities promoting different ranges in the media.

Products designed for men have evolved to take into account that the skin is more resistant but, conversely, may also be more fragile through neglect, misuse or total lack of protective products such as moisturisers and sun blocks.

Most men's basic product needs are for the daily routine of washing, shaving and moisturising. Calming products may also be needed for the specific treatment of blocked pores, irritation from shaving and razor burn or folliculitis (inflammation of the hair follicle in the skin, commonly caused by an infection).

Men who shave daily are automatically exfoliating the upper epidermal cells, so the skin stays healthy looking and clear. There are many products available for sensitive skins, both for dry and wet shaving, to avoid shaving rash, which can be very sore and unsightly.

Healing and soothing products, creams that reduce razor bumps, products that reduce the possibility of ingrown hairs are popular. Anti-ageing creams (although the name is misleading – nothing stops the ageing process) are also a fast-selling line. Although the signs of ageing appear later on a male face, when they do arrive the wrinkles are more intense and visible – men have fewer small lines but more deep wrinkles.

Some men use salon treatments to enhance their natural good points – eyelash tinting and the application of tinted moisturiser are very common. Manicures and pedicures are also a favourite with male clients. (Refer to Provide facial skincare for information on how to prepare for a facial on a male client, page 270.)

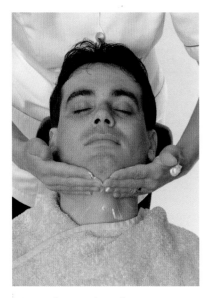

A growing number of men are visiting salons for treatments such as facials and manicures

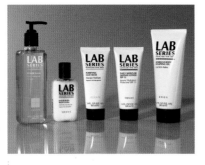

Many product ranges are designed specifically for men

Factors affecting the skin-ageing process

Along with the skin type your clients inherit, the care they take of it and their general health, age has to be the other greatest influence on the skin, not only because of the hormonal impact. Ageing is a natural part of the life cycle of a human being – it cannot yet be stopped or reversed, and is part of our evolution to keep the species going.

Unfortunately, western culture is geared up to the young and growing older is not seen as a desirable trait, unlike eastern cultures where age is equated with wisdom and knowledge. Western society tries to push back the ageing process and this has led to a marked rise in the demand for face lifts and extreme beauty treatments, such as Botox® injections and collagen infills, to delay the ageing process. However, we are genetically programmed to age, and temporary solutions are expensive, although they may provide a mental boost to the client. But we should celebrate ageing and enjoy the wisdom that age brings with it.

Ageing happens to us all and at generally the same rate, unless we have a disease that interrupts these natural processes. The inherited factor comes into play again – if your parents age well, enjoy good health and have good skin, the chances are you will too.

As well as the inheritance factor, the environment has a big impact on the ageing process. During normal metabolism, your cells make small electrically charged molecules called free radicals. These are very reactive and will react with proteins, DNA and some minerals. They can interfere with normal cell function, often causing irreversible damage that accumulates as we age. It is not yet known which chemicals within our environment stimulate free radical production: crop sprays, pesticides and household cleaning items are some of the products under investigation. Those people living in a built-up area, with exhaust fumes and lots of chemicals in their environment, are likely to have more free radicals in their body than country dwellers, who live in a less-polluted environment and on a diet of freshly grown organic fruit and vegetables.

The ageing process affects the skin in the following ways.

- Cell renewal is always faster in youth. The older we get, the slower the renewal process becomes, until it stops altogether.
- The genetic information in each cell gets a little diluted every time the cell reproduces, so the body cells of an 80-year-old do not have the same information as a young baby's.
- Hormone production in both sexes varies with age and contributes to the skin's development, health and deterioration.
- Fewer skin cells are being reproduced as a person gets older.
- The underlying structures supporting the skin begin to offer less support – the collagen and elastin fibres in the skin degenerate, muscular tension diminishes and wrinkles appear.
- The adipose tissue (the fat) supporting the skin diminishes and the skin starts to sag and gravity begins to win!
- Sun damage and pigmentation disorders become more noticeable as the melanin production within the skin lessens. Age or liver spots (lentigo) may appear on the surface of the epidermis.
- The face shape may alter if extensive dental work has been done or teeth are replaced with false ones – this causes the contours to drop and may make the face age.

Age grouping of the skin

Teenage years, 13–20 years

Just as the body is changing at puberty and getting ready for the reproduction stage of the human life cycle, so the emotional development also begins, making teenagers acutely aware of themselves and their relationships with their peers.

In females puberty is beginning earlier, often by the age of ten or twelve, which is largely due to better nutrition. Raging hormones dictate the development of the body, causing both the sexual development and the emotional highs and lows that accompany this dramatic change.

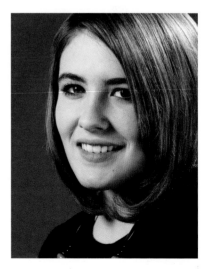

Teenagers have firm, compact skin

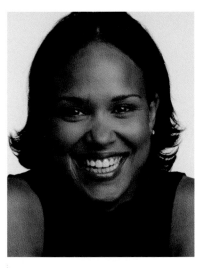

Skin is at its peak in the twenties

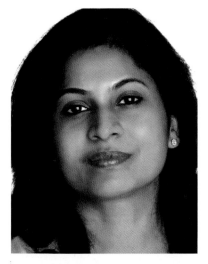

In the thirties, skin begins to dry out and fine lines appear

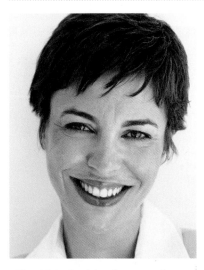

The skin's elasticity disappears in the forties

At this age the skin should be firm and compact, with a good supporting structure of collagen and elastin to give it a smooth feel. Unfortunately, the hormone levels can be unbalanced and the sebaceous glands can produce too much sebum, leading to blackheads and congested skin. Acne is common in this age group and may be directly related to high progesterone levels, so is more common in boys than girls.

Teenage boys may also cause skin problems by neglect — regular skin cleaning with the correct products can diminish skin problems but can be perceived as not a masculine pastime. However, with males accounting for a larger proportion of retail skin care sales than ever before, there is no reason for a teenager not to use a foaming facial cleanser designed for the male skin to help keep the skin clear.

A proportion of late-teen skins are not as clear as they could be for reasons that are self-inflicted. A poor diet of fast food, few vegetables and an excessive alcohol intake, combined with smoking, do nothing to enhance the skin. The only advantage is that this age group has youth on its side and the skin will recover more easily.

Adulthood, 20–30 years

This is when the chubbiness of the teenage years and the raging hormones disappear, or at least settle down, so the skin is at its peak. It looks fresh, radiant and glowing. The underlying structure is good, there are no fine lines developing yet, and providing good health is enjoyed and a healthy diet gives the body the correct nutrients, the skin is good.

Tiredness in young parents, bad lifestyle choices and simply 'burning the candle at both ends' will take its toll on this generation if care is not taken. Good choices in the appropriate skincare range and protection with a moisturiser, along with correct use of sunscreens, will be an investment for the future.

30–40 years

The skin begins to dry out and slows its reproduction down, with fine lines appearing, usually on the neck area first. The jawline is firmly defined at the beginning of the decade but can show signs of change. It may lose its definition, or if the client puts on weight, it will fill out and a double chin may form. Puffiness may be found in the cheeks — any weight gain in the face or body is instantly ageing.

The facial tissues begin to lose their fatty layer and tiredness can creep into the eye area. Creases and wrinkles remain after the depressions that form them have disappeared. Correct use of skincare products and protection against UV damage is essential in this age group as prevention is better than cure. A neck and hand cream will prevent dehydration, that is water loss. Many clients forget this — they may spend a fortune on their faces and forget that hands and neck areas are the true age reflector.

40–50 years

There is still a good clear definition of features, but 'temporary' double chins and wrinkles developed in the late thirties become a permanent feature. Elasticity and the supporting structures of collagen and elastin fibres are diminishing, especially if the client is female and is undergoing the menopause, which may start towards the fifties. Oestrogen levels start to fall and this affects bone density, elasticity in the tissues and skin thickness.

The skin becomes thinner and more prone to damage from UV and the environment. Blemishes, broken capillaries and pigmentation changes begin to occur.

50–70 years

All women will have begun the menopause in this age group and the skin will be loose and thin. It may feel coarse to the touch, and the eyes are lined and puffy. The muscle tissue around the eyes and mouth develops depressions, seen as wrinkles around them, and the lip line loses definition. The sebaceous glands have slowed down the production of sebum and care must be taken to keep the skin lubricated and free from infection. With ageing the skin loses some of its ability to fight infection and heal itself quickly. Facial hair growth may start to be obvious around the mouth and chin. This hair is coarse and thick because of the influence of the male hormone testosterone which is not being balanced by oestrogen.

Over 70 years

At this stage the skin has the appearance of being soft. There may be very little underlying fat to support the facial structure, and deeper furrows appear from the corner of the nose towards the lips and from the outer mouth down to the chin. Darkened patches may appear, or loss of pigment may be seen, especially on the hands and arms. The throat, neck and chest are very lined and like tissue paper, with very little sebum to lubricate the skin.

Can we slow the rate of ageing?

Evidence suggests that genes affect how long people live: long life seems to run in families. It is also known that cells have a programmed maximum number of divisions before they die off, so your life span is, to some degree, predetermined.

However, there are some sensible precautions you should be advising your clients to take.

- **Eat healthily** – people on lower calorie diets tend to live longer and meeting the body's additional demands as you age is important, e.g. a female who has heavy periods throughout her life will need more iron, a menopausal client will need more calcium to help keep bones healthy.

- **Keep physically active** – three half-hour aerobic sessions a week will help to keep circulation and metabolism going and will stimulate the body to repair itself (a brisk walk or swim will get the cardiovascular system working).

- **Get enough sleep or rest** – rest allows the body to repair and heal itself and the brain activity to slow and so the brain can sift through all the stimulation it has received during the day. Sleep deprivation is very harmful to the body in the long term.

- **Remain mentally active** – the more you use your brain, the better it works and the longer you remain alert. Doing a crossword, mental arithmetic, music and learning poetry is an ideal brain activity as you get older.

- **Remember good health maintenance** – this includes avoiding smoking (very ageing on the skin), moderate alcohol intake and low medication levels.

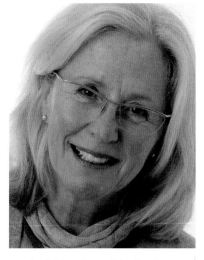

In the fifties, skin will be lined around the eyes and the mouth

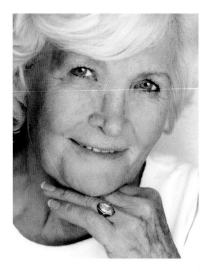

When we reach sixty, care must be taken to lubricate the skin

Anti-ageing treatments

The key here is 'prevention is better than cure'. In other words, encourage the client to look after their skin as early as possible, rather than waiting until the signs of ageing have begun to show. Looking after the skin in the twenties and thirties and developing good skincare habits, using sun protection and maintaining a work/life balance will pay dividends for a client in their sixties.

Anti-ageing treatments cannot turn back years of poor skin care and neglect, nor can they stop the ageing process. Some can significantly enhance the skin's appearance immediately. However, continuous treatments are needed for a long-term effect. The only true anti-ageing creams are sun protection creams with a high SPF factor – these prevent the skin from being harmed by the sun's rays.

Moisturisers

Contrary to popular belief, moisturisers do not add moisture to the skin, but rather they prevent moisture from being lost. This is achieved with the use of non-irritating oils and emollients such as lanolin, or vegetable-based or petroleum-based oils, which form a thin layer on top of the epidermis and stop water from literally evaporating out of the body. The result is that the outermost layers of the skin absorb the water being released by the deeper layers, so small wrinkles are filled out and the skin looks and feels a lot softer. Moisturising the skin also helps protect it from air pollution, harsh weather conditions and the drying effect of air conditioners. Most importantly, the majority of moisturisers contain ingredients that provide UV protection, which can affect the skin throughout the year, not just in the summer months.

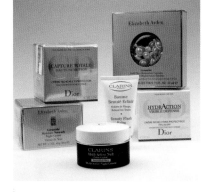

Moisturising products prevent moisture loss from the skin

Recommending good skin care products

Don't be afraid to offer your own salon range as a retail sale to your client. They have come to you in your role as a professionally trained therapist and will be looking to you for a recommendation for skin care that works! The over-the-counter products bought in a local store are fairly weak and diluted, so will not be as effective as those sold in the salon.

Salon strength moisturiser and serums, especially those in the 'cosmecutical' range – that is with more active ingredients in them – will work far better and penetrate further down into the epidermis and rehydrate the lower layers, where the cells are forming. Don't think of it as selling a product: think of it as recommending the best for the client.

Salon treatments

Any treatment which helps the desquamation process, that is the old cells of the epidermis being shed and new cells coming to the surface, is going to help the skin look clean and fresh. Combine a treatment that deep cleanses and then rehydrates the skin using an electrical current, such as in a galvanic facial, and the result is instant: the skin looks plump and refreshed and very, very clean. However, as we have already discovered, nothing prevents the ageing process, so all salon treatments will only last as long as the treatments are carried out on a regular basis. Scrubs, face masks and electrical treatments will work on the outer layers of the epidermis and will improve the look and feel of the skin. However, under the Trade Descriptions Act, a salon would be liable to prosecution if advertising these treatments as anti-ageing.

Alpha-hydroxy acids (AHAs) and skin peels

These treatments work by applying a chemical agent or acid (e.g. AHAs or vitamin A in the form of retionic acid) to the skin which dissolves the outermost layers, thus temporarily reducing fine lines and other superficial signs of ageing. A full consultation is essential as occasionally the client may have an adverse reaction, particularly if the concentration of the active ingredient is quite high, or if the product is left on the skin for too long. Timing is crucial. Always carry out a patch test and always do this treatment in the salon – it is not for home use as it is a professional treatment. Peels also leave the skin far more susceptible to damage from UV rays and so sun protection is essential following treatment. However, peels are very effective in making the skin heal faster and therefore cell production is speeded up, something that happens naturally in young skin. This is not a treatment to be given immediately before a special occasion, such as a wedding, and needs careful planning so the skin is healed and blooming at the right time.

These treatments should only be carried out by trained professionals and a full aftercare programme is recommended as the skin is left vulnerable.

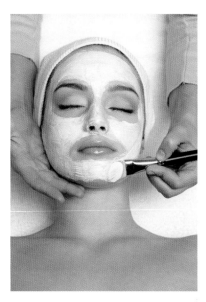

Salon treatments such as a facial mask help the skin look fresh and clean

Micro-dermabrasion (MDA)

Micro-dermabrasion (MDA) is the professional exfoliation of the top layer (stratum corneum) of the epidermis, using minute aluminium oxide crystals which are smoothed onto the face using a negative vacuum suction unit. The crystals are used once across the skin and disposed of as they contain all the dead skin cells, old make-up and accumulations from the skin. Some machines use a diamond head for the same effect which can be sterilised and reused on different clients. The removal of the top cells of the epidermis will encourage new cell formation and give the skin a renewed look; it encourages the skin to replace the stratum corneum and go into 'hyper repair' mode. MDA can be used as a one-off treatment to perk up the skin prior to a special occasion, but is best given as a course of six treatments with a maintenance programme once a month after that.

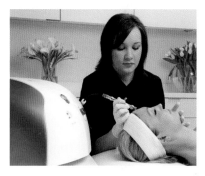

A micro-dermabrasion treatment taking place

This treatment needs to be carried out by a professionally trained therapist, with a full consultation and aftercare given. Some medical treatments make this unsuitable: for example, if the client has been taking medication such as Accutane to treat acne, then the skin is already thin and dermabrasion is not suitable. If the client has recently had filler of collagen injected or Botox® injections, again do not treat. It may mean that the filler is dispersed through the tissue, and spreads. Skin conditions such as psoriasis are also unsuitable as the skin's cells' replacement time is already speeded up from an average of 28 days to 5 or 6, so this treatment would accelerate the problem.

MDA is especially effective on scarring and stretch marks as it stimulates new cell growth.

Laser skin resurfacing

The word 'laser' is an acronym for Light Amplification by Stimulated Emission of Radiation, and laser therapy for the skin is becoming a very popular salon treatment. Laser treatment can be used for skin ageing and wrinkles, as the light stimulates the capillary level, so improving the circulation. Acne and cellulite also respond well to laser treatment, as do pigmented lesions and the removal of tattoos. The pigment is broken down into minute particles and removed through the lymphatic system.

You and the skin

Hair removal is also carried out in salons using impulse light. The heat travels into the melanin within the hair and goes down into the dermal papilla which is destroyed. A course of treatments is very effective in hair removal. Although expensive, it is worthwhile.

Full aftercare and support should be given as sunlight can be very damaging to a skin following laser treatment. Full training and a competent certificate are required for insurance, as laser work is specialised.

Collagen treatments

Collagen is a protein that is the principal ingredient of white fibrous connective tissue found within tendons, skin, bone, cartilage and ligaments. Despite any claims made by the manufacturers of collagen-containing products, it is said that the skin cannot absorb artificial collagen.

However, one collagen treatment that is temporarily effective and growing in popularity is collagen replacement therapy (CRT). This involves collagen being injected directly into the dermis to improve the appearance of fine lines and pockmarks. Collagen injections to the lips to create a 'bee sting' pout to the lip shape are common, but can go wrong if the client has an allergic reaction to the injection, leaving the lips very swollen and sore.

Avoid treating a client after a collagen treatment as there is a danger that massage movements could move the implant to another area.

Botox® treatments

Botox is a protein produced by a bacterium, Clostridium botulinum, which can relax and paralyse muscles located at the site where it is injected, thus reducing lines and wrinkles in that area. It is often used to treat frown lines and crow's feet around the eyes. It originated to help sufferers with muscular eye problems but doctors noticed a side effect of minimal lining in the area. Once again, the effects are only temporary, and regular treatments are required. These should only be carried out by someone trained in injectable treatments. Spas often employ a nurse or doctor to administer these injections. Side effects can include dropped contours or a raised eyebrow, headaches and flu-like symptoms. Too much and the face looks expressionless, but for a client with a permanent frown line (or nasal labia lines) it will help retrain the muscle and prevent the skin folds from becoming worse.

The long-term effects of this botulinum-based treatment are not yet known. A recent report in the *Journal of Cosmetic Dermatology* suggests that people using Botox® to defeat the signs of ageing may simply be developing more wrinkles in nearby areas, as neighbouring muscles try to compensate for those that are paralysed.

Cosmetic surgery

Surgery is an invasive treatment and carries all the risks of any other medical operation. It is, however, considered an affordable treatment by many, and it can be very successful. Sagging contours and wrinkles can be removed by tightening the eye area or chin or having a complete face-lift, and this will reduce the signs of ageing. However, there is a danger of the skin looking too tight and not in keeping with the rest of the body — many film stars may look good in pictures of their face alone, but the neck and hands reflect their true age when a larger picture is taken. This can look most odd. Too much or poor surgery procedures can make the face look frozen, which is not a good thing for an actor who relies on expression to portray emotions.

Cosmetic surgery should only be considered after a great deal of research and through a recognised medical referral. The newspapers often report that so-called 'clinics' cause a lot of pain and distress to 'patients' as they are not medically qualified to carry out procedures for cosmetic surgery, or because the post-operation care is so poor that secondary infection may occur.

In some cases, corrective surgery can be very successful and most beneficial, especially if the physical problem causes psychological distress too. The correction of a hare lip, reshaping of a broken nose or pinning back ears that protrude can give back client confidence and improve a person's self-image.

Stop the clock!

In conclusion, the ageing process is inevitable. Some treatments can suspend the process, but they cannot stop it. Take time to explain to your clients a little about the ageing process, and be honest about the limitations of any treatment they may be considering as well as its benefits. Having integrity means being honest and honouring your personal relationship with your clients. Rather than mislead or give false information about ageing and related treatments, discuss the lifestyle changes that will encourage clients to be active in preserving their quality of life: advise them to give up smoking, eat a healthy diet, drink plenty of water, take regular exercise and embark on a good skincare routine, including protection from the sun.

The skin and the sun

Coco Chanel introduced a tanned skin into high society in the 1930s when she was one of the first travellers to the South of France in the summer months. It became a sign of wealth and social standing if you could afford a tan as it meant you were rich enough to travel abroad. Going back through history the reverse is true: ladies and gentlemen of the 'upper classes' had very light faces and used powder to emphasise their whiteness. Only manual farm labourers had a tan, and this meant you had a job working outside in the sun. Unfortunately, we now think of a healthy skin as being a tanned one. This is, of course, not true. (Tanning is the name of the process used to dry out a cow's hide in the sunshine to turn it into leather!)

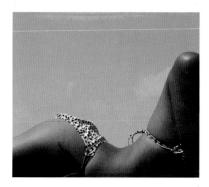

Remember – a tanned skin is a damaged skin

We all need a little sunlight to help with the production of vitamin D; the recommendation is half an hour per day of gentle exposure to ensure good manufacture. However, the possibility of skin cancer has made people aware of the dangers of sun exposure and, ironically, there have been cases reported in the media of people using too much sun cream and not getting enough vitamin D resulting in poor bone and joint functioning.

Sunlight also helps to relieve certain conditions like asthma, aching joints and psoriasis, and remember that, along with aiding health, sunlight gives a real psychological boost. However, we all know that too much sun can be positively harmful to the skin.

The immediate result of too much sun is severe sunburn, and many of us have experienced the painful blisters, fever and swelling that come from too much sun too fast. Another result of sun exposure is prematurely aged skin. The sun causes the skin to thicken and gives it a leathery, coarse appearance. With enough time, the sun weakens the skin's elasticity by cross-linking the collagen fibres in the dermis. This results in sagging and wrinkles on all sun-exposed areas.

The sun also causes dark pigmentation patches and scaly grey growths known as keratoses, which are often pre-cancerous. Sunburn and prematurely aged skin are not the worst results of constant exposure to the sun; skin cancer is. Almost all of the 300,000 cases of this disease that develop annually are considered to be sun-related. Some people are more at risk than others. Britain is fast catching up with Australia in numbers of skin cancer patients — in fact the promotion of skin cancer awareness in hotter countries is bringing down their skin cancer rate as ours is growing.

People with black skins are relatively safe because the darker skin provides good protection against UV light. Those with light skin, notably redheads and blondes, are at the greatest risk due to less melanin in the skin.

Certain drugs, such as antibiotics, medicated soaps and creams, and even barbiturates and birth control pills, can make the skin more susceptible to damage.

All clients concerned with premature ageing should be advised on the dangers of sun exposure, and a sunscreen or sun block should be recommended to them. Those clients who are avid sun worshippers should be educated to understand the relationship between the sun and skin cancer.

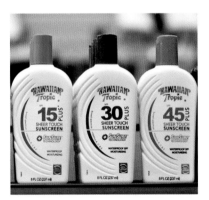

Always use a good sun cream to protect your skin

Once the UV light has caused cross-linking and thickening in the dermis and has predisposed the skin to premature ageing, there is no reversal of the damage. Plastic surgery techniques can help disguise the sagging by re-draping the skin, but this does not compensate for the damage that has occurred. It is, therefore, the first topic that must be discussed with the client who expresses concern about ageing. Advice on sun protection should be given verbally and in a written fact sheet. Indeed, the only cosmetic product that can legally be labelled 'anti-ageing' is a sunscreen or sun block preparation.

Concern is growing in the medical world for 'tanorexia', where young girls are becoming addicted to the use of sunbeds in tanning centres. Often, the use of these machines is not monitored and the client pays for the time on the sunbed, so they go several times a week to top up their tan. Unfortunately, this has resulted in a large increase in the incidence of skin cancers in young people, where it would not be expected under natural circumstances.

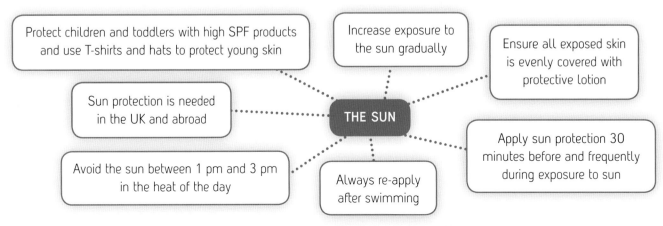

Protect children and toddlers with high SPF products and use T-shirts and hats to protect young skin

Increase exposure to the sun gradually

Ensure all exposed skin is evenly covered with protective lotion

Sun protection is needed in the UK and abroad

THE SUN

Apply sun protection 30 minutes before and frequently during exposure to sun

Avoid the sun between 1 pm and 3 pm in the heat of the day

Always re-apply after swimming

While sun preparations are not included in the normal facial routine in a salon, lots of clients need the right information for homecare advice and use of the correct products, especially if going on holiday either in the UK or abroad. Remind clients who are heading off on skiing holidays that they should consider taking sun protection; sunlight bounces off snow and, even though it may be cold, they should still use a sunscreen or sun block.

Sun protection can come in the form of lotion, cream or milk, and some large manufacturers have now designed a spray-on application of sun protection.

Sunscreens filter the harmful ultraviolet rays, UVA and UVB, for a period of time. Most are water resistant and contain moisturisers to help nourish the skin. They come in various strengths, measured by a sun protection factor (SPF) ranging from 2–35. The higher the SPF number, the better the protection. The wearer can stay out in the sun for a longer time depending on the number: for example, SPF 6 permits sun exposure six times longer than with unprotected skin without burning; an SPF of 30 allows sun exposure 30 times longer. The choice of SPF depends upon the skin type and the strength of the sun. The nearer the equator, the hotter the sun, so a higher protection factor would be needed in, say, the Mediterranean than in the UK. The sun's rays are also reflected so there is a risk of getting sunburnt when sailing or skiing, even when the temperature is low.

Sun blocks are total blocks and will screen out all the sun's rays. They have become essential in some countries, for example in Australia, where there is a high incidence of skin cancer. Sun blocks are seen as coloured strips of cream that sit on the nose and forehead – very popular with cricketers.

Skin products for different types of skin

See individual products and follow individual recommendations as products do vary. As sun on the face accelerates the ageing process, clients should be advised to wear a hat or cover the face liberally with the correct SPF cream.

Most manufacturers recommend the following:

Skin type	Recommended sun preparation
Fair skin or redhead with fair skin burns easily after 30 minutes' exposure	20–35 SPF or sun block for complete protection
Sallow-skinned person who is fair will tan, but feels sore after 30 minutes	10–20 SPF
Darker skins that tan easily but tend to get sore initially	10–15 SPF

Self-tanning creams

This is a very popular salon treatment for both face and body, and the safest way to get a tan. After exfoliation and moisturising, the tanning lotion is applied. It will develop over several hours and last for several days. Most large cosmetic houses make self-tans for the face, which are not as strong as the body self-tan. These are often in the form of an impregnated tissue, which just wipes over the facial area and leaves a residue which develops into a tan. There are also spray guns which deliver a fine mist of the product all over the body, for a speedy application.

The active ingredient is a chemical, dihydroxyacetone, which reacts with the keratin in the skin to produce a golden colour through oxidation. This has become a very popular salon treatment to offer clients. It looks very natural and lasts about a week, depending upon the depth of the application.

Think about it

Self-tanning application will only be as good as the surface it goes onto – a bit like nail varnish! If the skin is dry or rough, then the colour will come out patchy and darker in some places.

You and the skin

An increasingly popular treatment in the salon is to offer a complete body spray application, where the client stands in an open cubicle with three sides, and tan is literally sprayed all over the body. This application is carried out with a commercial tanning gun, which pumps the liquid tan through a nozzle turning it into a mist. The tan must be allowed to dry on the skin. A setting time is required, so the client relaxes in a reclining chair and then showers the residue off. The tan is visible immediately and develops into a deeper tan over the next 24 hours.

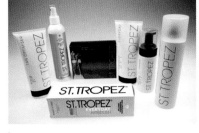

Self-tanning products

For your portfolio

When out shopping, pick up several samples of self-tanning preparations and try them out at home. Remember to exfoliate first and then apply moisturiser before applying the tan. Follow the manufacturer's instructions and apply the tan to your legs.

Note the different textures and smells. Which one did you prefer? Which one gave the most natural colour? (Do remember to scrub your palms if you did not wear gloves, otherwise they will be tanned too!)

Check your knowledge

1 AHA stands for:
 a) alpha hydrogen acids
 b) alpha hydro acids
 c) alkaline help acids
 d) alpha hydroxy acids.

2 Chloasma is easily recognised as:
 a) white patches of skin
 b) pink patches of skin
 c) yellow patches of skin
 d) brown patches of skin.

3 Which of these is NOT a contra-indication to a treatment?
 a) Leucoderma
 b) Cancer
 c) Impetigo
 d) Dermatitis

4 Acne vulgaris is caused by a:
 a) fungal infection
 b) bacterial infection
 c) congenital condition
 d) viral infection.

5 Eczema is a:
 a) fungal infection
 b) bacterial infection
 c) congenital condition
 d) viral infection.

6 A Wood's lamp gives off:
 a) ultraviolet light
 b) infrared light
 c) green light
 d) orange light.

7 The Fitzpatrick classification system measures:
 a) blood flow in the skin
 b) tanning properties of skin types
 c) the acid mantle of the skin
 d) muscle tone of the skin.

8 Intrinsic ageing of the skin means:
 a) the internal body clock of cells
 b) the external factor of pollution
 c) the effect of sunlight on the skin
 d) the importance of diet as you age.

9 Blepharitis is an infection of the:
 a) mouth
 b) ears
 c) eyes
 d) nose.

10 The function of the acid mantle is to:
 a) control blood flow to the skin
 b) produce histamine
 c) control bacteria on the skin
 d) plump up collagen levels.

You and the skin

Related anatomy and physiology

What you will learn

- Bones of the head, face, neck and shoulder girdle
- Bones of the arm and leg
- The skin – structure and functions
- Structure of the nails
- Muscles of the face, neck and shoulder area
- Muscles of the arm and leg
- Hair
- Blood
- The lymphatic system
- Structure of the heart
- Cell

Introduction

As a beauty therapist you should have an understanding of the body and its basic functions so that you can give the most effective treatments to your client. When you can look at the body with knowledge and understanding you will be able to identify any problems and treat them with suitable products, and make recommendations to help your client.

The information in this section is compatible with the new standards for VRQ Level 2 Beauty Therapy. It can, however, be used to support other qualifications within the beauty therapy framework.

The depth of knowledge for VRQ at Level 2 is very defined; the requirements for this section have been taken directly from the standards for each unit. Therefore no other anatomy or physiology is required to complete these qualifications. The related knowledge, to support anatomy links to a specific treatment given, is contained within the book.

A Try it out activity is included at the end of each topic. You may like to undertake this either with your study group or independently.

Bones of the head, face, neck and shoulder girdle

This section will teach you about the position of the bones of the head, face, neck, shoulders and bones of the forearm, hand and lower leg and foot.

The arrangement of bones that are joined together is known as a **skeleton**. The skeleton gives the body shape; it provides **attachment** for muscles and protects delicate organs. For good facial work the therapist needs to identify the bones of the head, neck, face and shoulders.

Bones that form the skull (cranium)

The skull, also known as the cranium, is a very hard structure that protects the brain. Although it looks like one bone it is actually made up of 22 separate bones. Ten bones make up the skull and 12 form the face. These bones are fused together at ridged joints called **sutures**. The sutures are classed as fibrous joints because they only allow movement in the head of babies for ease of the head coming through the birth canal. A baby's skull has soft spots called the fontanelles. Over a period of about 18 months the bones gradually join together. During this time, care should be taken to protect the baby's head.

There are many openings in the skull to allow blood vessels and nerves to enter and leave. The largest of these is at the base of the skull and this is called the foramen magnum. This opening allows the spinal cord and blood vessels to pass to and from the brain.

Key terms

Skeleton – the bony framework of the body which supports and protects the tissues and organs. It allows movement through specially designed joints and provides an attachment for muscles. It is also a store for minerals and blood cells. Erythrocytes (red blood cells) and leucocytes (white blood cells) are formed in bones. From birth to late teenage years bones continue to grow and have the ability throughout life to repair themselves, although with age this process takes longer.

Attachment – where the muscle is attached to the bone. The origin is where the muscle is attached and does not move. Where it joins and is moveable, it is called the insertion.

Sutures – ridged, fibrous joints of the skull.

Think about it

Skulls vary in size and shape. Your genes can dictate many features of your face shape, such as prominent cheekbones. A bigger skull does not necessarily mean a person is more intelligent.

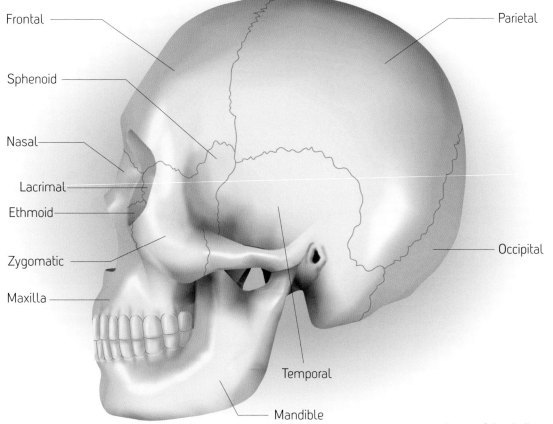

Frontal

Sphenoid

Nasal

Lacrimal

Ethmoid

Zygomatic

Maxilla

Parietal

Occipital

Temporal

Mandible

Bones of the skull

Bone	Position
Occipital bone (1)	At the back of the skull
Parietal (2)	Positioned at the back of the head and forms the roof of the skull
Frontal (1)	Forms the front of the skull, forehead, and upper eye sockets
Temporal (2)	At the side, around the ears
Sphenoid (1)	At the base of the skull, wing shaped, forms the temple
Ethmoid (1)	Positioned between the frontal and sphenoid bones and forms roof of the nasal cavities
Lacrimal (2)	One in each eye orbit These bones are fused together to form the shape of the skull, and their joins are known as sutures

The skull is attached to the body via the **vertebral column**. The vertebral column enables the head to turn and tilt. The weight of the head is supported by the neck, the shoulder girdle bones and muscles.

Key terms

Vertebral column – the spine or backbone which runs from the cranium (head) to the coccyx. It keeps the body upright and supports it, as well as protecting the spinal nerves and spinal cord.

The bones of the face

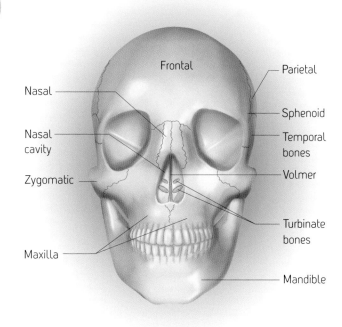

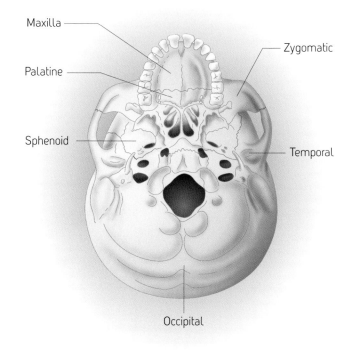

Bones of the face

Bones of the face from below

Bone	Position
Zygomatic bones (2)	These form the cheek bones
Maxillae (2)	These form the upper jaw, most of the side wall of the nose and the front part of the soft palate
Mandible (1)	This is the lower jaw and is the only moving bone in the face, allowing movement of the mouth for chewing and talking
Nasal (2)	These form the bridge of the nose
Turbinate (2)	The bones inside the nose
Vomer (1)	This forms part of the nasal septum
Palatine (2)	These form part of the side walls of the nose and the hard palate

The openings in the base of the skull provide spaces for the entrance and exit of many blood vessels, nerves and other structures. Projections and slightly elevated portions of the bones provide for the attachment of muscles. Some portions contain delicate structures, such as the part of the temporal bone that encloses the middle and internal sections of the ear. The air sinuses provide lightness and serve as vibrating chambers for the voice. There are four sinuses: the frontal, ethmoidal, sphenoidal and maxillary.

Bones of the shoulder girdle, upper vertebra, upper arm and chest

The bones of the shoulder girdle allow the arms to move freely. The **clavicle** is more commonly known as the collar bone, and you can feel it in the area where the collar of a shirt or blouse would sit. The **scapula** is commonly referred to as the shoulder blade. The scapula is only secured to the skeleton by muscle, so it is fairly free to move about.

Bone	Girdle
Clavicle (2)	Across the front of the chest, going from each shoulder to the breast bone
Scapula (2)	At the back of the shoulder girdle, sitting on top of the rib cage
Sternum (1)	This is often called the breast bone; it forms part of the rib cage
Cervical vertebra (7)	The vertebrae which form the neck; the first two are called the Atlas and Axis, and support and allow free movement of the head
Humerus (2)	These bones form the top of each arm; they move in a groove in the clavicle by a joint called a ball and socket
Hyoid (1)	This is a U-shaped bone at the base of the tongue that supports the tongue muscles.

Key terms

Clavicle – the collar bone.

Scapula – the shoulder blade.

Try it out

Draw your arms back, and look in the mirror. Can you see your scapula? It may be easier to identify this on a partner.

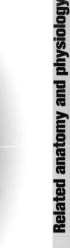

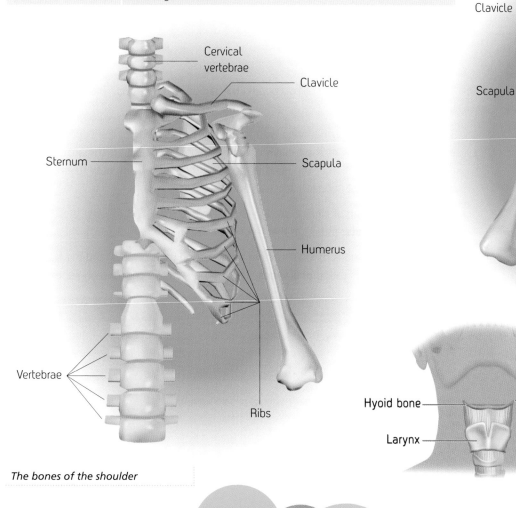

The bones of the shoulder

Related anatomy and physiology

Bones of the arm and leg

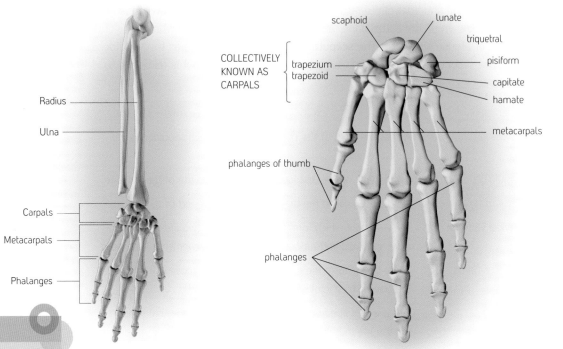

Bones of the forearm and hand

Bones of the hand and wrist

Key terms

Radius – bone on the outer side of the forearm; smaller of the two bones in the lower arm.

Ulna – bone on the inner side of the forearm; larger of the two bones in the lower arm.

Humerus – bone of the upper arm; called the 'funny bone'.

Ligament – strong bands of fibrous, connective tissue binding bones together.

Carpals – bones that make up the wrist joint, consisting of hamate, capitate, pisiform, triquetral, lunate, scaphoid, trapezium and trapezoid.

Metacarpals – bones that make up the palm of the hand.

Phalanges – bones that make up the fingers.

Pronation – rotation movement of the palm away from you (face down).

Supination – rotation movement of the palm to face you (face up).

The lower arm is made up of two bones: the **radius** and the **ulna**. The ulna is the larger of the two bones.

The radius and ulna form a hinge with the **humerus** (the bone of the upper arm sometimes referred to as the funny bone). This hinge joint enables the arm to flex and extend. The rotation of the hand is made by the radius being able to cross over the ulna. A **ligament** connects the two bones.

The wrist is made up of eight individual bones in two rows. Collectively these bones are known as **carpals**, although they each have individual names.

The palm of the hand is made up of five bones called **metacarpals**, and the fingers are made of three bones called **phalanges**. The thumb contains only two phalanges bones.

Try it out

Have the palm of your right hand facing you. Now rotate your palm so it turns away from you. This rotation movement is known as **pronation**. Now rotate your hand so your palm faces you again. This is called **supination**.

Think about it

A simple way to remember which forearm bone is which: ulna contains the letter 'l' and this bone goes to your little finger.

Bones of the lower leg and foot

The bones that make up the lower leg are the **tibia** and **fibula**. The tibia is often called the shinbone. This bone is the stoutest in the body and transmits body weight directly to the ankle joint. The fibula forms part of the ankle joint.

The foot is constructed in a similar way to the hand. Seven bones, all with individual names, make up the **tarsals** (like the wrist). Five **metatarsals** together support the major arches of the foot.

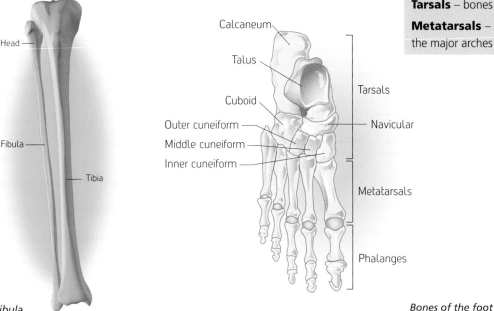

The tibia and fibula

Bones of the foot

The foot has four arches: two **transverse** (across the foot) and two **longitudinal** (from heel to toe). The function of these arches is to:

- provide support for the body
- act as shock absorbers
- aid posture.

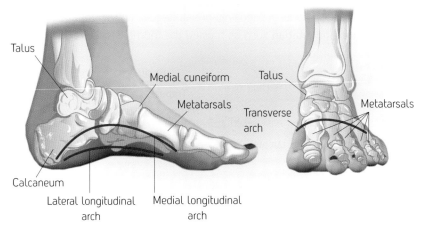

The major arches of the foot

Like the fingers, the toes are made of phalanges. The big toes have two phalanges each and the other toes have three.

Related anatomy and physiology

Types of joints

To enable movement in various ways the body has a number of different types of joint that allow different types of movement to occur. There are three basic joint types:

- ⦿ fibrous — this type of joint is fixed and you will see this in the sutures of the skull
- ⦿ cartiligaginous — this type of joint gives a limited amount of movement as in the vertebrae
- ⦿ synovial — this type of joint allows free movement. There are a number of types of synovial joint located around the body:

ball and socket — found in the hip and top of the humerus

hinge — the elbow and knee joints are hinge joints

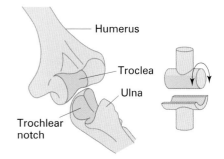

pivot — the head is a pivot

gliding joint — found in the wrist and ankles

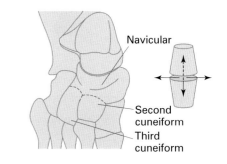

condyloid and saddle — condyloid or saddle joints allow for **abduction**, **adduction** and **rotation** such as moving the thumb.

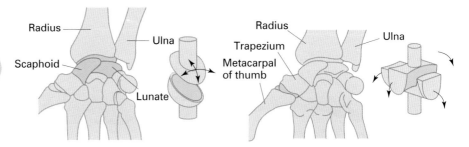

Key terms

Adduction – taking away from the mid line of the body.

Adduction – bringing back to the mid line of the body.

Rotation – a motion that occurs when a part turns on its axis. The head rotates on the neck when we shake it.

The skin – structure and functions

Refer to You and the skin, pages 181–226 for further information on the skin.

The skin's structure

Skin is a remarkable organ that is able to adapt and perform various functions. It can mould to different shapes, stretch and harden, but can also respond to delicate touch, feel pain, pressure, hot and cold, so it is regarded as an effective communicator.

Skin makes up about 12 per cent of an adult's body weight and consists of three layers: the **epidermis**, **dermis** and the **subcutaneous layer**. You can think of these layers like clothing. The epidermis is the outer skin, like a breathable waterproof jacket – this is the skin we see. Our skin, or dermis, is under this and could be thought of as a blouse or shirt with lots of pockets containing many different items. Underneath this is a cushioned soft layer for protection, like a soft thermal vest. This bottom layer (the subcutaneous layer) contains fat which helps to insulate and keep in warmth. The layers vary in thickness over different areas of the body. The thickest layers are over friction and gripping areas, such as the palm of the hand and soles of the feet, and the thinnest are over the eyelids, which must be light and flexible.

Key terms

Epidermis – outer layer of the skin.

Dermis – layer of skin below the epidermis.

Subcutaneous layer – the fatty tissue found beneath the dermis which contains fat cells that act as both insulation against heat being lost and protection for the internal organs.

Think about it

Even though on average skin is just 2 mm thick, it receives about one eighth of the blood supply for the whole body. In some areas, such as the soles of the feet, the skin can be 6 mm thick while on the eyelids, it's just 0.5 mm thick.

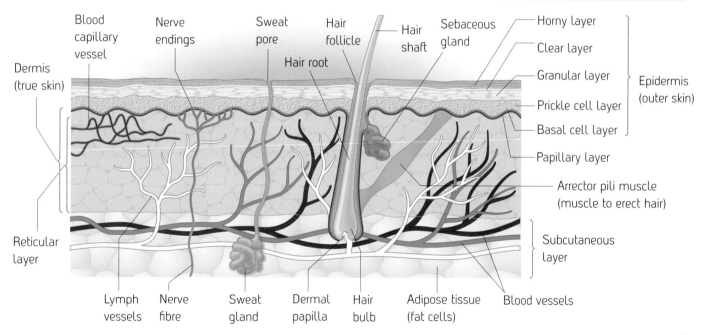

The structure of the skin

The epidermis

The epidermis is the outermost layer of the skin. It is made up of five layers.

1 Horny layer (**Stratum corneum**)
2 Clear layer (**Stratum lucidum**)
3 Granular layer (**Stratum granulosum**)
4 Prickle cell layer (**Stratum spinosum**)
5 Basal cell layer (**Stratum germinativum**)

Key terms

Stratum – layer.

Stratum corneum – horny layer, top layer of skin.

Stratum lucidum – clear layer, layer of skin beneath the horny layer.

Related anatomy and physiology

Key terms

Stratum granulosum – granular layer, layer of skin between the clear and prickle cell layers.

Stratum spinosum – prickle cell layer, layer of skin between the granular and basal layers.

Stratum germinativum – basal cell layer, bottom layer of skin.

Bacteria – single-celled micro-organisms found everywhere; can be either pathogenic (capable of causing disease) or non-pathogenic (not capable of causing disease).

Keratin – a fibrous protein that forms in the body. It is found in the skin, hair and nails.

Keratinisation – the production of keratin that occurs in the Stratum spinosum (prickle layer). The keratin is further formed in the Stratum granulosum (granular layer).

Hair – a fine thread-like filament; an appendage growing out from the skin, found on all parts of the body except the palms, soles of the feet and lips.

Desquamation – a natural process of shedding dead skin cells from the top, horny layer of the epidermis.

Melanocytes – pigment containing cells, which are responsible for the synthesis of melanin, and provide the different colours to the skin, including yellow, black and brown pigments in various strengths.

Melanin – pigment or colour found in skin or hair that protects us from the sun. It determines our colouring and is determined largely by hereditary influences and location in the world.

Basement membrane – a thin layer of connective tissue that joins the epidermis and dermis together.

Layers 1 to 3 – the stratum corneum, stratum lucidum and stratum granulosum – are dead and are constantly being shed. But the prickle cell and basal cell layers – layers 4 and 5 – are still living because the cells contain a nucleus and can therefore reproduce. Skin renews itself every 28 days.

For assessment you should know both the Latin and English names for the layers of the skin.

The layers of the epidermis need to be looked at in order of formation.

The five layers of the epidermis, or our outer skin, begin at the *Stratum germinativum* or basal cell or bottom layer (5). This skin is constantly being reproduced, as the cells contain a nucleus or seed. As the cells reproduce the layers get constantly pushed up into the next layer. Each of the layers has its own specific function.

The *Stratum spinosum* or prickle cell layer (4) is called this because the cells have spines, which prevent **bacteria** entering the cells and moisture being lost. These cells also have a nucleus and so reproduce.

The next layer is the *Stratum granulosum* or granular layer (3). The prickle cells lose their spines and become flatter. The nucleus dies and a protein is formed called **keratin**. The formation of keratin is called **keratinisation**. This protein prevents moisture loss and is found in skin, nails and **hair**.

The next layer is the *Stratum lucidum* or clear layer (2). This layer is for cushioning and protection and is found only on the palms of the hands and soles of the feet.

The final layer is the *Stratum corneum* or horny layer (1), where the cells are dead and ready to be shed. If you look at flakes of skin under a microscope they would resemble flakes of almond. The name for the shedding of the skin is **desquamation** (refer to You and the skin, page 191). This process speeds up as we age.

Layer	Function
1 Horny layer **Stratum corneum**	Made up of many flattened dead skin cells which contain the tough keratin This is the final top layer of skin. These cells are shed continuously to allow the new cells through.
2 Clear layer **Stratum lucidum**	3 to 4 rows thick of dead flattened cells. Only found on the palms of the hands and the soles of the feet, above the granular layer. These cells act as protectors in areas of friction.
3 Granular layer **Stratum granulosum**	2 to 4 layers thick, the cells begin to die and flatten. The middle layer of the epidermis. Waste and other substances from the cell get squashed together and harden.
4 Prickle cell layer **Stratum spinosum**	10 to 20 cells thick, with spines that connect with other cells. Sits on top of the basal layer. This layer of cells, called **melanocytes**, starts to harden and produce keratin. **Melanin** is also produced here which determines our colouring and helps protect against ultraviolet light. Macrophages sometimes referred to as Langerhans cells carry bacteria and foreign bodies from the epidermis to the dermis which sit in this layer to the lymph nodes to be destroyed and removed from the body.
5 Basal cell layer **Stratum germinativum**	A single layer of column-shaped cells. The deepest layer of epidermis. Continuously produces new cells. These cells are loosely attached to the dermis by a thin supportive layer called the **basement membrane**.

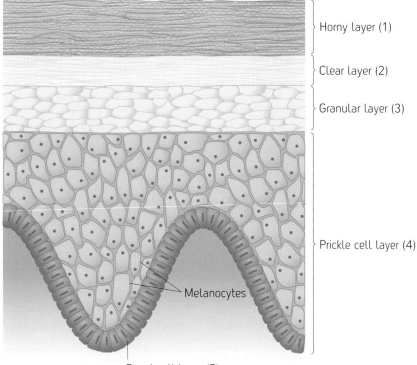

Horny layer (1)

Clear layer (2)

Granular layer (3)

Prickle cell layer (4)

Melanocytes

Basal cell layer (5)

The layers of the epidermis

You may be required to label this diagram for a written skin assessment.

The dermis

The dermis or true skin contains many structures. It can be subdivided into two parts.

1   Papillary layer

2   Reticular layer

The dermis contains the main components of the skin such as nerve endings (for pain, pressure, hot and cold), the blood supply and the lymph vessels, **hair follicles** and our sweat glands for temperature **regulation**.

Papillary layer

◉ Undulating wavy tissue, rich in blood and lymph vessels and nerve endings.

◉ Joins the dermis to the epidermis (the basement membrane).

◉ Area of cell reproduction, provides lots of nourishment and aids waste removal via lymph system.

Reticular layer

◉ Dense and fibrous, contains main components of dermis.

◉ Found beneath the papillary layer.

◉ Contains **collagen**, **elastin** and reticulin tissue.

◉ Contains fibroblast cells that produce collagen fibres.

◉ Contains mast cells which are found in the connective tissue nearer the outside of the body such as nose, skin and eyes. They are best known for their role in allergy by producing histamine, a protein that causes allergic reactions (hayfever) and heparin (which is used to treat and prevent blood clots).

Key terms

Hair follicle – threadlike growth of the epidermis.

Regulation – control.

Papillary layer – connected to the underside of the epidermis; a connective tissue that contains nerve endings and a network of blood and lymphatic capillaries.

Reticular layer – situated below the papillary layer; formed of tough, dense, fibrous connective tissue which contains collagen, elastic and reticular fibres for support and elasticity within the skin.

Collagen – protein found in white, fibrous connective tissue. In the skin it provides strength and resilience.

Elastin – allows the skin to stretch easily, and then regain its original shape.

Related anatomy and physiology

Key terms

Sudoriferous glands – found in the dermis; excrete waste products through sweat and help to control body temperature; classified as apocrine and eccrine.

Eccrine glands – sweat glands with ducts opening directly on to the surface of the skin; linked to the sympathetic nervous system, they help to regulate body temperature and are found all over the body, but more abundantly on the soles of the feet, palms of the hands and forehead. They produce sweat that is composed mainly of water and salts.

Apocrine glands – sweat glands that occur on hairy parts of the body, especially armpits and groin. They develop during puberty and produce sweat that contains fatty materials. It is the activity of these glands that causes body odour due to bacteria breaking down the organic compounds in the sweat.

The subcutaneous tissue

This is the fatty layer of the skin, underneath the dermis. Cells called adipocytes (sometimes called lipocytes) produce lipids, which are the fat cells from which we form subcutaneous tissue.

The job of the subcutaneous tissue is to:

- protect the muscles, bones and internal organs from being damaged
- provide insulation against the cold and provide a source of energy if the body should need it.

Functions of the skin

You can help yourself to remember the functions of the skin by the word 'shapes'.

S = Sensitivity

There are five types of nerve ending within the skin to help identify pain, touch, heat, cold and light pressure.

H = Heat regulation

The skin helps regulate the body's temperature by sweating to cool the body down when it overheats and shivering when it is cold. Shivering closes the pores. The tiny hairs that cover the body stand on end to trap warm air next to the skin and therefore prevent heat loss, when cold.

A = Absorption

Absorption of ultraviolet (UV) rays, from the sun. The skin synthesises vitamin D when exposed to UV light: modified cholesterol molecules in the skin are converted by the UV to vitamin D. The body needs vitamin D for the formation of strong bones and good eyesight. However, the skin has limited absorption properties. Only fat-soluble substances, such as oxygen, carbon dioxide, fat-soluble vitamins and steroids, along with small amounts of water are allowed through. Some creams, essential oils and some medication may be absorbed through the skin.

P = Protection

Too much UV light may harm the skin, so the skin protects itself by producing a pigment, seen as a tan, called melanin. Bacteria and germs are prevented from entering the skin by a protective barrier called the acid mantle. This barrier also helps protect against moisture loss. (Refer to You and the skin, page 190, for more information on the acid mantle and the pH of the skin.)

E = Excretion

Waste products and toxins are eliminated from the body through the sweat glands.

S = Secretion

Sebum and sweat are secreted on to the skin's surface. The sebum keeps the skin lubricated and soft, and the sweat combines with the sebum to form the acid mantle.

Structure	Location	Function
Sudoriferous glands There are two types: 1 **Eccrine glands** (sweat glands) 2 **Apocrine glands** (post-puberty sweat glands)	Eccrine glands are found all over the body but dense on the palms of the hands and soles of the feet. Apocrine glands are fewer in number and larger than eccrine. Only found in hairy parts of the body, i.e. armpits, nipples, anal and genital areas.	Eccrine glands produce sweat, water and urea, so help to regulate body temperature, remove toxin accumulations and help with the acid mantle. Apocrine glands are under the control of the nervous system and respond to sexual attraction, emotional demands and psychological factors.
Hair follicle A threadlike outgrowth of the epidermis	Found in the dermis but not present on the soles of the feet or the palms of the hands or lips.	Produces and contains the hair during its life cycle.
Hair Not present on the soles of the feet and the palms of the hand or on the lips	Grows in the follicles in the dermis and is then seen growing out through the epidermis.	Believed to be connected to the production of body warmth. It is also a sexual characteristic.
Sebaceous glands Not found where there are no follicles present – see hair follicles	In the dermis, adjacent to hair follicles.	Produce sebum to lubricate the hair and the skin. Combine with sweat to form the acid mantle. Help to waterproof the skin.
Arrector pili muscle (also spelt erector) Muscle tissue	Attached to the hair follicle at the base of the epidermis.	Raises the hair follicle to close the pore and so trap warmth in the body. Gives that goose pimple look to the skin.
Nerves Sensory nerve endings	Found on the dermis and subcutaneous tissue.	Respond to pain, pressure, heat, cold and touch. The nerves carry impulses to the brain for response by the body for protection.
Blood vessels These consist of **arteries**, **veins** and **capillaries**	Found in the dermis and subcutaneous layer.	Arteries carry nutrients and oxygen to the skin via capillaries. Veins remove waste products. Capillaries also help with heat regulation.
Lymph vessels	Found in the dermis and subcutaneous layer.	The body's secondary circulation system, they collect germs, bacteria and waste from the system that the blood supply cannot take. The lymph is filtered and returned to the bloodstream.

Location and function of structures found in the dermis and subcutaneous layer

Key terms

Sebaceous glands – exocrine glands found all over the body, in the dermis, apart from the soles of the feet and palms of the hands; secrete sebum and are situated adjacent to hair follicles.

Arrector pili muscle – fan-shaped, smooth muscle in the dermis attached to the base of each hair that contracts when the body surface is chilled causing the hair to stand erect.

Blood vessels – arteries, veins and capillaries that carry blood to and from the heart and body tissues.

Arteries – the largest blood vessels with thick muscular walls that carry blood away from the heart (except the pulmonary artery which carries deoxygenated blood to the lungs).

Veins – blood vessels conveying blood towards the heart (except the pulmonary vein which carries oxygenated blood from the lungs to the heart).

Capillaries – the smallest blood vessel in the body; has thin walls and is located between an arteriole and venule. A capillary is one cell thick, allowing the exchange of substances, such as oxygen, water and lipids, between blood and body cells.

Related anatomy and physiology

Additional knowledge

The specialised nerve endings in your skin all have different functions and are named after the people who discovered them.

- Pacinian corpuscles and Meissner's endings react to sudden pressure.
- Krause's bulbs, Merkel's discs and Ruffini's corpuscles respond to steady pressure.
- Krause's bulbs are sensitive to cold.
- Ruffini's corpuscles react to temperature changes.

Cells

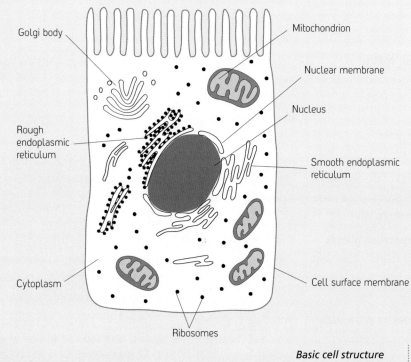

Basic cell structure

Cells are the basic building blocks of the body. There are about 200 different types of cells. Cells that group together form tissue, and several tissues grouped together form the organs of the body.

A cell is a parcel of complex chemicals that have a basic structure.

- **Cell membrane** – this is the outer wall of the cell. It consists of two layers of membrane with a thin fatty layer between. The membrane is slightly elastic and **porous** to allow nutrients in to feed the cell and waste products to be removed.

- **Cytoplasm** – this is a semi-solid, jelly-like substance that is made of approximately 70 per cent water.

- **Nucleus** – this is located in the middle of the cell. This is where the genetic information about the cell is interpreted. It is otherwise known as DNA (Deoxyribonucleic acid) which gives the body instructions on development and function.

- **Nucleolus** – this the control centre of the cell. It provides the genetic information.

Cells are living structures; therefore they exhibit the properties of all living things. In order for a cell to function it must have the following properties.

- **Mitochondria** – this generates energy for all the cells' activities and is vital for cell reproduction or **mitosis**.

- **Metabolisation** – this is essential for life. Metabolism involves taking in and using nourishment. The cell receives nourishment from the bloodstream, which passes through the porous membrane walls. Metabolism refers to the basic working of the body's cells and concerns the continuous chemical changes that occur to sustain life. Energy released is a by-product of the reactions within the cells.

- **Respiration** – this process allows oxygen and nutrients to pass into the cell and waste products to pass out of the cell.

- **Sensitivity** – this means that the cell is able to respond to a stimulus, which could be either physical, chemical or thermal: for example, the **contraction** of a muscle fibre when it is stimulated by a nerve impulse would cause movement.

- **Growth** – cells have the ability to grow until they are mature enough to reproduce.

- **Reproduction** – when growth in a cell is complete, reproduction takes place. The cells of the human body reproduce by division, making identical copies. This process is known as mitosis.

- **Excretion** – during metabolism the cell produces waste products that it can no longer use. If allowed to build up, these products will become harmful, so they are passed out through the cell wall via the porous cell membrane to be excreted.

- **Movement** – the cell needs to be able to move either fully or in part: for example, white **blood cells** (**macrophages**) move freely so that they are able to move quickly to the site of an infection.

Nerve cells are some of the biggest cells as they have tails that can be up to a metre long and can be seen without the aid of a microscope. Unlike other cells in the body that are continually being replaced, nerve cells have a long life and are rarely replaced.

Key terms

Mitosis – a complicated method of cell division occurring in specialist cells; the process involves four stages: prophase, metaphase, anaphase and telophase.

Contraction – tightening (tension in a muscle – the opposite is relaxation in the muscle).

Blood cells – known as corpuscles; they are red cells called erythrocytes and white cells called leukocytes.

Macrophages – the white defence cells that ingest bacteria and regulate immunity.

Related anatomy and physiology

Structure of the nails

The nails are the hardened growth on the ends of the fingers and toes. Their cell formation is similar to that of the skin and hair follicle, based on the protein keratin. The purpose of the nails is to protect the fingers and toes by providing a hardened covering. The nails contribute to the daily functions of the fingers and toes, and in the instance of finger nails many people use their nails as tools.

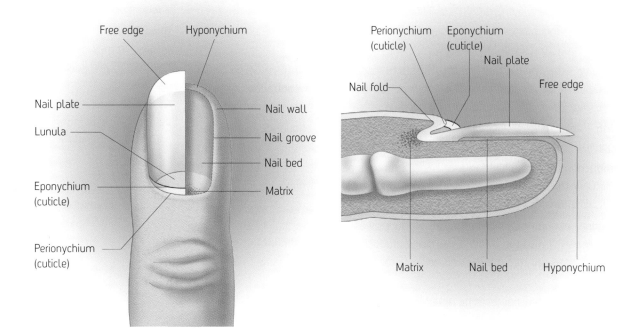

Structure of the nail unit

Key terms

Matrix – root of the nail; produces cells that form the nail plate.

Mantle – the area of tissue that contains the matrix.

Nail bed – underneath the nail plate.

Lunula – often called the 'half moon' as that is what it looks like; found at the base of the nail, often hidden by the cuticle.

Structure	Location	Function
Matrix	Situated in the dermis in an area of dense fibrous tissue called the mantle.	The reproductive part of the nail, where new cells are formed. It contains nerves, blood and lymph vessels. The continual process of cell renewal is called mitosis. If the matrix does not get enough nutrients, the nail may not grow correctly.
Mantle	An area of tissue that contains the matrix.	Helps protect the matrix cells from damage.
Nail bed	Underneath the nail plate.	Continuation of the matrix, similar to ordinary skin, with a good nerve supply and blood vessels. The nail bed gives a healthy nail its pink appearance.
Lunula (half moon)	At the base of the nail, linked to the nail plate. Sometimes hidden by the cuticle.	Visible part of the matrix. It is crescent-shaped with translucent appearance.

Lateral nail fold	An extension of the cuticle.	To prevent bacteria entering the matrix.
Nail groove	These are deep ridges like train tracks that run under the sides of the nail.	As the nail grows it runs along the grooves which help the nail to grow straight.
Nail plate	Lies on top of the nail bed.	The compressed keratinised cells produced by the matrix form the nail. They lie in three layers and are held together by moisture and fat.
Nail wall	Around the three sides of the visible nail plate.	The framework of skin to support the nail plate.
***Cuticle**	The barrier that protects the matrix by preventing bacteria entering the nail.	The horny layer of epidermis around the nail. It is constantly discarding old cells and producing new ones.
***Eponychium** (pronounced ep-on-nik-ee-um)	The extension of the cuticle around the nail.	To prevent bacteria entering.
***Perionychium** (pronounced peri-on-nik-ee-um)	Surrounds the entire nail border.	A framework of skin to support the nail plate.
Hyponychium (Pronounced hy-po-nik-ee-um)	Underneath the nail plate where the free edge is formed.	A horny layer of the epidermis for protection.
Free edge	An extension of the nail plate which grows over and beyond the finger tip. It does not adhere to the nail bed, so therefore it lacks the colour of the nail plate.	For protection of the nerves at the fingertip. This is what we shape during a manicure. It is the hardest part of the nail. The nail plate and therefore the free edge are dead so there is no pain when they are cut and shaped.

* These are often collectively referred to as the cuticle rather than by their individual names. The cuticle is an extension of the horny layer of the epidermis.

Key terms

Lateral nail fold – the flap of skin which cushions the cuticle and covers the matrix.

Nail groove – the border of the nail bed which allows the nail plate to grow upwards.

Nail plate – the tough protective coating of cells on top of the nail bed, which grows up, and we then paint with nail varnish.

Nail wall – around the nail plate along the three edges of skin.

Cuticle – a barrier around the nail plate to protect the matrix and prevent bacteria from entering.

Eponychium – extension of cuticle around the nail to prevent bacteria from entering under the cuticle.

Perionychium – surrounds the entire edge of the cuticle, to support the nail plate.

Hyponychium – under the free edge.

Free edge – the white part of the nail plate which grows up and is seen over the top of the finger when the palm is facing you.

Try it out

1 Look at your hands and finger nails. Can you identify your lunula? Do your cuticles overgrow your nail plate and is your free edge growing over your finger tip?
2 How much does a healthy nail grow each month and what should your nails look like?
3 Are your nails healthy? For further information on the skin and nails, refer to You and the skin, pages 181–226.

Related anatomy and physiology

Key terms

Voluntary muscles – muscles we can control with conscious thought such as skeletal muscles for movement.

Involuntary muscles – muscles we do not control with conscious thought such as digestion and respiration.

Extensor – straightens the muscle, or increases the angle between the joint, e.g. when the hand touching the shoulder then moves out so the arm is in a straight line.

Flexor – shortens the muscle, or decreases the angle between the joint, e.g. when the hand comes up towards the shoulder, the elbow joint is made smaller.

Tension – muscle will appear tight. This can be caused by over work or repetitive strain. A muscle could also be considered tense when preparing for exercise.

Fatigue – decrease in oxygen and nutrients to the muscles leading to stiffening/cramp.

Nail growth

The cells in the matrix reproduce to form the nail plate. As the cells multiply they are gradually pushed up, before they die and harden. This process is called keratinisation. For cells to reproduce, the matrix needs a good supply of oxygen and nutrients.

The growth of the nail can be influenced by:

- poor diet – through lack of vitamins and minerals
- illness – nails can also provide medical professionals with indications of general health and certain diseases
- medication – some medication can enhance or slow down growth rates
- age – cellular regeneration declines with age
- time of year (more growth in summer)
- injury to the matrix or nail bed
- neglect – if nails are looked after, their growth rate and appearance can be enhanced
- pregnancy – increases nail growth by up to 20 per cent
- poor circulation – affects the blood supply to the matrix, restricting cellular regeneration, which will affect growth.

If the cells in the matrix are damaged by illness or injury, the thickness of the nail plate can vary, showing itself as a furrow ridge or overgrowth of the nail plate.

A healthy nail grows at an average of 1 mm per week for finger nails, and 0.5 mm for toe nails, so it takes approximately six months for the nail to grow from matrix to free edge.

A healthy nail should have:

- supple unbroken cuticle
- no inflammation
- a natural sheen
- a pink glow from beneath the nail bed
- no ridges or spots
- an unbroken free edge.

Muscles of the face, neck and shoulder area

Muscles

The body is made up of more than 600 **voluntary muscles** (that is muscles we can control). They make up 40 per cent of a person's body weight. The contraction (or tightening) of these muscles causes body movement: it can be a large movement, e.g. for bending or running, or a small movement which brings about a change in facial expression.

Most muscles are arranged in pairs because, although they can shorten themselves, they cannot make themselves longer, so a muscle known as a **flexor** works with a muscle called an **extensor**: the flexor shortens the muscles and the extensor straightens the muscle out again, for example doing a bicep curl.

All practical units require knowledge of muscular structures and functions for underpinning knowledge, so an understanding of the position and the action of these muscles is vital for beauty therapists.

Facial muscles

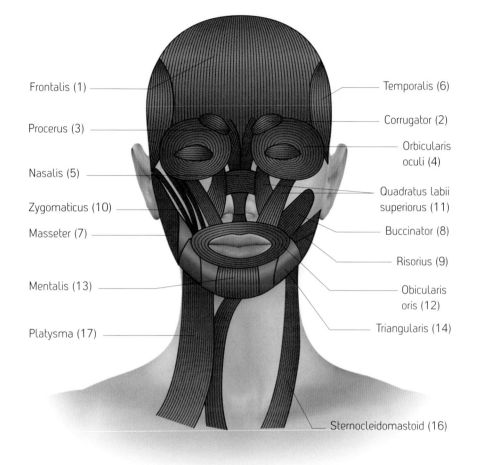

Frontalis (1)
Procerus (3)
Nasalis (5)
Zygomaticus (10)
Masseter (7)
Mentalis (13)
Platysma (17)

Temporalis (6)
Corrugator (2)
Orbicularis oculi (4)
Quadratus labii superiorus (11)
Buccinator (8)
Risorius (9)
Obicularis oris (12)
Triangularis (14)

Sternocleidomastoid (16)

Forehead muscles

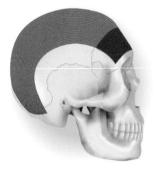
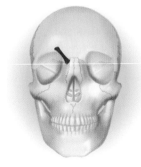
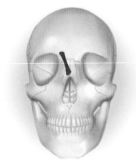

1 Frontalis
- Upper part of the cranium
- Scalp moves forward, raises eyebrow

2 Corrugator
- Inner corners of the eyebrows
- Draws eyebrows together – as in frowning

3 Procerus
- Top of nose between eyebrows
- Depresses the eyebrows, forming wrinkles over the bridge of the nose

Related anatomy and physiology

Eye and nose muscles

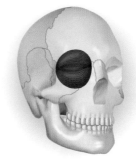

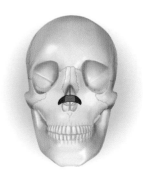

4   Orbicularis oculi
- Surrounds the eyes
- Closes eyes, blinking

5   Nasalis
- Over the front of the nose
- Compresses nose, causing wrinkles

Side of face muscles

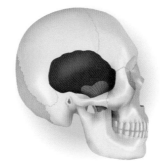

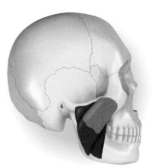

6   Temporalis
- Runs down side of face towards upper jaw
- Aids chewing and closing mouth

7   Masseter
- Runs down and back to the angle of the jaw
- Lifts the jaw and gives the teeth strength for biting

Cheek muscles

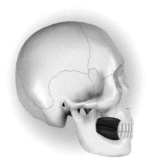

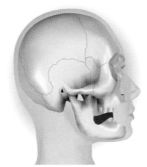

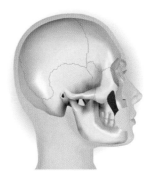

8   Buccinator
- Forms most of the cheek and gives it shape
- Puffs out cheeks when blowing, keeps food in mouth when chewing

9   Risorius
- In the lower cheek. It joins to the corner of the mouth
- Pulls back angles of the mouth — smiling and in grimace

10   Zygomaticus
- Runs down the cheek towards the corner of the mouth
- Pulls the corner of the mouth upwards and sideways

Mouth muscles

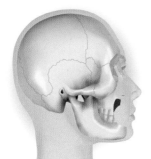

11 Quadratus labii superiorus
- Runs upward from the upper lip
- Lifts the upper lip and helps open the mouth
- The collective term is levators labatis

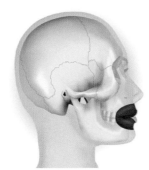

12 Orbicularis oris
- Surrounds the lips and forms the mouth
- Closes mouth, pushes lips forward. Pulls the corner of the chin down

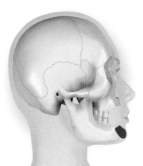

13 Mentalis
- Forms the chin
- Lifts the chin and moves the lower lips outwards

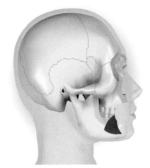

14 Triangularis
- Corner of the lower lip, extends over the chin
- Pulls the corner of the chin down

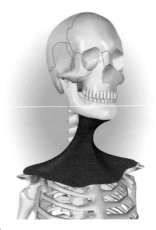

15a Depressor labii inferioris
- Runs from the outer surface of the mandible to the lower lip
- Pulls lower lip downwards and laterally

15b Depressor anguli oris
- Runs from the platysma to the corner of the mouth
- Pulls the corners of the mouth downwards, when sad or frowning

Neck muscles

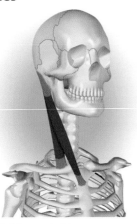

16 Sternocleidomastoid
- Either side of the neck
- Pulls head down to shoulder, rotates head to side and pulls chin onto chest

17 Platysma
- Front of throat
- Pulls down the lower jaw and angles of the mouth

Upper body or trunk muscles

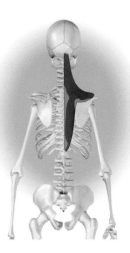

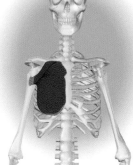

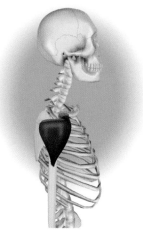

18 Trapezius
- The upper back and sides of the neck
- Rotation of shoulders, draws back the scapula bones, pulls head back, assists in rotation of head

19 Pectoralis
- Front of chest, under the breast
- Pulls arms forwards and assists rotation of the arm

20 Deltoid
- Caps the shoulder
- Raises arm from the side, pulls it back and forward

Think about it

The occipitalis is linked to the frontalis by a tendon called the epicranial aponeurosis which covers the skull like a tight swimming cap. A tendon joins muscle to bone.

Think about it

It takes less effort to smile than frown: 17 muscles are involved in smiling while over 40 can be used in a frown.

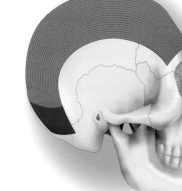

21 Occipitalis
- At the back of the skull
- Helps with the movement of the head

22 Pterygoids
- Two pairs of pterygoid muscles – lateral and medial
- Lateral allows the jaw to protrude
- Medial works with masseter muscle to aid mastication

23 Llevator anguli oris
- Located just above the upper lip on each side of the face
- Help raise the corners of the mouth

24 Llevator palpebrae
- Thin sheet of muscle located across the eyelid
- Elevates the eyelid

Muscles of the arm and leg

Muscles of the forearm and hand

There are 12 muscles that allow us to move our forearms, hands and fingers, and they are referred to as flexors and extensors. These muscles allow us to **supinate** and **pronate** the hand and arm, and flex and extend the fingers, thumb and wrist. The muscles allow the fingers to be spread apart (**abduction**) and to close together (**adduction**). A band of tendons holds all these muscles together at the wrist.

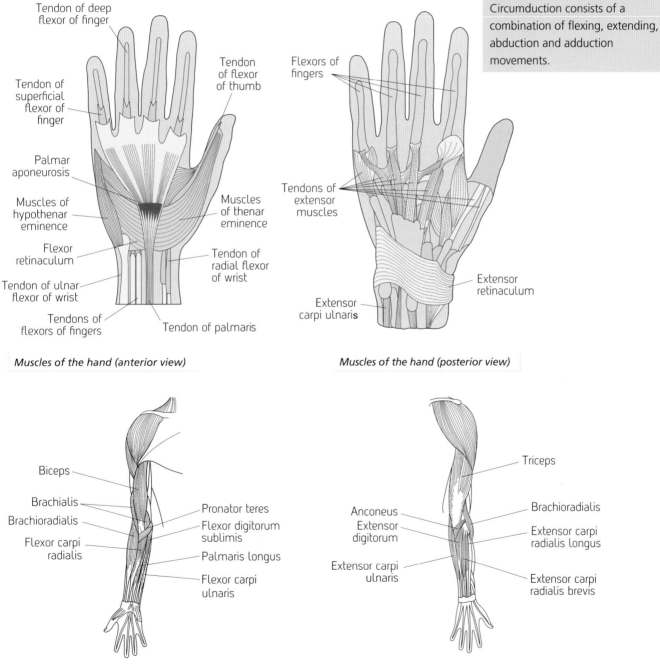

Muscles of the hand (anterior view)

Muscles of the hand (posterior view)

Muscles of the lower arm (anterior view)

Muscles of the lower arm (posterior view)

Related anatomy and physiology

Name of muscle	Action of muscle
Hypothenar muscles – below the little finger on the palm of the hand	Flexes, abducts and adducts the little finger
Thenar muscles – below the thumb on the palm of the hand	Flexes, abducts and adducts the thumb
Flexor carpi radialis – anterior side of the forearm	Flexes and abducts the wrist
Flexor carpi ulnaris – along the ulna side of the forearm (towards the little finger)	Flexes and adducts the wrist
Palmaris longus – medial side of the forearm on the anterior surface	Flexes wrist
Flexor digitorum sublimis – medial side of forearm	Flexes the fingers
Pronator teres – across the elbow joint on the anterior side of the forearm	Pronates the forearm, flexes the elbow and turns wrist down
Anconeus – small triangular muscle that lies on the elbow joint	Stabilises the elbow and abducts the ulna
Extensor digitorum – back of the forearm on the radial side	Extends the fingers
Extensor carpi ulnaris – back of the forearm on the radial side	Extends and adducts the wrist
Extensor carpi radialis brevis – radial side of the forearm	Extends and abducts the wrist
Extensor carpi radialis longus – thumb side (radial) of the forearm	Extends and abducts the wrist

Muscles of the lower leg and foot

There are four main superficial muscles of the lower leg that you will be concerned with when carrying out a leg massage. Many more muscles also work to move the leg. Two of the main superficial muscles are at the back of the leg: the gastrocnemius (often referred to as the calf muscle) and the soleus, which sits slightly underneath the gastrocnemius. The third muscle of the lower leg is the tibialis posterior and acts in conjunction with the tibialis anterior at the front of the leg. They act to flex and extend the foot, are often referred to as flexors and extensor muscles, and work in harmony when we move.

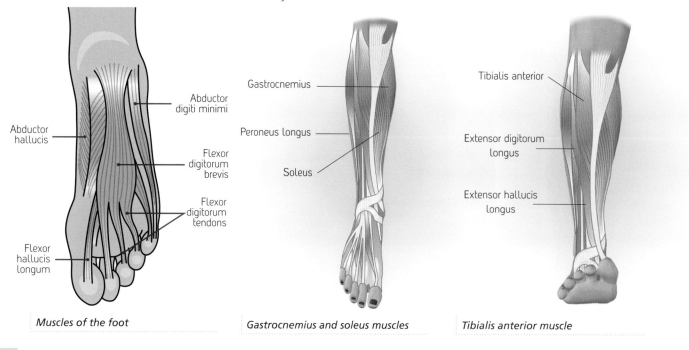

Abductor digiti minimi

Abductor hallucis

Flexor digitorum brevis

Flexor digitorum tendons

Flexor hallucis longum

Muscles of the foot

Gastrocnemius

Peroneus longus

Soleus

Gastrocnemius and soleus muscles

Tibialis anterior

Extensor digitorum longus

Extensor hallucis longus

Tibialis anterior muscle

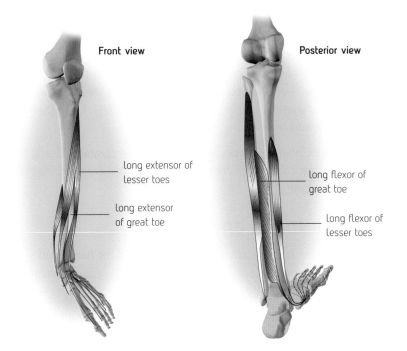

Front view

Posterior view

long extensor of lesser toes

long extensor of great toe

long flexor of great toe

long flexor of lesser toes

Flexors and extensors of the foot

Name of muscle	Action of muscle
Gastrocnemius	**Plantar flexes** the foot (points toes), pushes body forward when in motion
Soleus	Plantar flexes the foot, maintains standing position
Tibialis anterior	**Dorsi flexes** the foot (bends ankle) and inverts the foot (turns sole inwards)
Extensor digitorum longus	The lateral (outside) part of the shin bone Bends the ankle and pulls the foot upwards, turns the feet to face outside and extends the toes
Extensor hallucis longus	Situated partly behind the tibialis anterior down the shin bone Extends the big toe
Flexor digitorum longus	Inside the back of the calf (gastrocnemius) Plantar flexes and inverts the foot Flexes the toes and supports the inner longitudinal arch of the foot
Abductor hallucis	Runs along the medial border of the foot A muscle of the foot that adbucts the big toe
Flexor hallucis longus	Runs from the back of the fibula along the sole of the foot to the big toe Flexes all joints of the big toe, plantar flexes the foot
Flexor digitorum brevis	Runs down the middle of the sole of the foot Flexes the four toes laterally
Abductor digiti minimi	Down the lateral side of the sole of the foot Flexes and abducts the little toe

Key terms

Plantar flex – the flexion of the entire foot as if pushing down onto the floor. This action comes from the ankle.

Dorsi flex – the extension of the entire foot as though pointing the toes.

Achilles tendon – band of tendons in the ankle.

Inversion – the movement of the sole of the foot towards the median plane (as when an ankle is twisted).

Eversion – the movement of the sole of the foot away from the mid line of the body.

Related anatomy and physiology

The muscles of the lower leg and foot are also held in place by a band of tendons at the ankle – known as the **Achilles tendon** – like those of the wrist. A tendon is made up of white fibrous connective tissue which attaches muscle to bone.

Hair

Humans are one of the few land mammals with almost bare skin, but we have a coating of downy hair all over the body, and in certain places the hair grows thicker and more densely. The average human head has approximately 120,000 hairs, which grow about 3 mm per week.

The colour of hair is dictated by the pigments melanin and **carotene**. Black, brown and blond hairs get their colour from melanin, while red or auburn get their colour from the pigment carotene.

Types of hair found on the body

Hair is found all over the body except on the lips, palms of the hands and soles of the feet. Before birth the body is covered in a soft, downy hair called **lanugo**. This has mostly disappeared at birth.

Different areas of the body have different types of hair growth. These can be divided into two types:

- **vellus**
- **terminal**.

Vellus

This is soft, downy hair, covering most of the body. Normally without colour, it rarely grows longer than about 2 centimetres in length. Regardless of ethnic origin, vellus hair is usually straight due to the fact that the follicles are not very deep.

Terminal

Terminal hair grows from deep follicles which go down to the subcutaneous layer of the skin. They are strong hairs, which contain pigment, and grow on the scalp, eyebrows, under the arms and pubic areas.

Terminal hair can be curly, wavy or straight depending on ethnic origin, hereditary factors and chemical hair treatments, such as perms. If a cross-section was taken of a terminal hair for Europeans, the hair would be oval in shape, and would tend to be wavy. Asian hair would appear round in shape and tend to be straight, and African-Caribbean hair would appear flattened and tend to be very curly.

Key terms

Carotene – a pigment found in the granular layer of the epidermis.

Lanugo – soft, downy hair covering most of the body before birth.

Vellus – soft, downy hair covering most of the body.

Terminal – strong hairs which contain pigment; found on the scalp, eyebrows, under the arms and pubic areas.

Structure	Function
Connective tissue sheath	Surrounds the hair follicle and sebaceous gland. It has a rich blood and nerve supply to feed the hair.
Outer root sheath	Forms the hair follicle wall – made of basal cells.
Inner root sheath	The cells in the inner root sheath run in the opposite direction to the cells in the outer root sheath. The inner root sheath consists of three small layers: the Henle's layer, the Huxley's layer and the cuticle layer. They act like Velcro™ to anchor the hair into the follicle. They grow upwards with the hair. The outer root sheath stops where it meets the sebaceous gland.
Dermal papilla	This is the vital blood supply for the hair cells providing food and oxygen.
Hair bulb	The hair bulb is where the cells grow and divide by mitosis.
Matrix	The lowest part of the hair bulb where the cells grow.

Sebaceous gland	Produces sebum which lubricates both the hair and skin.
Arrector pili muscle	Attached to the hair to trap warm air next to the body when we are cold.
Cuticle	Gives the hair its elasticity. Made of transparent scales that interlock with each other like roof tiles. The cuticle protects the cortex.
Cortex	The middle layer of tightly packed keratinised cells that contain the pigment. The cortex gives hair strength.
Medulla	The middle of the hair consists of loosely connected keratinised cells and tiny pockets of air. The air spaces allow light to be reflected through them, giving the hair both colour and sheen.
Vitreous membrane	This is a thickening in the basal membrane. It forms a connective sheath that surrounds the whole follicle.

Structure and function of hair

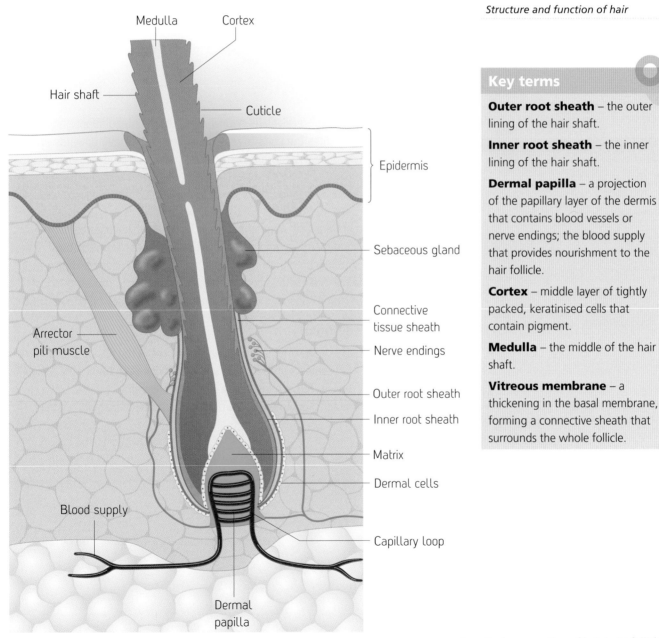

A vertical cross-section of hair in its follicle

Key terms

Outer root sheath – the outer lining of the hair shaft.

Inner root sheath – the inner lining of the hair shaft.

Dermal papilla – a projection of the papillary layer of the dermis that contains blood vessels or nerve endings; the blood supply that provides nourishment to the hair follicle.

Cortex – middle layer of tightly packed, keratinised cells that contain pigment.

Medulla – the middle of the hair shaft.

Vitreous membrane – a thickening in the basal membrane, forming a connective sheath that surrounds the whole follicle.

Related anatomy and physiology

Key terms

Anagen – a stage of growth in the life of a hair: the growing phase.

Catagen – a stage of growth in the life of a hair: the changing phase.

Telogen – a stage of growth in the life of a hair: the resting phase.

Think about it

Here is an easy way to remember the different stages of hair growth:

A – active (anagen)
C – change (catagen)
T – tired (telogen).

Think about it

- We lose between 50 and 100 hairs a day!
- People with blond hair have more hairs per square centimetre than people who have other hair colours, although no one knows why.
- One eyebrow contains approximately 900 individual hairs.

Hair growth

A normal hair in the body is contained in a tube-shaped pocket called a follicle. These follicles consist of an inner sheath and an outer sheath which are similar in structure to the cells of the epidermis.

The hair is made of hardened protein called keratin. The outside of the hair is a scaly layer called the cuticle. The hair grows from the bottom of its follicle by cell division, being fed by a good blood supply from the dermal papilla.

Hair growth is a continuous cycle of events that is repeated as long as nourishment is available, or until the hair follicle is damaged through illness or the ageing process. Hair does become thinner in old age due to hormonal changes which occur within the body.

The life of a normal hair is divided into three stages of hair growth:

- **anagen** – the growing phase
- **catagen** – the changing (transition) phase
- **telogen** – the resting phase.

Anagen

In the anagen stage the hair receives its nourishment via the blood supply from the dermal papilla. This enables the cells to reproduce. The cells move upwards and form the different structures of the hair shaft. Melanin cells are also produced and this forms the hair colouring.

Catagen

This is the changing or transition stage of hair growth. During this stage the dermal papilla breaks away and the lower end of the hair becomes loose from the base of the follicle. The hair is still being fed from the follicle wall and is sometimes known as a club-ended hair. The hair gradually becomes drier and continues to move up to just below the sebaceous gland. Here it is very vulnerable and can easily be brushed out.

Telogen

This is the final stage of hair growth and is the resting period. The follicle rests until stimulated by hormones to return to the anagen phase. Telogen lasts for a few weeks, with the club hair often being retained until new hair is produced – pushing the club hair out.

The hair growth cycle

Blood

Blood is the transport system for the body to deliver and remove vital ingredients needed by the cells in the body. It is pumped around the body by the heart. (Read pages 260–261 about the structure of the heart to aid your understanding.) Arteries, veins and capillaries are the vessels that carry the blood to their destination.

Arteries:

- have thick elasticated walls
- carry blood under pressure
- contain oxygenated blood (except the pulmonary artery)
- tend to lie deep in the body.

Veins:

- have thinner walls
- contain valves to prevent a back flow of blood
- rely on muscular contractions to push the blood back towards the heart
- carry deoxygenated blood
- are more superficial than arteries.

Capillaries:

- are tiny vessels one cell thick
- carry both oxygenated and deoxygenated blood to and from the cells and tissues
- do not work under pressure
- can be both deep and superficial.

Composition of the blood

Oxygenated blood flows from the heart through the arteries and deoxygenated blood flows back to the heart through the veins. Capillaries are very small vessels which form a network to get into tiny cell spaces to allow delivery (of oxygenated blood) and removal (of deoxygenated blood) to take place.

Blood is a slightly sticky fluid that is composed of:

- 55 per cent **plasma**
- 45 per cent blood cells.

Plasma is a yellow, transparent fluid made up of mostly water, with a small amount of protein present. There are three types of blood cells.

1 Red blood cells (erythrocytes) transport oxygen to the cells and take away carbon dioxide.

2 White blood cells (leucocytes) protect the body against invading bacteria and help form the immune system.

3 **Platelets (thrombocytes)** play an important role in blood clotting.

Related anatomy and physiology

Functions of the blood

The blood has three main functions in the body:

- transport
- regulation
- protection.

Transport

Blood transports or carries:

- oxygen from the lungs to the body cells
- carbon dioxide from the cells to the lungs
- nutrients from digestion to the cells
- waste products from the cells to be excreted
- hormones sent from the endocrine gland to regulate the cells
- medication, which can be passed into the cells.

Regulation

Blood regulates:

- water content of cells
- body heat.

Protection

Blood protects against:

- infection and disease
- blood loss by clotting.

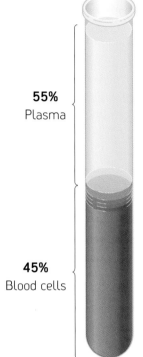

55%
Plasma

45%
Blood cells

The structure of blood

Blood circulation to the lower arm and hand, and lower leg and foot

After picking up oxygen in the lungs, oxygenated blood is pumped from the heart via the arteries, which work under pressure to supply all the extremities (the fingers and toes). Once the blood has delivered food and oxygen to the cells, the veins return waste matter and carbon dioxide. The veins do not have the same pressure as the arteries, so it is the pressure of the muscles on the veins in the hands and feet which aids the blood's return. Veins have valves to prevent the blood flowing back, and they can become enlarged, as in varicose veins.

The main arteries that deliver blood to the forearm are the radial and ulnar arteries (the same names as the bones in the forearm). These arteries bring blood to the palm of the hand and branch on still further to the metacarpal and digital arteries that bring blood to the hand and fingers.

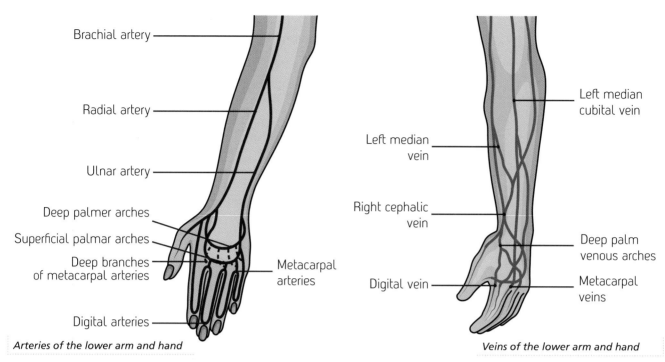

Arteries of the lower arm and hand

Veins of the lower arm and hand

The blood to the lower leg and foot is supplied by the anterior (front) and posterior (back) tibial arteries which take their name from the large bone in the leg. When the anterior artery reaches the ankle the artery forms the dorsalis pedis artery. The posterior artery also divides at the ankle into two branches — the medial and lateral plantar arteries. These go on to further connect with the dorsalis pedis artery and continue to form the digital arteries.

The digital veins in the toes drain into the dorsal and plantar venous arches. These arches connect into the dorsal pedis veins and then into the saphenous veins which join the iliac vein. These are the more superficial veins. The deeper veins in the leg are the posterior tibial vein, which links to the peroneal vein and the anterior tibial vein which connects at the knee to the popliteal vein.

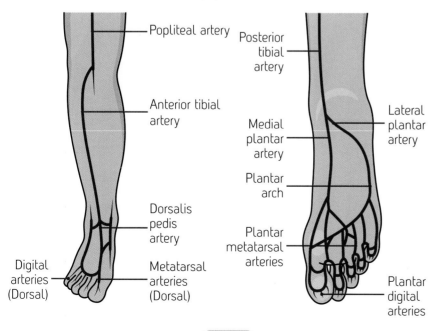

Anterior view of arteries of the lower leg and foot

Related anatomy and physiology

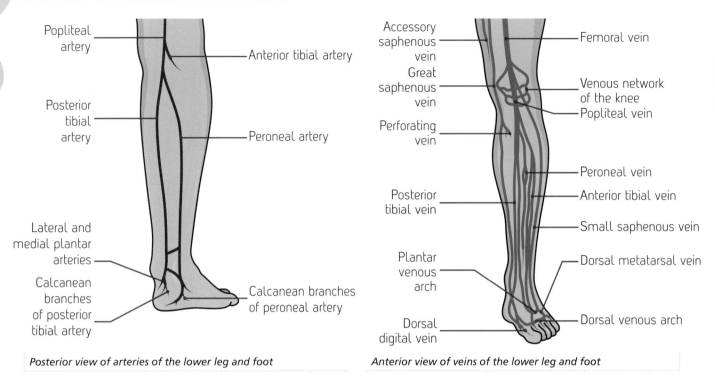

Posterior view of arteries of the lower leg and foot

Anterior view of veins of the lower leg and foot

All clients benefit from massage to the hands and feet: it stimulates blood flow and enables oxygen and nutrients to get into the area more quickly, the blood warms the tissues and muscles, so muscles relax and circulation is improved. When massaging, remember that you must always work towards the heart, so that you work with the natural flow of the blood, instead of against it.

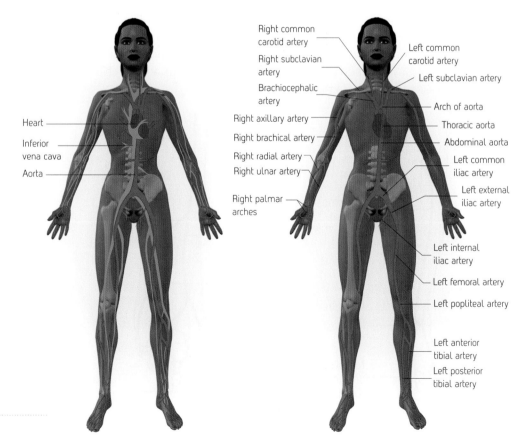

The heart and blood vessels

The effects of massage on blood circulation

Massage increases the amount of blood flow into the area, which is seen as an **erythema** or reddening of the skin. It has a number of beneficial effects.

- It speeds up the flow of blood through the veins and therefore helps with the metabolic waste being carried away.
- It increases the fresh blood to the area, bringing oxygen and nutrients to the cells and so helping with cell growth and repair.
- Warmth is created by the increase in blood flow, which is relaxing to the client.
- Because of the increase to the cells of oxygen and nutrients the skin will look and feel softer.
- Muscle efficiency and response is improved due to the increased oxygen and nutrients.
- The removal of waste products gives a more **toned** appearance to the muscles and makes them more relaxed.

Blood flow to the face and head

Arteries of the head

The blood is pumped to the head via the common carotid artery, which has two branches. The internal carotid artery passes through the temporal bone of the skull behind the ear and takes blood to the brain. The external carotid artery remains outside the skull and divides into facial, temporal and occipital arteries which supply the skin and muscles of the face, side and back of the head.

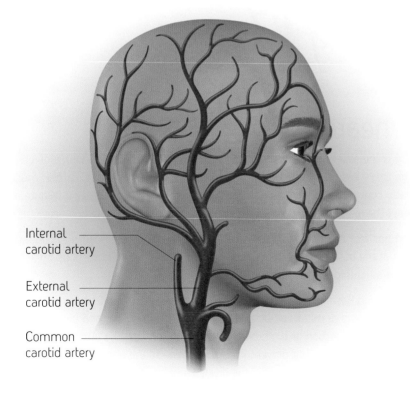

Internal carotid artery

External carotid artery

Common carotid artery

Arteries of the head

Key terms

Erythema – vasodilation of the blood capillaries, causing surface reddening of the skin.

Tone – the constant contraction of some of the muscles all of the time for the maintenance of posture, often dictated by fitness and age.

Try it out

1 Test your pulse rate. First take your pulse for 15 seconds and multiply by 4. This tells you your pulse rate at rest (multiplying by 4 gives you the rate per minute). Do this again after jogging on the spot for two minutes.

2 Has your skin developed any reddening?

3 What is this reddening called?

Related anatomy and physiology

Veins of the head

Blood is collected up from the scalp capillaries by the facial, occipital and posterior veins, which run alongside the similarly named arteries. These join to form an external jugular vein behind and below the ear on both sides.

The external jugular veins go down the neck and enter the **subclavian veins**. An internal jugular vein brings blood from the brain, goes down on either side of the neck and enters the subclavian vein. The subclavian veins carry on towards the heart and eventually the blood enters the superior vena cavae.

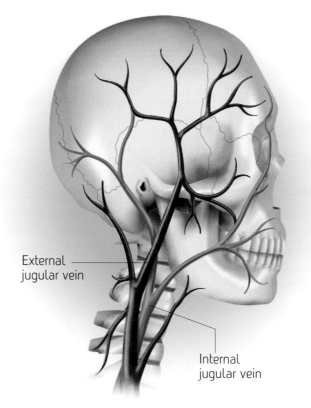

External jugular vein

Internal jugular vein

Veins of the head

The heart

The heart is the size of a clenched fist. It has a lung each side of it and is protected by the rib cage. It is made of **cardiac** muscle – unlike normal muscle, cardiac muscle continually contracts. These contractions occur approximately 70 times a minute and throughout the average life span the heart contracts roughly three billion times.

The heart has four chambers: two smaller **atria** at the top of the heart and two larger **ventricles** at the bottom of the heart. The heart is divided into two sections by a muscular wall called the **septum**.

To prevent blood flowing back into the other chambers, the heart contains four valves – tricuspid, bicuspid or mitral, aortic and pulmonary. The bicuspid and tricuspid valves help maintain the direction of the blood flow through the heart by allowing blood to flow into the ventricles but prevent it from returning to the atria. The aortic and pulmonary valves are semi-lunar, that is divided into halves. They control the blood flow out of the ventricles into the aorta and pulmonary arteries respectively without any back flow into the ventricles.

Each of the four chambers of the heart ejects about 70 ml of blood with each beat.

The left ventricle wall is thicker than the right because it pumps blood all round the body – the right ventricle only pumps blood as far as the lungs.

Deoxygenated blood is brought back to the heart by the veins and enters the heart via two larger vessels – the superior and inferior vena cava – which flow into the right atrium. The blood then passes into the larger right ventricle and is pushed into the pulmonary artery, which takes the blood to the lungs where the exchange of carbon dioxide and oxygen takes place.

Blood then re-enters the heart via the pulmonary vein into the left atrium. It passes to the left ventricle and is then pushed into the aorta. From here the blood is carried into the arteries of the body, and so the cycle continues.

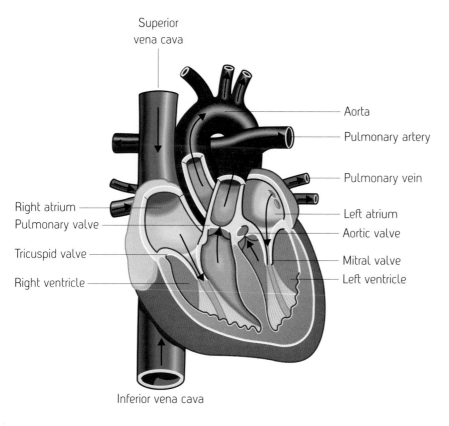

Chambers of the heart

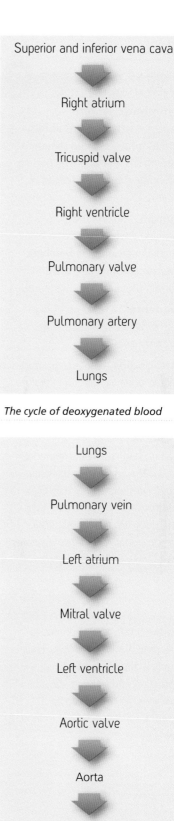

The cycle of deoxygenated blood

The cycle of oxygenated blood

Think about it

- Arteries carry oxygenated blood away from the heart – except the pulmonary artery, which carries deoxygenated blood.
- Veins carry deoxygenated blood to the heart – except the pulmonary vein, which carries oxygenated blood.
- Arteries always *leave* the heart and veins always *go to* the heart.

Related anatomy and physiology

The lymphatic system

The **lymphatic system** is the body's second circulation system for collecting waste products. It carries away waste from the tissues that the blood cannot manage to take. For example, you could think of it as a second bus that collects all the passengers the first bus left behind.

The fluid that is left behind is known as **lymph** and is straw coloured. It is emptied back into the blood system via the subclavian vein, which is in the upper chest. The removal of the lymph from around the body prevents the tissues from becoming clogged and swollen. If tissue fluid builds up, swelling occurs and this is called **oedema**. People who are pregnant, ill or have very sedentary lifestyles can suffer from oedema. Gentle massage can aid the removal of the stagnant fluid. Lymph, like blood in veins, relies on muscular movement to push it around the body, so the healthier and fitter a person, the better their lymphatic system is at dealing with waste.

The lymphatic system also plays an important role in protecting the body against infection. At various stages along the route that the lymph travels are glands or nodes; you could think of these as bus stops. It is here that the lymph is filtered of bacteria and germs, and **antibodies** are produced to fight infection. When someone is ill the doctor often feels the glands in the neck and looks in the mouth. This is to find out if the glands are filtering the bacteria properly. If the glands are very swollen, antibiotics may be needed to help the **lymph nodes** and antibodies fight infection.

The main lymph nodes in the leg are the popliteal, at the back of the knee. The lymph then travels to the inguinal nodes in the groin. The supratrochlear nodes in the crook of the arm lead to the axillary node in the underarm. If any of the nodes are swollen, treatments can be painful.

Composition of lymph

Lymph is made up of:

- plasma
- proteins
- waste products
- toxins
- fats
- oxygen
- carbon dioxide
- urea
- lymphocytes.

Function of the lymph system

The purpose of lymph is to collect germs, bacteria and waste in the system, then to carry these to the lymph glands to be filtered and made harmless. The lymphatic system uses different methods to do this.

- The lymphatic system drains tissue fluid from the spaces between the cells.
- It transports the tissue fluid and proteins back to the bloodstream via the subclavian vein.
- It transports fats from the small intestine to the blood.
- It produces lymphocytes which protect and defend the body against infection and disease.

Key terms

Lymphatic system – a separate system of vessels that comes from the blood stream to filter toxins and waste by passing lymph fluid through a series of glands.

Lymph – fluid in the lymphatic system derived from tissue fluids; circulates around the lymphatic system removing bacteria and certain proteins from the tissues.

Oedema – a build-up of fluid in the tissues causing the area to become swollen.

Antibodies – proteins produced by the body to fight an infection.

Lymph nodes – small structures made of lymph tissue, located at intervals along the lymphatic system particularly at the neck, under the arm and in the groin. They filter bacteria and foreign particles from lymph fluid. When the body is fighting infection lymph nodes may become swollen with activated lymphocytes.

Think about it

By the time your lymph nodes become swollen and sore, your body is already fighting the infection and filtering harmful bacteria, so this would be a contra-indication to any treatment.

Benefits of treatments on the lymph system

As a therapist the treatments that you can perform can greatly assist the lymphatic flow. This is because:

- massage stimulates the flow of lymph, so removing the toxins and fluid from the area faster
- general swelling can be reduced
- absorption of waste matter can be speeded up
- skin will be smoother and softer because cell renewal is helped
- muscles will be relaxed and work more efficiently.

Lymphatic flow to the head and neck:

- **Left side** – lymph from this side of the head and neck passes through the thoracic duct and empties into the left subclavian vein (the thoracic duct is situated in the upper chest under the rib cage).
- **Right side** – lymph from this side of the head and neck passes through the right thoracic duct and empties into the right subclavian vein.

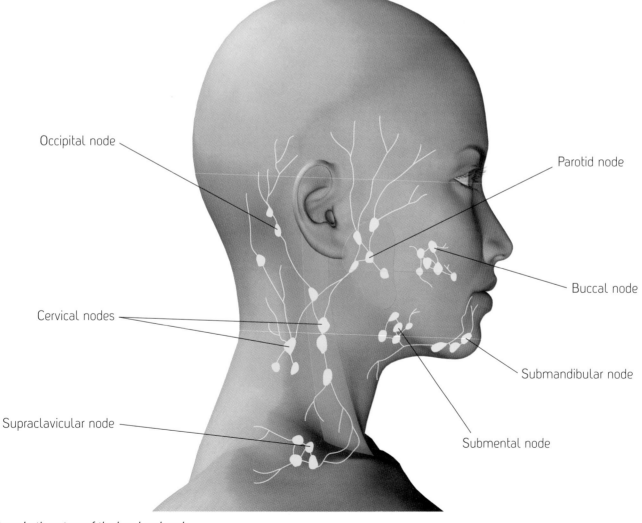

Lymphatic system of the head and neck

Occipital node

Parotid node

Buccal node

Cervical nodes

Submandibular node

Supraclavicular node

Submental node

Related anatomy and physiology

Check your knowledge

Bones

1 How many bones make up the skull?
2 What is the name of the fibrous joints that join the bones of the skull together?
3 What is the clavicle commonly called?
4 Where would you find the zygomatic bone?
5 Name the bones of the shoulder girdle.
6 What are the functions of the arches of the foot, and how many are there?
7 Where would you find the tibia?
8 Where would you find carpals?
9 What is the function of a ligament?
10 What is the upper part of the vertebral column called?

Skin

1 Name the five layers of the epidermis.
2 What is the function of the arrector pili muscle?
3 What is desquamation?
4 What is a melanocyte?
5 What is the function of a sebaceous gland?
6 Name the four senses that can be detected by the sense receptors in the dermis.
7 What are sudoriferous glands?
8 Name the hardened protein that is found in the skin.
9 In what layer of the epidermis do cells start to die?
10 Name the two living layers in the epidermis.

Nails

1 What is the reproductive part of the nail called?
2 What is the function of the nail groove?
3 What type of protein is the nail plate made of?
4 How many layers is the nail plate made of?
5 Where would you find the perionychium?
6 Is the nail living or dead?
7 What is the function of the cuticle?
8 State the appearance of a healthy nail.
9 State four factors that can affect nail growth.
10 What is the purpose of finger and toe nails?

Muscles

1 Approximately how many voluntary muscles are there?
2 Where would you find the gastrocnemius?
3 What is the action of the buccinator muscle?
4 Where would you find the platysma muscle?
5 What does supinate mean?
6 State the action of the orbicularis oris.
7 How many muscles make a smile?
8 What is the action and position of the deltoid muscle?
9 Is the triangularis a happy or sad muscle?
10 What action does the masseter muscle have?

Hair

1 What are the two pigments that give hair colour?
2 Name the resting stage of hair growth.
3 Which hair type is found on a foetus?
4 Which type of hair forms the eyebrows?
5 What protein is hair made of?
6 What is the function of the matrix?
7 Where would you find the medulla?
8 How many connective tissue sheaths does a hair have?
9 What type of hair covers the body?
10 Where do humans not have hairs?

Blood

1 What is the function of platelets?
2 Blood is a sticky fluid composed of blood cells and _____?
3 What are the three main functions of blood?
4 What do arteries carry?
5 What do veins carry?
6 When carrying out massage in which direction must you go?
7 List five products that are transported in the blood.
8 Which bone does the internal carotid artery pass through?
9 Which vein does the external jugular vein join?
10 List three effects massage can have on the blood supply.

Lymph

1 What colour is lymph?
2 What important role does lymph play in protecting the body?
3 List three substances that you will find in lymph fluid.
4 State four benefits of massage on the lymphatic system.
5 Name the vein where lymph joins the blood supply.
6 Name the lymph nodes in the mouth.
7 The lymph system is often referred to as the body's _____?
8 Name the lymph node in the back of the knee.
9 Name the lymph node under the arm.
10 If lymph builds up, it will cause swelling in the tissues. What is this called?

Section

4

Practical skills

Provide facial skincare

What you will learn

- Prepare for facial skincare treatments
- Provide facial skincare treatments

Introduction

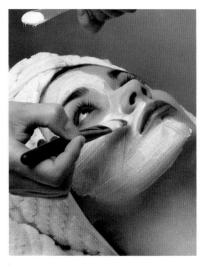

A facial is a lovely treatment to give and receive

A facial is a lovely treatment to offer any client: it is both extremely relaxing and very beneficial. In fact, for a professional beauty therapist, a facial can be as relaxing to give as it is to receive. The client is cocooned on the couch, wrapped warmly and securely, with the luxury of knowing that expert hands are cleansing, massaging and improving the skin's condition. Many clients fall asleep during a facial, as the relaxation is so deep.

A facial makes a perfect gift, and vouchers for the treatment can be purchased in most salons. For many women a facial is the height of luxury; for a beauty therapist it rates very highly on the scale of favourite treatments to give. Many beauty therapists decide to specialise only in facials and call themselves facialists. The majority of their bookings will be for top-of-the-range facials and little else — and with a celebrity endorsement and/or a write-up in a woman's magazine, the facialist can be booked up months in advance!

This unit is about preparing for and providing facial skincare treatments. All of these treatments will be carried out on a variety of skin types, age groups and conditions. It is also important to remember that you need to maintain your health and safety, along with rigorous hygiene practices throughout.

Prepare for facial skincare treatments

In this outcome you will learn about:

- preparing yourself, your client and your work area for facial skincare treatment
- using suitable consultation techniques to identify treatment objectives
- carrying out a skin analysis
- providing clear recommendations to the client
- selecting products, tools and equipment to suit client treatment needs, skin types and conditions.

Think about it

No client is going to feel comfortable in a dirty environment. She probably won't even stay if she feels it is unhygienic. Would you?

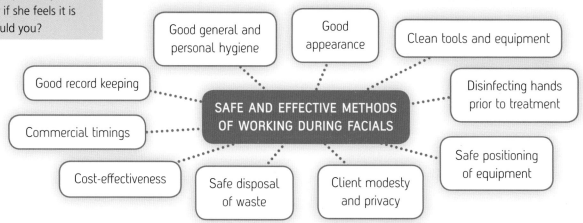

SAFE AND EFFECTIVE METHODS OF WORKING DURING FACIALS

- Good general and personal hygiene
- Good appearance
- Clean tools and equipment
- Good record keeping
- Disinfecting hands prior to treatment
- Commercial timings
- Safe positioning of equipment
- Cost-effectiveness
- Safe disposal of waste
- Client modesty and privacy

For facials, as with all other beauty treatments, you must work within the legal, hygiene and treatment requirements as set out by your Awarding Organisation to meet industry standards. This will ensure the health and safety of the client and puts them in the centre of your focus — exactly where they should be. Preparation is the key to giving a relaxed and flowing treatment. All aspects of the treatment need to be carefully prepared to enable you to give the client your full attention and a super-pampering treatment.

Preparing for the treatment

Be fully prepared. This allows you to concentrate on your client and to give a relaxed treatment without the distraction of having to leave the area to get products, equipment or towels. A little preparation time should be built into each appointment slot, so that each client feels special. It is also important to ensure that your working area is kept clean to ensure good health and safety and that the **environmental conditions** are conducive to a relaxing treatment.

Good habits to stay tidy

- Organise the layout of the trolley in an ordered fashion – have all the labels of products facing you so you can easily see which is needed. Arrange the products in order of use, and replace them back in their slot when you have finished with them. They will always then be at hand, and you will always look tidy and controlled. Have a space for everything and everything in its place. Have a system where all necessary tools are in a jar or pot (even a plastic beaker is easy to clean), the tissues and cotton wool in their own plastic bowl or tub.

- Tidy as you go along – put used tissues and cotton wool into a small pedal bin (lined with a bin liner) as you finish with them, rather than leaving them on the trolley.

- If you can, wash up mask brushes and bowls while the mask is setting on the client's face. This may not be possible if you do not have a sink near the workstation, as you should not leave the client unattended.

- Minimise waste by using only the amount of product required. This is not only cost-effective, but it also means there is very little product left over to clear up.

- Always put lids back on to pots if decanting products. This avoids the possibility of a spillage, which is time-consuming to clear up. It also stops alcohol-based products from evaporating.

- Mop up spills as they occur and do not allow them to endanger others.

If you follow these tips, you will not need a major tidying session at the end of your treatment. Becoming tidy is a skill that comes with experience. Always ask yourself if you could have been tidier as you went along. Unless the client is the last one of the day, you will not have the luxury of time to clean and tidy the area. If your next client is due straight away, you could be in trouble if you have to spend a long time tidying and preparing for your next treatment.

Ensuring the client's clothing, hair and accessories are protected or removed

The client's modesty and privacy must be preserved. In a closed cubicle ask the client to remove all outdoor and top clothes and put on a gown.

The client should remove all jewellery, accessories, wig, if worn, and glasses. Clients wearing contact lenses may prefer to remove them during the written consultation stage if they have suitable storage for them. Some clients prefer to keep them in, even though make-up will be removed and the eye area will be massaged. Be guided by the client's choice, as only the client will know which is most comfortable.

A headband or turban should be used to remove all hair from the face.

Key terms

Environmental conditions – the conditions that are appropriate for a facial treatment, including warmth, ventilation, privacy, volume and type of music/sounds, and a pleasant aroma.

Think about it

Always complete the client record card at the time of treatment. If you leave it for later you may forget, and vital information may not be recorded. See the Professional skills section of this book for more on client record keeping.

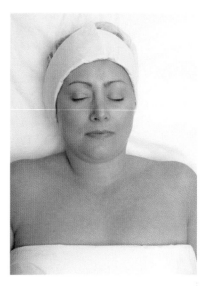

Preparation of the client

Provide facial skincare

For the female client	Tights and half-slip may be kept on, but shoes should be removed. Bra straps may get oily and should be dropped off the shoulder, or the bra may be taken off altogether, depending on client preference. If the client chooses to push her straps down on to the top of her arms, there is still a danger they will get massage medium on them, as you will be going halfway down the upper arm with your movements. Above all, you want the client to be comfortable and she will not be if she has a bra clasp digging into her.
For the male client	Facial massage includes the upper back and shoulders, and these therefore need to be free of clothing. The shirt or T-shirt of the male client should be removed, and his chest covered with towels and/or blankets to prevent his upper body getting cold.
For all clients	Assist the client on to the couch and remove the gown. Depending upon the time of year, wrap the client in either a blanket with towels or just towels, so that he or she is comfortable and warm. There is nothing more distracting than clients feeling insecure or cold – they need to unwind and feel relaxed.

Using consultation techniques to identify treatment objectives

A full consultation is vital before the treatment can begin. Refer to the Professional skills section of this book for further information on how to conduct a consultation. Anatomy and physiology relating to the head and neck are covered in the Related anatomy and physiology chapter.

Always use a consultation sheet to record all the client details during your analysis.

It should be in three parts:

- the client's history
- skin analysis
- client treatments and retail recommendations.

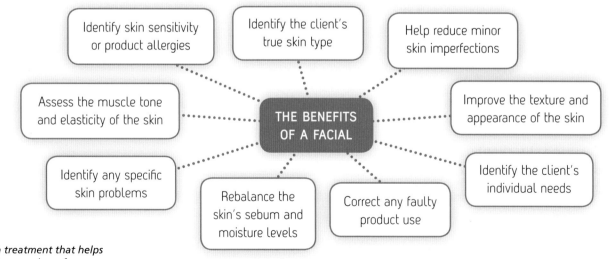

A facial is a treatment that helps the client in a number of ways

Before you can decide upon your treatment objectives you need to carry out a skin analysis to tailor make a bespoke facial for your client's needs.

Carrying out a skin analysis

A good skin analysis takes time and practice. Eventually, you will be able to:

- identify the correct **skin type** and **skin condition**
- evaluate and decide which products are most suitable
- evaluate and determine which treatments are most appropriate
- clarify which home care routine to recommend
- recommend a personal skincare routine to retail.

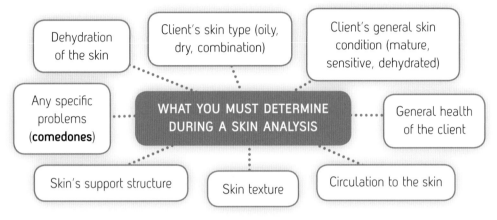

When examining the face and neck it is important to consider the following:

- **Contra-indications** – check the skin prior to the treatment for any condition present that would prevent treatment or any adaptation that may be necessary. For more information on contra-indications see, pages 274–5, and the chapter in this book called You and the skin.
- **Client's skin type** – identify the client's skin type correctly. This is essential, both to enable the therapist to give the right treatment, and to recommend the most suitable products.
- **Minor skin problems** – look for any problems that can be given specific treatment for improvement.
- **Client's work/life balance** – take into account the client's age, lifestyle, nutrition and general health. These will be reflected in the colour and texture of the skin, muscle tone in the face, elasticity, the number of wrinkles present and skin discolouration. Stress, alcohol, dehydration, smoking and central heating are also reflected in the skin's condition. Record the client's colouring and pigmentation, as well as any other facial features: this will help with a make-up application and when recommending other treatments such as eyebrow shaping.
- **Medication** – if the client is taking regular medication, has been under a consultant within the last year or has had surgery in the last nine months, this should be noted. Many different types of drugs affect the skin and need to be taken into account.
- **Hormone levels** – the client's age will give a good indication of her hormone levels. Teenagers' hormone levels may be erratic and unsettled causing acne and breakouts, pregnancy will have an effect on the skin, and older women going through the menopause may be lacking in the vital hormones that help the skin's collagen and elastin levels, which support underlying structures (refer to You and the skin, pages 216–19).

Key terms

Skin type – a means of classifying the skin during skin analysis.

Skin condition – the appearance, texture and state of health of the skin including classification of skin type and any problems.

For your portfolio

Many salons provide skin analysis as a free service prior to the facial. Specialist facial therapists offer a one-hour service, which is chargeable. Do some research and find out which large commercial companies offer a stand-alone skin analysis and how much they charge. Compare prices and find out what the process involves. You may even decide to have one done yourself as a hands-on investigation!

Think about it

Product houses or companies have their own facial diagnosis and consultation techniques. Therapists working for them are trained to use these techniques: for example, one company may start with a back **massage** and diagnosis, then turn the client over and diagnose any facial problems; another company may include a hand and foot massage in the facial, which is carried out while the mask is on! So, once you are qualified be prepared to learn new techniques, but first you need to learn the basics.

Key terms

Massage – manual manipulation of the skin and muscles for a therapeutic purpose using different massage techniques.

Comedones – blackheads.

Provide facial skincare

271

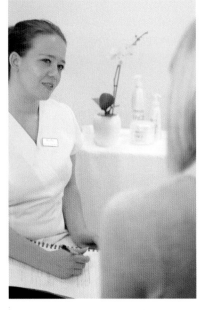

Fill out a client record card and ask the client to sign it prior to treatment

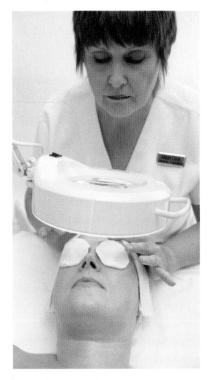

Visual examination using a magnifying lamp

Facial examination techniques

There are four techniques to a facial examination:

- questioning
- visual
- manual examination
- reference to client records.

Questioning

Follow your consultation form when questioning the client before their facial. This will establish the factors that contribute to the skin's condition. Gentle questioning should help identify the client's normal skincare routine and products used as well as the client's expectation of the treatment – clients do need to be realistic. Encourage the client to ask questions to clarify any points they do not understand. It is important that the client understands that a skin condition may take several treatments to clear. A realistic treatment plan, with both time-scale and cost, should be discussed prior to the treatment taking place.

Visual

Visual examination should be done under a strong light with a magnifying glass to determine the client's skin type and condition. The skin should be clean and free of make-up. Any areas of sensitivity, problem areas such as comedones or an oily T-zone can be recorded on a facial record card.

Look at the colour of the skin, so that you can see pigmentation levels and patches, sun damage, capillary damage and the circulation of the skin. The efficiency of the skin cells for respiration, elimination of waste products and blood flow to the epidermis are all indicated by skin colour (see the chapter in this book called You and the skin). Colour changes are also caused by fluctuating hormone levels, exposure to chemicals, allergic reactions, some skin conditions such as eczema, certain drugs and extremes of temperature. It may also be something which is inherited – a client with high colour and a tendency to blush or have a flushed appearance may have just been given that in the gene pool with their DNA! You will also be able to look at the skin and see if it looks naturally oily or has a drier or irritated appearance.

Manual

This should be gentle, and will give some indication about the elasticity of the skin, its warmth and texture. After a gentle pinch of the skin in the main facial areas the skin should spring back to its original shape. Poor elasticity of the fibres will mean that the skin takes longer to recover from the pinch test and this could be due to age. The warmth of the skin will indicate how good the circulation is, and the texture will be felt as smooth, coarse or rough. Lumps under the skin may need further investigation.

There are some excellent skin diagnosis devices available which can be incorporated into the skin analysis. Until recently, the Wood's lamp was the prime diagnostic equipment, but there are also skin scanners and skin analysers which measure hydration levels, fat content, melanin levels and erythema levels of the skin. These are all tools for an experienced therapist once you have developed a trained eye! (Refer to You and the skin, pages 205–206, for a full explanation of Wood's lamp and skin scanners.)

Referring to client records

If the client is a regular customer, always have the record card with you so that you can view previous treatments, talk about how successful they are/were, if there were any contra-actions, allergies, anything the client was particularly pleased with, or anything she did not particularly like. Not only is this a good ice breaker if the client is new to you, it is also important to continue the good work that the previous therapist has done. For more information on record cards, refer to Essential professional knowledge, pages 24–26.

Additional knowledge

Some skin scanners are able to measure the density of the skin, the pH of the skin and pigmentation levels. These are very good tools and valid for a clinical examination of the skin. However, there is no substitute for touch, looking under the magnifying lamp and massaging the skin, to feel texture and depth. All leading commercial companies agree that the scanners, even in the hands of experts, will never replace the touch of an experienced therapist!

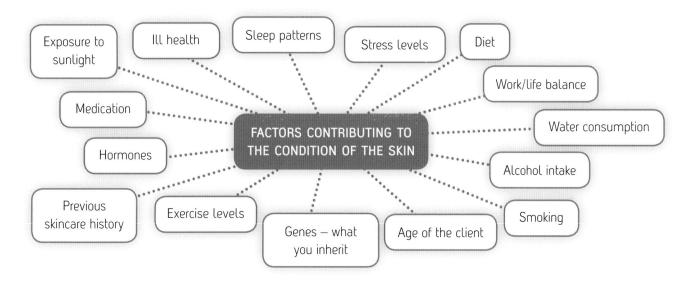

Preparing the client for examination

Initial discussion with the client will take place while the client is still clothed and sitting with you. The discussion will cover contra-indications, her expectations of the treatment and your treatment plan. Obviously, a full treatment plan cannot be given until you have closely examined the skin, but you may not get that far if the client has an infectious condition and the treatment cannot go any further. It is much better to terminate the treatment with the client at that point, rather than place her on the couch and remove the make-up, if appropriate, only to find that the treatment cannot go ahead as a contra-indication is present.

Provide facial skincare

Identifying contra-indications

Contra-indications to a facial treatment

- Cuts and abrasion of the skin's surface
- Scar tissue less than six months old
- Recent sunburn
- Any undiagnosed lumps or swellings
- Severe eye infections
- Any bacterial, fungal or viral infections
- Conjunctivitis
- Bruising to the area
- A known allergic reaction
- Any loss of sensation in the face, dropped muscle contour or speech impediments
- For a visual reminder of the various contra-indications, refer to You and the skin, pages 208–213.

Other skin conditions

Although not commonly seen, you need to be aware of these skin conditions.

Pseudo folliculitis

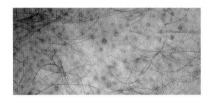

Folliculitis is an inflammation of a follicle: usually referring to infection around the hair follicle as in barbae, which is an infection of the hair follicle of the beard. Pseudo means false or a deceptive resemblance, or an illusion. So, pseudo folliculitis means the follicle is inflamed, but there may not always be an infection present.

Keloids

A keloid is a scar which has overgrown and developed into a shiny, firm, usually raised, benign (non-malignant), thickened mass of fibrous tissue. It is often seen at the site of a burn, skin wound or surgical incision, and is mostly found on the trunk or face. It is more common in pigmented skin.

Ingrowing hair

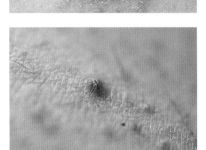

An ingrowing hair is one that grows abnormally under the skin having been covered by an overgrowth of skin cells. There are several reasons for this: some people are genetically predisposed towards them; waxing or tweezing often causes them when the hair breaks at the weakest point just below the surface of the skin. If the hair continues to grow under the skin, it can often be seen and may develop into an infection. If not infected, the hair can be freed using a sterile microlance and an antibacterial wipe.

Papule

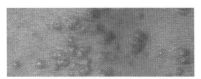

A papule is a small, solid, round, rising of the skin – in other words, a pimple. It can be quite large and sore.

Pustule

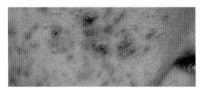

A pustule is a papule with an infection present as in acne, eczema, smallpox, chicken pox or impetigo. Pus forms and will need to be treated with antibiotics. If the papule becomes infected and red, then pus is present.

Taking action if a contra-indication is found

Treating a client with a known contra-indication has consequences. The client could experience pain and discomfort if the treatment went ahead and the condition could be made worse, or spread to other parts of the body. The therapist could be found to be negligent, both by her insurance company and by her professional body, and the expected support may not be forthcoming should the client decide to take legal action. Any client with a suspected infection should be referred to her GP. But be careful — it is not a therapist's job role to give a medical diagnosis.

If no contra-indications are present, continue the skin analysis.

Examining the face and neck

When examining the face and neck there are many points to consider:

◉ A full picture of the skin can only be seen in a good light, with the skin free of make-up, which may mask the skin's true condition. The client is usually laid on the couch, wrapped up and then eye make-up and lipstick removal and a full cleanse takes place. Only then can you look at the skin in detail, under a magnifying lamp with the light on. However, that is an unnatural position for the client to be in — the human body is usually upright (vertical) and you should look at the client's skin when they are standing or sitting, too, so that you can allow gravity to show how the skin behaves naturally. This shows what muscle tone is like and how the contours of the face dictate the face shape, how lined the skin is and the firmness of the jaw line.

◉ Carry out the first part of the client's history when you are sitting face to face with the client. The eye contact you have gives the client the feeling that you are interested in her, that you are listening and she can see exactly what you are writing on her card.

◉ Try not to be too judgemental when talking to your client about skincare and their existing routine. They will not want to be made to feel like a naughty child who has not used the correct products.

◉ Skin conditions may not be what they at first appear. You may have to dig slightly deeper than your initial skin-type judgement. There are lots of factors which may lead you to make an incorrect diagnosis. Skincare products used wrongly and which may not be appropriate for the skin type can mislead the client into damaging the skin. For example, if strong products are used on an oily skin, it can look very dry on the top of the epidermis, with lots of sebum still being produced by the sebaceous glands. The client then adds more oil-based moisturiser as she thinks her skin is dry, and the problem gets worse. A dry skin with a rich moisturiser applied can appear to be greasy and redness can be caused by an irritation or allergy to a food, product or chemicals. All of these mask the true condition of the skin.

Think about it

You should never diagnose a contra-indication as you are not qualified to do so. You can give advice without referring to a specific medical condition and always advise the client to see their GP for a diagnosis.

Think about it

Male grooming is big business and more men are booking facials. Ask male clients to have a close shave prior to their appointment. This stops the tissues or cotton wool dragging on the skin and the skin gets maximum benefit of the massage, mask and products used.

Provide facial skincare

Preparation for full facial, including massage

1 Couch and working area tidied and prepared:
- Couch prepared with blanket and towels
- Couch roll on headrest and foot area and on the floor for client to stand on

2 Trolley prepared with:
- products
- spatulas
- tissues
- wet and dry cotton wool
- sponges (if preferred)
- jewellery bowl for client
- headband

3 Ensure client record card (and client record number if known) and pen are to hand

4 Make sure there are two chairs, a magnifying mirror and a bin with a bin liner

5 Ensure your nails are short and you are not wearing jewellery

6 Greet your client

7 Carry out a full consultation and contra-indication check

8 Position client on couch with headband on and jewellery off

9 Wash hands prior to treatment

Before beginning the examination, remember the following.

- Wash your hands thoroughly.
- Remove any make-up a client may be wearing, and cleanse, deep cleanse, tone and pat dry the skin using a tissue.
- Ideally, a male client will have had a clean shave prior to the facial examination – otherwise the cotton wool may stick to the beard growth or stubble. Also the state of the skin may be camouflaged behind a day's growth of hair, and a true picture of the skin's condition may not be seen.
- The texture of the skin and the muscle tone will be felt as the cleansing movements are made.
- The warmth of the skin will indicate how good the circulation is.
- You need a pen and your record card so you can fill in all the client's details.
- Remember to include on the record card the client's current skincare routine and how successful it is (refer to page 398, for a sample record card).

Think about it

Obtain a signed, written consent form from the client prior to carrying out the treatment. If the client is under the age of 16, a signed parental or guardian consent is essential prior to treatment and a parent should be present.

Think about it

Facials make the skin look cleaner, refreshed and are relaxing for the client. However, many long-term skin conditions will need more than one treatment before you see a good result, so you must explain that to the client and manage her expectations of the results after only one facial.

Providing recommendations to the client

If the client is suitable for treatment, with no contra-indications, you can go ahead and prepare the client for the beginning of the facial and the full skin analysis.

The treatment plan should be agreed with the client and recorded on the personal record card, along with a suitable time frame for a course of treatments, a price and budget structure (payment planning or perhaps a discount for payment in full) and details of recommended treatments and products. Remember that if you are off sick, another therapist will not know what you have agreed with your client if you have not written it down fully on the record card.

My story

Salon life – understanding the assessment process

My name is Sophia and I have been working on my facial treatments for about six months now and our tutor says we are nearly ready for assessments. Over coffee all the girls in our group discussed how scared we were of the whole assessment process and our tutor overheard us talking.

When we got into class she made us do some role-play. One of us became the assessor, one the client, and one the therapist. Our tutor explained about looking for key things, and turning the practical skills and underpinning knowledge into questions. So, instead of 'communicate and behave in a professional manner' and 'use suitable consultation techniques', we had to ask 'Did the therapist have good communication skills and did the therapist use suitable techniques'? It's not that scary because it is all in the book and you just have to follow your outcomes. One therapist forgot to wash her hands before treatment so our tutor said that the assessor had to assess that treatment as non-competent for not following good health and safety practice. It was a really good lesson on how an assessor will be observing absolutely everything you do.

I understand what an assessor is looking for now because I have been one!

Above all, you want the client to be happy with your recommendations – your client is a valued customer, who you want to keep for a long time, and your professionalism and integrity will ensure this. Revisit Client care and communication (pages 67–98) to remind yourself how to agree services and treatment objectives with the client.

Your final treatment plan should be suitable for the client's skin type and condition and she must be happy with what you are planning to do.

All the findings from your consultation and skin analysis should be recorded on the client's personal chart. The style of the chart may vary from salon to salon, but the basic information recorded is the same (see Professional skills (pages 8–65)).

Refer to You and the skin (pages 181–226) to refresh your knowledge of skin types and how to recognise them.

It is important that all information is recorded – the client may not be booked in with the same therapist every treatment, and records of any allergies, reactions and favourite products will help keep the client safe and avoid duplication.

Think about it

During a facial treatment the client should feel warm and cosy under either a blanket and towels, or a quilt – often clients fall asleep when the mask is on. However, check with the client that they are not claustrophobic and are happy to be cocooned. It will detract from the treatment and add to their stress if they feel trapped and hot and bothered.

Provide facial skincare

Think about it

Never be persuaded to carry out a treatment on a client with any contra-indications present. They are asking you to compromise your professional standing and there could be serious consequences. There is both a risk of cross-infection and of cross-contamination. If the client then decides that you have caused further skin damage or made an existing condition worse, she could sue you, your insurance may be void, and you might be proven to be negligent in a court of law. It really is not worth risking your whole career to keep a client happy. Just say no.

When planning your treatment, you must consider the personal product preferences of the client. Some clients like the feel of water on the face, others do not; some like a cream, others prefer a lighter texture. Investigate different product houses – most produce specific lines for each skin type, and you can recommend a whole range which work together. Also remember to introduce the client to professional ranges of skincare which are for salon sales only – they are generally more effective than normal retail products and are part of the professional package of having treatments from a trained professional skincare expert – you!

Equipment and materials

As well as deciding on the type of products that will meet your client's needs when planning her treatment, you should give some thought to the equipment and supporting materials required – such as a magnifying lamp, skin warming devices, for example hot towels, and consumables – before beginning the facial.

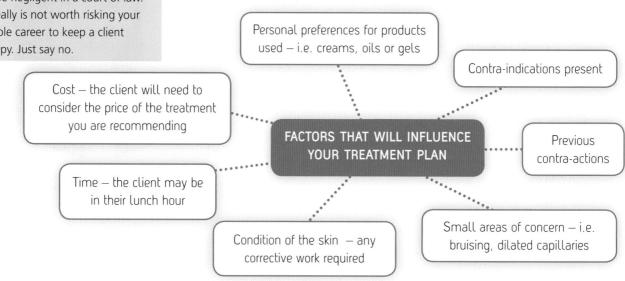

Personal preferences for products used – i.e. creams, oils or gels

Contra-indications present

Cost – the client will need to consider the price of the treatment you are recommending

FACTORS THAT WILL INFLUENCE YOUR TREATMENT PLAN

Previous contra-actions

Time – the client may be in their lunch hour

Condition of the skin – any corrective work required

Small areas of concern – i.e. bruising, dilated capillaries

For your portfolio

Most large product houses (e.g. Dermalogica, Decleor and Clarins) produce their own skin analysis and record cards. Investigate two of them and see how they differ from the one you use at college – which one is best and why? Should you devise one of your own?

How did you do?

You can check your facial cleansing techniques quite easily. To ensure that the eyes are grease free, go back to the eyelashes and run a dry cotton bud along the length of the lash. If the cotton bud is dirty, you will know you have not cleaned thoroughly enough.

You can repeat the exercise for the skin by running a dry cotton bud along the cheek bones.

Do not be disappointed if you haven't got it right the first time. Your technique will improve with practice.

Cleansing the client's skin prior to skin analysis

Step-by-step facial cleanse

1 Using damp cotton wool apply eye make-up remover, working around the eye, over lid, underneath and over lashes. Work from inner to outer area. Remove with damp cotton wool. Follow the same routine with the other eye. Be careful to support the eye area, and do not drag, or apply any pressure.

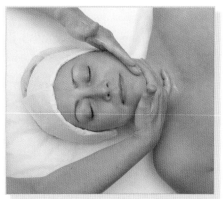

2 Apply a small amount of cleanser, using damp cotton wool, and remove the lipstick in small circular motions.

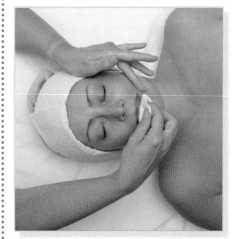

3 Apply dots of cleanser over the entire face and warm some in the palms of your hands. Working from the neck upwards, use upward movements towards the jaw line.

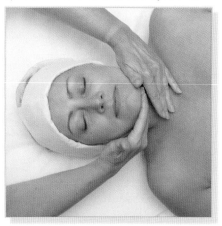

4 Work from the jaw line; use alternate hand movements to cover the entire cheek area.

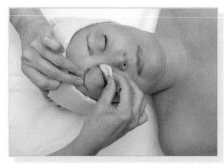

5 Using the index fingers, work into the nose, with small circular motions, without blocking the nostrils in! Use light pressure only.

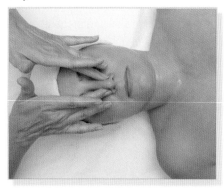

6 Travel over the bridge of the nose, on to the forehead working out towards the temple areas. Using index fingers, apply a little pressure to the temples.

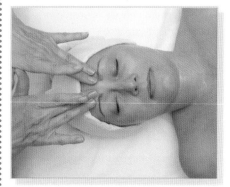

7 Sweep back down to the chin, working over the jaw line with alternate hand movements, to finish the cleanse routine.

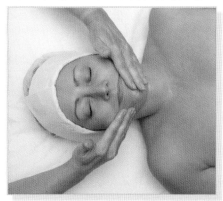

8 Remove cleanser, following the same routine direction as for the application of cleanser, with tissues, damp cotton wool or sponges.

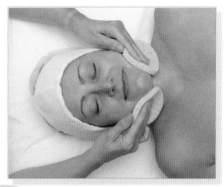

9 Blot the face with the tissue folded in a triangle. Pat gently with the hand, turn tissue over and repeat on the other side of the face.

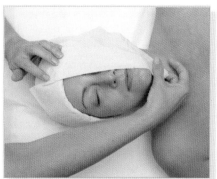

Selecting suitable products, tools and equipment

Before you can decide on any treatment plan or recommend suitable products, you have to know the treatments and products thoroughly. You should have experience of the treatments yourself, so you can talk about the sensations as well as the effects.

You need to have a full knowledge of products and treatments before you go on to facial massage techniques. This is so you can decide upon oil or cream and which massage medium and movements are most suitable for the skin type. You will need to refer back regularly to the planning section as you work through the massage techniques.

Facial products

To improve the facial skin condition, there are many **facial products** available on the market that can be used to good effect within the facial treatment:

- eye make-up remover
- cleansers
- toners
- moisturisers
- exfoliants
- masks
- specialist skin preparations
- massage mediums – usually oil or cream
- specialist products – serums or eye creams

The cosmetic and skincare preparation market is huge. The range of manufacturers producing good-quality products both for salon use and for retailing is ever-growing. Your salon or teaching establishment may have their own particular favourite which, from experience, they prefer.

Reasons for skin damage	Signs or symptoms
Ultraviolet radiation – excessive exposure to the sun or artificial sunlight (sunbeds)	The skin ages prematurely because of free radicals (highly reactive chemicals that attack molecules by capturing electrons and thus changing chemical structure) causing breakdown of collagen and elastin that supports the skin Uneven pigmentation – either brown spots (hyperpigmentation) or loss of pigmentation (hypopigmentation) Blood and lymphatic flow to the skin cells may be impaired due to loss of structural support of the connective tissue Cellular reproduction is slowed down through damage to the DNA in each cell Loss of strength and resilience in the skin Skin looks lined and wrinkles appear prematurely Skin feels thick and may be dry to the touch
Insufficient fluid intake	Poor blood flow and sluggish lymph drainage to the skin resulting in lack of oxygen to the skin cells and reduced removal of water products Impaired epidermis enzyme activity resulting in loss of strength in the skin's fibres

Key terms

Facial products – therapeutic beauty treatments using manual techniques and a variety of cleansers, toners, moisturisers and masks designed to improve all skin conditions.

For your portfolio

Do some research to discover the latest trends in techniques. Today's discerning skincare and massage clients are often quite knowledgeable and expect the latest massage techniques and anti-ageing preparations. The eastern-influenced Ayurveda treatments are also very popular and skincare companies are trying to match the trends. Many clients will be interested in Fairtrade and organic products, so research the best ones to offer.

Think about it

Skincare products must, by law, display their ingredients on the outside of the package, with the ingredient with the highest percentage of content appearing first. Check for products which your client might be allergic to. There may also be a rabbit sign which means the product has not been tested on animals – but be careful, as although the finished product might not have been tested on animals, individual ingredients might have been. This may be important to your client.

Reasons for skin damage	Signs or symptoms
A fat-free diet and/or general poor nutrition	Lack of essential fatty acids in the diet weakens the acid mantle resulting in slow healing and poor nerve reactions to stimulus
Impaired defence against disease and infection
Poor cell division for healing and a higher likelihood of scar tissue forming because of lack of vitamins
Lack of protein in the diet (protein promotes growth and repair of cells). A very narrow food intake will mean vital minerals and vitamins may be missing
Hyperpigmentation
Vascular conditions forming and developing earlier such as spider naevus or couperose conditions
Reactive skin conditions more likely, e.g. acne rosacea
Excessive lines and wrinkles from alcohol intake and smoking	Contamination of skin, clogged and blocked pores, irritations occur and a tendency to comedones. Skin is more prone to allergic reactions. Lack of oxygen makes the skin yellow with sallow tones often with nicotine residue left on the skin
Pollution from chemicals, traffic and thinning of the protective ozone layer	Leads to dehydration and over activity of the sebaceous glands causing congestion problems
Heat and steam	Overstretches the skin, causing damage such as permanent open pores
Incorrect use of skincare products	Inappropriate products can cause comedones to form or skin becomes oversensitive. Using products with a high alcohol content will dry out the surface but with sebum coming through from the sebaceous glands, so greasy skin has dry patches
The acid mantle may be disturbed as it tries to rectify the damage caused by incorrect skincare

How to recognise skin damage

Think about it

In a salon you will need to have all equipment to hand while talking through the client's needs. You will choose the equipment you need according to the results of your skin analysis. So, while you may think you do not need equipment information at this stage in your training (as you have yet to learn a facial cleanse routine), you will need the information to make an informed decision at the consultation stage in a proper client situation.

For your portfolio

All beauty therapists need to use a variety of different products until they find their own personal preference. You should attend the various trade shows and exhibitions to experiment and try the vast range available. Go to your nearest large perfumery and approach the various cosmetic houses for free samples of products, until you find one you most like. Try at least three each of cleansers, toners and moisturisers. Collect price lists and advertising leaflets for your portfolio.

Provide facial skincare

Procedure	Action on the skin	Products available
Pre-cleanse – a.m. and p.m.	Part of a double cleanse – mixed with water this liquefies sebum on the skin and helps dissolve make-up making the second cleanse more effective and deep	Emulsifying cleansing oil Facial washes
Cleanse – a.m. and p.m.	Removes dirt, sweat, sebum and make-up from the skin's surface and freshens the skin after sleep	Cleansing creams, lotions and milks, facial wash-off bars, gels Water-soluble creams with muslin cloths to remove
Tone – a.m. and p.m.	Tightens the skin, stimulates the circulation and eliminates any trace of remaining cleanser from the skin	Toning lotion astringent, skin tonic bracers and fresheners
Exfoliate – once a week (some product houses produce a mild exfoliant which can be used daily)	Sloughs off the dead cells from the top layer of the epidermis to improve texture and colour while stimulating circulation	Cleansing grains that form a paste when mixed with water, ready-mixed granular paste, fruit acid peels
Day cream – a.m.	A protective film to keep the skin soft and supple – it restores the oils to the skin after toning, helping to keep the outer layers hydrated – also forms a seal and a good surface for make-up	Moisturiser creams or milks and lotions
Night cream – p.m.	An absorbent, intensive, rich cream to restore the skin's well-being without leaving the skin feeling oily	Rich moisturisers, usually in cream form
Face mask – once a week	Deep cleanses, soothes and balances the skin	Clay masks, peel-off masks, thermal masks, fruit masks, biological masks
Eye make-up remover – p.m.	A very gentle eye make-up remover, finer than a cleanser for the delicate eye area	Lotions and creams, wash-off gels
Eye balm	A delicate balm for upper and lower lid area when needed – soothing, refreshing, reduces puffiness	Moisturising lightweight creams or lotions

A good skincare routine

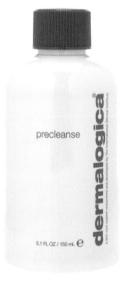

Pre-cleansers help to dissolve make-up

Pre-cleanser wash/emulsifier

Key ingredients

- Oils – olive, apricot kernel and nut oils
- Vitamin E
- Caprylic/capric triglyceride emulsifier

What they do

- Olive oil acts as a rich emollient to smooth and soften.
- Vitamin E is a rich, antioxidant vitamin to soothe.
- Capric triglyceride is an emulsifier which releases bonds into the skin when mixed with water.

Summary of action

- Liquefies sebum deposits from the skin's surface.
- Forms part of a double cleanse for a clean skin.
- Dissolves make-up.
- Removes grime and pollution without affecting the acid mantle.
- Helps smooth and nourish skin.

Method of use

- Mix with water in the palms of the hands and spread evenly over the face and neck, avoiding the eye areas.
- Lather up and massage in, using small circular motions, then rinse off with wet sponges and warm water.

Cleansing creams

Key ingredients

- An emulsion of oils, usually mineral oil or olive oil
- Waxes, usually beeswax or paraffin
- Water and water-soluble ingredients
- Emulsifiers
- Fragrance
- Preservatives

What they do

- A mineral oil will dissolve grease and oil-based products on the skin, i.e. make-up.
- Waxes provide a creamy firm texture to the product.
- The water content cools the skin and provides slip to allow easier spreading.
- Emulsifiers prevent the ingredients separating, i.e. oil and water.
- Fragrance makes the cream more appealing.
- Preservatives provide the product with a good shelf life and prevent deterioration.

Summary of action

- A deep efficient cleansing action, removes even heavy make-up.
- Leaves skin smooth and supple.
- Ideal for dry or normal skin types; too rich for an oily skin.

Method of use

- Decant a small amount onto a spatula, close lid, spread from spatula onto fingertips and massage over face and neck area using upward circular movements.
- Remove with tissues or damp cotton wool.

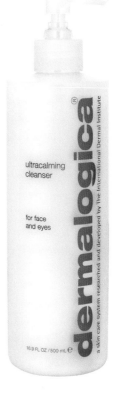

Cleansers leave skin smooth and supple

Cleansing milks

Key ingredients

- An emulsion of oils, usually mineral oil
- A smaller proportion of waxes than in a cleansing cream
- A higher proportion of water and water-soluble ingredients than creams
- Detergent
- Emulsifiers
- Fragrance
- Preservatives

What they do

◉ Detergent will act as a surface-active agent, which helps emulsify and create foaming action.

◉ For other ingredients, see above.

Summary of action

◉ A light cleansing lotion, which is easier to remove than a cleansing cream.

◉ Some cleansing milks can be worked into lather with water to wash off the skin.

◉ Ideal for most skin types except the very dry.

◉ Preferred by people who like a lighter feel to their cleanser.

◉ Also ideal for younger or greasier than normal skins.

Method of use

◉ Either apply directly on to the skin on damp cotton wool pads stroking in an upward motion, or apply with the fingertips in small circular movements.

◉ Remove with tissues or damp cotton wool.

Cleansing lotions

Key ingredients

◉ Detergent solution in water

◉ Emulsifiers

◉ Fragrance

◉ Preservatives

◉ Anti-bacterial ingredients

What they do

◉ Anti-bacterial ingredients help a greasy or problem skin.

◉ For other ingredients, see above.

Summary of action

◉ A light cleansing lotion, which can be applied on cotton wool pads.

◉ Ideal for most young skins, especially problem or blemished skins.

Method of use

◉ Apply directly on to the skin on damp cotton wool pads, stroking in an upward motion.

Facial washes and gels

Key ingredients

◉ A mixture of cleansing and wetting agents (often derived from palm oil)

◉ Water and water-soluble ingredients

◉ Fragrance and foaming agents

◉ Preservatives

◉ Conditioners and colour

What they do

◉ Cleansing agents will absorb the oil particles of dirt.

◉ Conditioners will match and balance the natural pH of skin.

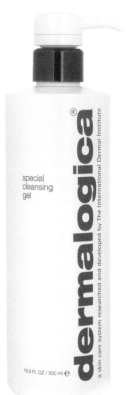

Encourage clients who like to wash with soap and water to use a cleansing gel instead

- Colour and fragrance will give appeal: for example, tea-tree may be added to give an anti-bacterial, healing property to a wash that is enhanced with a colour additive.
- For other ingredients, see page 283.

Summary of action

- Use a small amount on a moist skin, massage lightly over face and neck, and rinse off with water.
- Foaming properties will vary depending on hardness or softness of water.
- This method of cleansing can be used with a facial soft bristle brush for added stimulation.
- This is ideal for use with a brush cleanser unit (a small motor rotates the brush) and can be applied to the chest and back. This makes a very good salon treatment for a congested skin, and is very popular with male clients who suffer with problem skin.
- Some gels can also be used as shaving foam, cleansing at the same time. Check individual manufacturer's instructions for use – there are many preparations that can be bought over the counter.

Method of use

- Apply directly onto moist skin in circular motions, avoiding contact with the eyes.
- Rinse off.

Toners and skin fresheners

Key ingredients

- Alcohol, usually ethanol
- Astringents, such as witch hazel
- Antiseptic, such as hexachlorophene
- Humectants, such as glycerine
- Additives, such as cucumber, althea extract (from plants)
- Preservatives and perfume

What they do

- The alcohol removes traces of grease on the skin and helps with the drying action.
- The water content cools the skin and dilutes the alcohol content.
- Fragrance makes the toner more attractive and hides the alcohol smell!
- Antiseptic properties help heal a congested skin.
- An astringent tightens the skin and makes pores appear smaller.
- Additives such as cucumber and plant extracts soothe and soften skin.
- Humectants attract water and help rehydrate the skin.
- Colour and fragrance give appeal: for example, cucumber may be added to give a soothing property to the toner and it may be enhanced with a colour additive – blue or green are associated with cooling and calming properties.

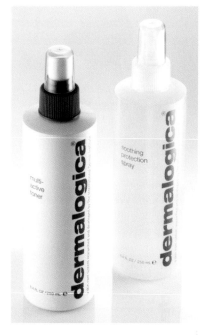

Toners and fresheners cool and refresh the skin and remove any make-up residue

Summary of action

- Toners cool and refresh the skin, and are available in differing strengths depending upon skin type.
- Strong toners for oily skins contain more alcohol, which dissolves grease; the astringent properties tighten the skin.
- All toners contain mostly water and humectants, which help with moisture retention.
- Fresheners are available which contain only soothing agents, such as azulene or camomile. As no alcohol is present, they are not as good at removing grease from the skin but are ideal on a sensitive skin.

Method of use

- Apply to the skin with damp cotton wool pads, stroking in a firm but gentle rhythm all over the face and neck.
- Toners can help smooth, soften and heal skin, increasing cell regeneration.
- They prepare the skin to receive a moisturiser by removing any trace of grease left by the cleanser.

Exfoliants

Key ingredients

- Abrasive powders such as finely ground olive stones, nuts, oatmeal, corn-cob powder or synthetic micro-beads
- Detergent
- Water and water-soluble ingredients
- Kaolin, or other clay-based ingredients
- Sodium lactate
- Added moisturisers and vitamins

What they do

- An abrasive will act as a gentle buffer to remove the dead skin cells, felt as small grains on the skin.
- Detergent continues the cleansing process.
- Water and water-soluble ingredients help provide slip so that the cream or paste flows over the skin easily and does not pull or drag the skin.
- Kaolin or other clays will absorb grease and dirt particles, gently cleansing and bleaching the skin slightly.
- Sodium lactate is an excellent humectant to regulate moisture content within the skin.
- Added moisturisers and vitamins impart a light, smooth feel to the exfoliant without being sticky or greasy.

Summary of action

- The definition of exfoliate is to peel, flake or scale, in this case the skin's cells.
- As the top layer of the epidermis is constantly shedding, an exfoliant helps the process along.
- Helping the skin clear the accumulation of dead cells brightens the complexion, softens the skin and makes the skin very receptive to receiving moisture.

Think about it

Skin toners contain 20–60 per cent alcohol.

Skin fresheners contain up to 20 per cent alcohol.

Some gentle toners for use on dry or sensitive skins do not contain any alcohol.

Skin toners with more than 25 per cent alcohol can only be used on an oily skin.

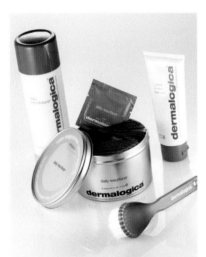

Exfoliants help to brighten the complexion by removing the dead cells sitting on the stratum corneum

Think about it

Exfoliation can be done in the shower over the whole body and is an ideal pick-me-up for the skin, for a special evening occasion, make-up application or fake-tan application. Because exfoliants remove old skin cells, other skin preparations will be able to penetrate more effectively. Many salons use exfoliants instead of steamers as they are quicker, take up less space and are economical to purchase.

- Exfoliants come in many commercial forms: a powder, which must be mixed with water, a ready-made paste, or in a suspension (with water) that can also be left on to form a face mask.
- Exfoliating face masks usually have a higher proportion of clay to make the mask dry and set on the face.
- All skin types benefit from **exfoliation** providing care is taken.

Method of use

- Apply a thin layer onto damp, cleansed skin in circular motions, avoiding the eyes. Work upwards with light pressure. Care must be taken over the delicate cheek area; if sticking or dragging of the skin occurs, add more water without soaking the client.
- Rinse off.
- Follow manufacturer's instructions. Some exfoliants can also be left on the skin as a face mask, which is left to dry and then rinsed off.
- Some face masks double as a peel, and the mask is removed by using dry fingers in a circular motion to slough off the remaining cream before rinsing.

Fruit acid peels

Key ingredients

- Available as lotions or masks containing alpha hydroxy acids (AHA)
- AHAs are fruit acids from citrus fruits, bilberries and sugar cane

What they do

- The fruit acids help dissolve the surface skin cells while stimulating the blood supply.
- They soften the skin cells and give the skin an appearance of being smoother and brighter.

Method of use

- The products come as a mask or a lotion to be applied to the skin in an upward smooth motion.
- They are ideal for a dry, mature skin.

Summary of action

- AHA treatments can cause a slight contra-action after treatment. The skin may go pink, with a tingling sensation and mild itching. This is a normal reaction and the client should be advised to expect it.

Moisturising creams

Key ingredients

- An emulsion of oils and waxes such as coconut or jojoba oil
- Water and water-soluble ingredients
- Fragrance
- Preservatives
- Emulsifier
- Humectants such as glycerine or sorbitol

> **Key terms**
>
> **Exfoliation** – the manual or mechanical method of removing dead skin cells from the top layer of the epidermis, called the stratum corneum.

> **Think about it**
>
> There are many moisturisers on the market, with different prices and varying promises to work wonders on the skin. The brand name, the packaging and the promotional skills that go with the cream can dictate the price as well as the quality of oil used and whether other key selling ingredients are included, such as vitamins.

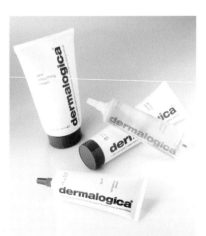

Moisturising creams

Provide facial skincare

Think about it

There are professional serums on the market for salon use which rehydrate the skin and work because they contain sodium hyaluronate which is an excellent dermal hydrator holding up to one thousand times its molecular weight. You do need to be a professional skin expert to use them as they can be full strength and for clinic use only. Serums are easily recognised by the skin and accepted at the live cellular level, allowing the active ingredients to be effective on the cells before they grow up through the epidermis and die off. Many over the counter products are greatly diluted for the general public, and cannot penetrate this far into the epidermis, working only on a superficial level. Which do you think is going to be the most effective?

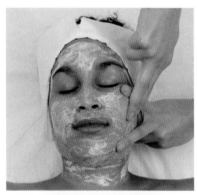

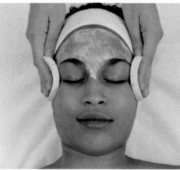

Some face masks are also peels and can be applied like a normal clay face mask but rubbed into the skin with the fingertips to aid exfoliation, then removed in the normal way with sponges and warm water

What they do

- Creams contain approximately 60 per cent water, which rehydrates the skin.
- Oils and waxes condition and improve the skin's natural water barrier; some oils such as jojoba oil prevent water loss so are ideal to add to a cream.
- Emulsifiers prevent the ingredients separating, i.e. oil and water.
- Preservatives provide the product with a good shelf life and prevent deterioration.
- Colour and fragrance will give appeal: for example, coconut oil has a very distinctive smell which appeals to most people.

Summary of action

- Moisturising creams can be used morning and evening depending upon skin type and cream used.
- Moisturising creams are recommended for dry skins that need the softening effects of the oil and waxes.
- Cream is especially good for skin in dry conditions, such as hot sun or central heating, and in very cold weather.
- Make-up application is made easier with a moisturiser underneath it. Be careful about applying cream too near the delicate eye area, which may absorb the cream and become puffy. Only eye cream should be used in the eye area.

Method of use

- Apply a light film to create a natural protective layer and prevent dehydration of the skin.
- To avoid too much cream sitting on the skin surface, check the amount applied by pressing a clean tissue to the face one minute after application. If grease is present on the tissue, too much cream has been applied, or the cream is too rich for the skin type.

Face masks

Key ingredients

- Varies depending upon type of mask used. Refer to pages 316–23 where all the products are discussed.

What they do

- Masks are deep-cleansing and draw any impurity to the surface of the skin.
- They may be slightly astringent to help dry up an oily skin, or rehydrating for a dry skin.
- Refer to specific mask information.

Summary of action

- Refer to specific mask information.

Method of use

- Refer to specific mask information.

COSHH considerations

- Health hazard: inhalation of fine particles can cause irritation when mixing powder.
- If inhaled, move to fresh air; if coughing persists seek medical advice.
- If mixing large quantities, a face guard is advisable.
- Store in a cool, dry place in a closed container.
- If in contact with eyes, rinse with plenty of water; if irritation continues, seek medical advice.
- If ingested, seek medical advice immediately.

Eye make-up removers

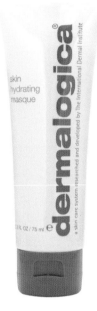

Face masks can either draw impurities from the skin or rehydrate it

Key ingredients

- Varies depending upon whether oil, gel, or lotion preparation.
- Most are prepared from a mild cleaning agent in a cosmetic base.

Typical ingredients may include:

- horse chestnut extract
- hydrolysed wheat proteins
- vitamins
- organic alcohol, e.g. PEG 200.

What they do

- Horse chestnut is used to decrease swelling and reduces puffiness in the eye area.
- Wheat proteins moisturise lids and lashes.
- Vitamins such as B5 increase cell regeneration.
- Organic alcohol is a solvent, which cleanses water and oil-based dirt.

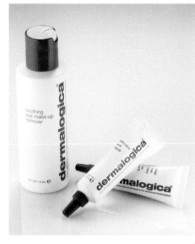

Eye make-up removers can be oils, creams or lotions depending upon the client's preference

Summary of action

- Eye make-up remover should be light, non-greasy and easily used without dragging the skin.
- Always ask the client if she is wearing contact lenses or false eyelash extensions. Both may require specialist removers, certainly one that is non-oily.
- Nothing is more irritating to the client than having a film left over the eye after removal of eye make-up. It must be thoroughly removed and not leaked into the client's eye.

Method of use

- Pre-soaked pads bought over the counter are usually lint pads soaked in remover.
- In a salon damp cotton wool pads are normally used. Gently move over the eye area with an upward and inward movement while supporting the eye area.
- Be careful to check that the client is not allergic to the metallic fibres present in cotton wool before commencing the treatment.
- A good eye make-up remover dissolves make-up immediately. Specialist oil-based remover may be needed to remove waterproof mascara.

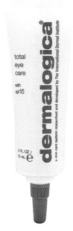

Eye cream should be used to delay the formation of wrinkles and lines – prevention is better than cure!

Eye creams, balms and gels

Key ingredients

Varies depending upon whether a cream or gel; may include:

- oil-in-water emulsions
- vitamins
- methyl cellulose
- collagen
- plant and herb extracts
- essential oils
- azulene, witch hazel, cucumber and camomile.

What they do

- Oil-in-water emulsion is easily absorbed by the skin so it moisturises and forms a good base for a daytime cream under make-up.
- Water-in-oil is a heavier solution and therefore only really good for the eye at night.
- Vitamins help with cell regeneration.
- Methyl cellulose thickens the suspension to give it a gel-like consistency, which dries on the delicate eye area firming and tightening the skin.
- Witch hazel and cucumber are mildly astringent and cooling to the eye, usually found in eye lotions.

Summary of action

- Eye creams should be used regularly to delay the formation of fine wrinkles and lines appearing with age.
- Prevention is better than cure, so eye protection should begin prior to lines forming.
- Lotions are better for oily skins and the richer, thicker-textured creams are suitable for drier, lined skin.

Method of use

- Less is more with eye creams. Application of too much is a waste of product and may cause swelling in the eye area if the soft tissue around the eye area has absorbed it.
- A small blob of cream should be warmed between your fingers before gently massaging the cream around the eye area. The ring fingers, i.e. the third fingers of each hand, have the lightest pressure and will avoid damage to the area.
- Work in small, circular motions from the bridge of the nose outward to the temples, across the top of the eye just under the eyebrow, and then underneath the eye towards the nose.
- Any excess can be blotted, but do try not to waste any of it.

COSHH considerations

For cleansing creams, milks and lotions; facial washes and gels; toners and skin fresheners; exfoliants; fruit acid peels; eye make-up removers; and eye creams, balms and gels:

- Non-hazardous, non-inflammable if less than 10 per cent alcohol.
- If ingested, drink milk or water.
- If in contact with the eyes, wash well with water; if irritation occurs, seek medical advice.
- If spilled, use absorbent towels to clean the area, wash with detergent and water to avoid slippery floors.
- No special handling and storage precautions are necessary.

Neck creams

While a lot of attention is given to the face, the neck area is a very clear mirror reflecting age and/or neglect of the skin. All facials should include the neck area, and some very good preparations are available.

Unfortunately, many clients do not bother with their necks — it is worth encouraging younger clients to pamper the neck area to prevent damage occurring.

Most neck preparations are very rich in formula, with high oil content to nourish and moisturise.

Hydrolysed collagen, elastin and vitamin E are common ingredients, which will moisturise, increase suppleness and firm the neck.

Instruct the client to apply a light film after toning at night. Encourage her to include the neck area in her morning cleanse, tone and moisturise routine even though make-up application will not go on to the neck. The neck still needs protection from pollution, the environment and the sun, and from the danger of dehydration.

Hand care

Hands often show the first signs of ageing (like the neck area), especially if neglected or unprotected.

Encourage the use of hand creams — again, prevention and protection are better than cure.

The client should rub in any excess moisturiser into her hands, rather than waste the product, and a hand cream should become part of a night-time routine.

Refer to Provide manicure treatments/provide pedicure treatments, for further information.

Lip care

Lips can be sadly neglected, until cold sores and chapped lips become a problem.

When you are removing the client's eye make-up the lipstick can also be removed, and the cleansing medium and massage motion will help keep the lips moist.

Lip balms, flavoured lip-gloss and lip creams are available to help dry or sore lips. Remember, the lips need protection against the sun, as they have no melanin of their own. While most lipsticks contain a sunscreen, naked lips will not be protected.

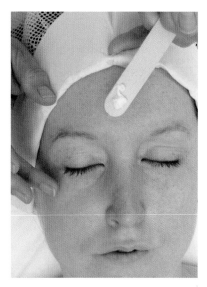

Applying eye cream: use a light touch and the ring finger to avoid too much pressure. Remember to decant the product first and use sparingly

Think about it

When carrying out a facial treatment the therapist should always include the neck area and the décolletage (chest area) as these areas are prone to ageing and lines in older clients. A face lift may make the face unlined and smooth but the ageing signs of the neck, décolletage and hands are often a giveaway to the client's true age!

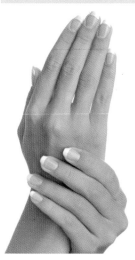

Keep hands well moisturised and use sunscreen to delay the signs of ageing such as age spots

Provide facial skincare

Product choices to suit client needs

Skin type	Products most suitable
Normal	Eye make-up remover lotion Light cleansing cream or lotion Facial wash if preferred Toner with 10–20 per cent alcohol content Light moisturiser cream or lotion Eye lotion
Dry	Eye make-up remover oil or cream Cream cleanser Low-alcohol-content toner, or no-alcohol if sensitive too Paraffin wax mask Non-setting (hydrating) mask Eye cream Cream moisturiser
Greasy	Eye make-up remover lotion Cleansing lotion or cleansing milk Facial wash or foaming gel Toner with 25–50 per cent alcohol content Cleansing grains or peel Clay-based masks Moisturiser milk Light eye gel
Combination	T-zone – follow greasy skin recommendations Dry cheek areas – follow dry skin recommendations Normal cheek areas – follow normal skin recommendations Young congested T-zone – follow congested skin recommendations with normal skin recommendations on cheeks Exfoliating cream/gel Balancing mask (two masks can be used, one on the T-zone and one on the cheeks)
Sensitive	As for dry skin Specialist products are available for hypersensitive skin Check for known allergies to products Check for allergies to cotton wool
Dehydrated	As for dry skin Specialist treatments are available in most salons using advanced techniques such as a galvanic facial (VRQ Level 3 work). Be aware and read the salon price list. Another therapist may be able to help the client's skin.
Congested	Eye make-up lotion Cleansing lotion or cleansing milk Facial wash or foaming gel Toner with 25–50 per cent alcohol content Cleansing grains or peel Clay-based masks Moisturiser milk Light eye gel

Provide facial skincare

Provide facial skincare treatments

In this outcome you will learn about:

- communicating and behaving in a professional manner
- following health and safety working practices
- positioning yourself and your client correctly throughout the treatment
- using products, tools, equipment and techniques to suit your client's treatment needs, skin type and condition
- completing the treatment to the satisfaction of the client
- recording the results of the treatment
- providing suitable aftercare advice.

Health and safety

Facials have many potential hazards. Remember to think of potential unsafe practice and to minimise risks prior to the client coming in for the treatment.

Health and safety considerations for facials

Hazards: only look for hazards that you would reasonably expect to result in significant harm under the conditions in your workplace. Use the following examples as a guide.

- **Environmental** risks such as slipping/tripping (e.g. poorly maintained floors or stairs) or spillage of massage oil, creams, etc.

- **Fire** from flammable materials or products (e.g. the magnifying lamp with no cap on it can be considered a fire risk if left by a window — the sun will come through the window, magnify the heat through the lamp and may set the couch cover on fire).

- **Equipment** The height of the couch, trolleys or stools could cause repetitive strain injury or a sore back through poor posture.

- **Reactions** Any products may cause irritation, swelling, redness of the skin, eye irritation or eczema. There may be a reaction between products, e.g. if a client has recently used a home hair colour and then uses her normal cleanser, one may trigger a reaction from the other.

- **Allergies** The most common ones are to nuts in almond-oil based products, cleansers and moisturisers and nickel, which is in some cotton wool as filaments, but clients can develop a sudden sensitivity to any product that they may have been using without problems for years.

- **Noise** Not necessarily a hazard unless the stereo is so loud it affects the eardrums, but certainly a distraction from relaxation if the noise disturbs.

- **Poor lighting** May cause accidents through not seeing a trailing lead or cable, and may cause the wrong products to be applied if the lighting is too low.

- **Low temperature** Not necessarily a hazard but this would certainly make the client uncomfortable and cause shivering, which is hardly relaxing.

Provide facial skincare

Disposing of waste materials safely and correctly

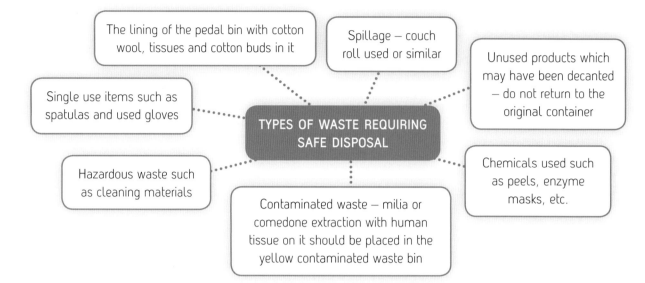

Important Acts of Parliament to take into consideration are:

◉ Environmental Protection Act, 1990

◉ The Controlled Waste Regulations, 1992 (as amended)

◉ Special Waste Regulations, 1996 (as amended).

All clinical waste must be kept apart from general waste and be disposed of in a licensed incinerator or taken to a landfill site by a licensed company.

This includes:

◉ waste which consists wholly or partly of animal or human tissue

◉ swabs or dressings

◉ syringes or needles.

Refer back to Professional skills, You, your client and the law, page 54, for further information.

The only human tissue you may be required to dispose of as contaminated waste during a facial treatment is the by-product of **extraction** (including milia extraction), or if you have made the client bleed during extraction. This human tissue needs special treatment. The probe should also be treated as contaminated waste, and be put into the sharps box for safe disposal by a registered firm.

Your legal and personal obligations are all covered in Professional skills, You, your client and the law (pages 42–64). The Health and Safety at Work Act (see pages 43–45) and Follow health and safety practice in the salon (pages 67–97) are also important, as the client's safety is a vital aspect of any facial treatment.

This outcome is all about performing the facial treatments: you have assessed all health and safety considerations, completed your skin analysis in a hygienic manner, prepared your products and equipment and the treatment plan has been agreed with the client. The client is in a safe and comfortable position, with the skin cleansed and ready to receive your attention.

Key terms

Extraction – the act of drawing or pulling out of the body a foreign body, blackhead or something from the eye.

Using a suitable skin-warming technique

Warmth applied to the face is a very good way of helping to maximise the effects of the treatment. Warmth will help relax the muscles, open the pores and soften the skin in preparation for further treatments. Extraction and nourishing the skin are extremely effective after **skin warming**.

There are several ways to warm the skin:

- hot towels
- facial steaming
- self-heating products such as thermal masks.

Hot towels

Hot towels are a very convenient method of warming the skin. They can be applied without equipment and are ideal for the mobile therapist who does not have access to a facial steaming unit.

Hot towels were always used in the old-fashioned barbershop when a close shave was offered with the haircut. A hot flannel would have the same effect but may make the client feel claustrophobic.

How do I do it?

- Fold a hand towel into four and immerse in hot water leaving an edge for the hands to grip.
- Alternatively, if you have a hot-towel steaming unit (a small oven that looks like a microwave), put in a damp towel and the heater will warm it up for you.
- Remember health and safety — if the towel is too hot to wring out with the hands, it is too hot to go on the face. It needs to be hand hot.
- Wring out and fold over the client's face, with the towel ends at the forehead. This will allow the nose to remain uncovered for claustrophobic clients.
- Press gently into the contours of the face until the towel cools. Do not allow the face to become cold again as this will negate the benefits of the treatment.

The hot-towel procedure can be repeated if needed.

Treatments can now be carried out on a beautifully clean, receptive skin.

Facial steaming

Face steamers are like big kettles — they boil water to create steam. Steam benefits the skin by opening the pores and allowing deep cleansing. They are nearly always used in conjunction with face masks and are classed as a special treatment.

Most facial steamer machines have the following characteristics:

- Vapour jets can be swivelled in all directions.
- Control panel has a warning light.
- Water capacity is 2 litres.
- Boiling time with 2 litres of water is nine minutes.
- Distilled water only must be used to maintain the life of the equipment and avoid limescale build-up on the heating element.

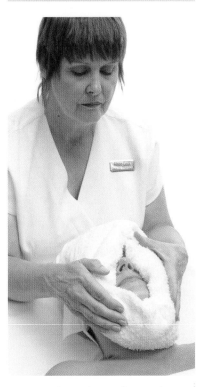

Hot towels can be used to apply heat to the skin, making it more receptive to further treatment

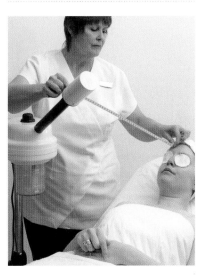

Always measure the distance of the steamer to your client's face to avoid scalding and drips which can burn the skin

Provide facial skincare

◉ Essential oils can be added by applying them to cotton wool, which is placed in the special filter basket located in the filling funnel. Oily liquids must not be poured directly into the steamer.

◉ The heater should be de-scaled periodically with acidulated water, following the manufacturer's instructions.

Caution

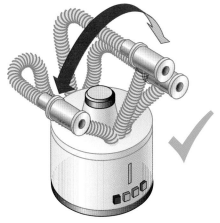
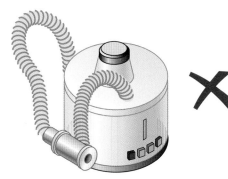

The illustration shows the maximum possible head swivel to prevent the vapour from spraying water during the treatment.

The vaporiser must under no circumstances be used with the head in the position shown on the left. This position stops the condensation returning to the heater and the vaporiser will spray water.

Contra-indications to a steam treatment

◉ Hypersensitive skins

◉ Open cuts – infection could set in

◉ Acne rosacea

◉ Split capillaries – increasing the circulation and heat will put extra strain on these delicate blood vessels, and in some cases will worsen them

◉ Bad streaming colds or hay fever

◉ Severe bronchial conditions or asthma

◉ Very high blood pressure or where the client suffers from dizzy spells

◉ Any eye infections, such as conjunctivitis, which could spread in the warm conditions

◉ Diabetes – the metabolic rate must not be increased

◉ Sunburn or previous ultraviolet exposure

◉ Claustrophobia

Benefits of steaming:

◉ The circulation is increased, causing the pores to open; the skin sweats, getting rid of impurities such as dirt, old make-up and dead skin cells, leaving the skin with a fresher, glowing appearance.

◉ Stimulates oil glands and improves moisture content in the skin.

◉ Comedones are more easily removed with less risk of scarring or marking the skin.

- Aids the process of shedding old skin cells – called desquamation.
- Helps with regeneration of skin cells in a dry, mature or dehydrated skin.
- A relaxing treatment for the client, because of the warmth and the essential oils if used.

Items required

- Distilled water (required for refilling machine).
- Cotton wool rounds (damp) for eyes.
- Tissue (this is used to wipe the client's face during treatment, avoiding drips which can lead to discomfort for the client).

Preparation of couch

- Check that the couch is stable and will not move during treatment.
- Place the couch in a semi-reclining position.

Preparation of client

- Prepare the client, as you would do for any facial treatment, paying special attention to the head and ensuring that there are no stray hairs around the face and neck.
- Ensure the client is comfortable and relaxed and all jewellery has been removed.
- Lay a towel across the neck area (if treating the neck and face, then lay the towel across the chest). Tuck the towel in at either end.
- Explain the treatment to the client – this will allay any fears she may have. Commence the treatment with a facial cleanse.

Safety precautions

- Check the machine, e.g. wires, flex, plug and on/off switch.
- Check the level of distilled water is correct.
- Check the machine is functioning correctly and producing ozone (before the client's arrival).
- Ensure the couch is stable and in the correct position.
- Ensure that the flex does not trail across the floor, endangering other clients, your colleagues and yourself.
- When the machine is not in use, make sure it is unplugged and in a safe area away from the main activity in the salon.
- During treatment the therapist must be in attendance at all times.
- Eye pads must be used throughout this treatment.
- While the machine is in use, ensure that it is the correct distance away from the client to avoid scalding.
- Take care when repositioning the machine, as it gets hot during use.
- Make sure there is a steady flow of steam coming from the nozzle before placing the steamer arm over the client's face. This will ensure the nozzle does not spit out hot water and burn the client.

Think about it

As a safety precaution for steaming, always place the client in a semi-reclining position. Never have the client lying flat with the face up and the steamer directly over the face – if the boiling water spits out or drips, it will fall on to the client and cause burns. If the steamer is parallel to the face, any drips will go on to the floor, which although potentially hazardous, will not harm the client. All spillage must be cleaned up, before an accident occurs.

Provide facial skincare

Face steaming – application

- Salon pre-treatment to facial steaming
- Manual cleanse
- Brush cleanse (depending on skin type)
- Facial vacuum (depending on skin type)

Aftercare to facial steaming

- Dry the skin with tissue before commencing other treatments.
- Continue with either massage or other electrical equipment that might be recommended for the client's skin type.
- A mask must always follow a facial steam treatment.

Steaming procedure

1 Check the tank is full and switch the machine on 5–10 minutes before it is required, to permit water heating to commence. The vapour switch is only required at this stage.

2 Ensure the client is well protected with towels and that her hair is covered.

3 Prepare the client for facial treatment by cleansing the skin, and at the same time discuss and explain the treatment and its effects, thus alleviating any fears she might have. Inform her that the machine will make a noise and that an unusual smell will be present – all of which is perfectly normal.

4 Ensure the client is in a semi-reclined position.

5 Place eye pads (damp) over the client's eyes. This will avoid irritation.

    When the client is fully prepared, position the steamer approximately 30–45 cm from the client's face, using at this stage only vapour.

6 Once the client is settled, inform her you are switching over to ozone, then switch on the ozone control. The steam changes its consistency, becomes ionised, cloud-like and very fine in appearance.

    (Refer to your professional body for directives about using ozone.)

7 Stay in attendance at all times and regularly check the client's skin reaction. Points to note are hot spots, erythema or client's discomfort – if any of these occur, discontinue treatment. Cool the skin with the application of a cool compress – not too cold as this will make the client jump.

8 Remember to wipe away with tissue any drips that might cause client discomfort.

9 Do not exceed the treatment time. This will vary between 10 and 20 minutes depending on skin type.

10 On completion of the treatment return to vapour, then switch the machine off completely.

11 Unplug the machine and place it in a safe area of the salon.

12 Remember to remove all surface moisture with a tissue.

13 If necessary, use your metal eradicator (comedone extractor) for blackheads.

14 Complete the treatment with a massage and face mask or continue with another electrical apparatus depending on the client's skin type or treatment plan.

Think about it

Before you start any electrical equipment application, you should carry out thermal and sensitivity skin tests to the face.

Thermal skin test – this involves the use of hot and cold to test the skin's sensitivity to heat. Fill two test tubes: one with cold water, the other with warm. Place the test tubes alternately on the client's skin and ask her to specify which one is cold and which one is warm. This test should be used before applying heat to the client's skin. It shows whether the nerve endings in the skin are working properly.

Sensitivity skin test – for this test the client should close her eyes. Touch her face alternately with a soft object, such as a smooth tissue or piece of cotton wool, and an object with a sharp edge, such as a spatula. If the client is able to distinguish between the two, then the sensory nerve endings are working in the skin and the treatment can take place.

General cleanse and tone	5 minutes on lower neck 5 minutes on lower face 4–5 minutes on full face
Disinfecting and antibacterial effect on oily and blemished skin	10 minutes on lower face and neck 10 minutes on full face
Regenerating effect on dry/dehydrated mature skin	2–3 minutes on lower face and neck 1–3 minutes on full face to achieve erythema

Recommended application time and treatments

Conclude this treatment with a nourishing massage to prevent irritation and overdryness.

Note: After treatment, surface moisture should be removed, then other treatments or a mask should be applied.

Risk assessment for steaming equipment

Refer to Follow health and safety practice in the salon, pages 68–90, for a complete discussion on risk assessment.

Hazards: only look for hazards that you could reasonably expect to result in significant harm under the conditions in your workplace. Use the following examples as a guide.

- **Fire** (e.g. from electrical flex or lead)
- **Burning of equipment** (through low water level in the tank)
- **Moving parts of machinery** (e.g. casing gets hot – use towel to protect hands)
- **Ejection of materials** (spitting hot water)
- **Electricity** (e.g. poor wiring)
- **Fumes** (e.g. from added aromatherapy chemicals)
- **Manual handling** (hot casing)
- **Falling machinery** (if not securely attached to base when moving steamer)

Salon after-treatment

- Extraction of blackheads – if required on oily skin. (Refer to page 300 for the procedure to use for comedone extraction.)
- Massage – all skin types.
- Massage including audio-sonic – dry or dehydrated skin.
- Mask – use appropriate mask for client's skin type.
- High frequency: direct – oily skin; indirect – dry or sluggish skin.
- Galvanic-iontophoresis – dry or dehydrated skin.

From this list and from the salon pre-treatment list for facial steaming, a treatment plan with variety can be compiled, offering maximum benefit to the client.

Provide facial skincare

Face steaming – suggested routines

A	B	C	D
Cleanse	Cleanse	Cleanse	Cleanse
Facial steam	Brush cleanse	Facial steam	Brush cleanse
Manual massage – either normal/dry or oily skin	Facial steam	Massage including audio-sonic – dry/dehydrated skin	Facial vacuum
Mask	Use of comedone extractor – oily/blemished skin	Mask	Facial steam – oily/blemished skin
Tone, moisturiser	Mask	Tone, moisturiser	Mask
	Tone, moisturiser		Tone, moisturiser

E	F	G	H
Cleanse	Cleanse	Cleanse	Cleanse
Facial steam	Facial steam	Facial vacuum	Facial steam
Direct high frequency	Massage	Facial steam	Non-surgical face lifting
	Galvanic iontophoresis – dry/dehydrated skin	Indirect high – dry/dehydrated skin	Galvanic cleanse
		Cleanse	Balancing programme
			Lifting
			Iontophoresis

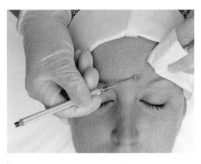

Extraction using a sterile comedone extractor

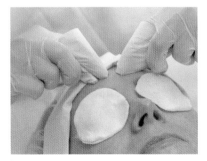

Extraction using fingertips covered with gloves and tissue

Awarding Organisation code of ethics on the use of ozone

The use of ozone can be very beneficial when administered in small quantities and under supervision, but it may also be destructive when used incorrectly.

Some public health authorities and beauty examination boards believe that the use of ozone can be bad for your health. Inhaling it in great strength can lead to respiratory infections.

Most Awarding Organisations do not recommend that ozone is used under any circumstances.

Self-heating products such as thermal masks

Refer to **mask treatments** (on pages 316–23) for the use of thermal masks to pre-heat the skin.

Carrying out comedone extraction

Some salons offer milia extraction during a facial, using a sterile probe to pierce the skin at the site of the milia. The milia are then safely squeezed out. Tissues should be used to protect the hands, and gloves should also be worn. There is often a small amount of blood spotting.

Using a sterilised comedone extractor, gently apply pressure to the comedone centre and ease the comedone out. Do not apply too much pressure, or squeeze, as this can cause scarring.

If a metal comedone extractor is not available, cover the fingertips with tissue and gently roll the skin around the comedone, to ease it out.

Brush cleansing

Brush cleansing is designed to give deep cleansing and a stimulating massage. It can be used to remove a mask or peel from the skin. It is essential to follow the individual manufacturer's instructions.

Most brush systems are supplied with a complete range of brush, sponge and pumice heads, which ensure perfect treatment on most skin types, providing no contra-indications are present.

To ensure there is no unnecessary pulling of the delicate facial or neck tissue, most machines have variable speed control and directional change for the heads.

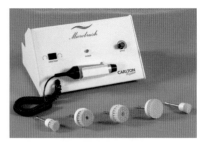

A brush cleansing machine

Pumice stone head (small 20 mm)

This pumice stone head will remove film or gel masks with a slightly abrasive action yet will cause very little skin drag. It can also be used for desquamation and treatment on scarred or pigmented tissue. It can be incorporated into a pedicure treatment for the removal of hard skin on the heel.

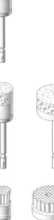

Sponges (small 20 mm, medium 40 mm)

When dampened, these very versatile heads can be used on the most delicate and sensitive skin types. For best results, they should be used in conjunction with a foaming, deep-cleansing product.

Brushes (small 20 mm, medium 40 mm)

Soft brushes can be used for all types of deep-cleansing treatments and stimulation massage on most areas of the face or body. The small head will easily treat areas around the ears, nose and eyes, while the larger head can be most successfully used on foreheads and cheeks.

Brush – bristle (medium 40 mm)

This bristle head gives a very stimulating treatment while desquamating the skin and cleansing blocked pores. It is a suitable treatment for those clients with firmer tissue, especially men.

Brush – medium goat hair (cylindrical 60 x 40 mm)

Used in conjunction with a foaming cleanser or any desquamating product, this cylindrical body brush will deep cleanse the back, arms or legs. As well as cleansing, the action provides a gentle, stimulating massage, increasing circulation and therefore improving skin texture and colour.

Contra-indications to a brush cleanse

- Broken skin
- Skin diseases or infections
- Hypersensitive skins
- Extremely loose tissue
- Broken veins
- Inflammation or irritation of the skin
- Diabetes

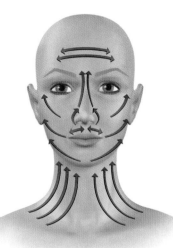

The direction of strokes when giving a skin brushing treatment

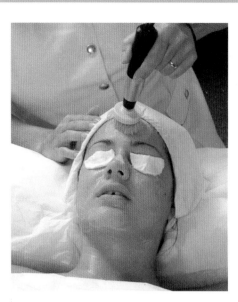

Brush cleansing of the face

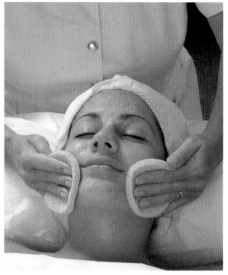

Sponges are used to remove the gel

Effects of a brush cleanse

- Aids desquamation.
- Stimulates deeper cell renewal.
- Removes surface cellular matter.
- Deep cleanses and refines skin tissue.
- Relaxes muscle fibres.
- Stimulates superficial and deeper tissues.
- Improves cellular function and regeneration.
- Aids the removal of waste products from the area.
- Increases blood and lymph circulation.

How do I do it?

1 Prepare the client for a normal facial procedure.

2 Remove eye make-up.

3 Give a superficial manual cleanse to the face and neck, using skin cleanser suitable for the skin type.

4 Select the recommended product suitable for the skin type to the face and neck. Decant a sufficient amount into a plastic bowl and replace the lid of the product. Application can be done with the brush head, mask brush, damp sponges or hands, depending upon recommendations. The product will either be a foaming cleanser or facial scrub, depending upon client needs.

5 Select the brushing head required, wet it in warm water (without it dripping) and insert it firmly into the black handle. Turn on the machine.

6 Make contact with the back of your own hand and ensure speed control is at minimum – always test the machine on yourself prior to using it on the client. Now switch on to confirm the machine is in good working order. Demonstrate the action to the client – she needs to be aware of the noise before the machine makes contact with the face.

7   Switch off, and remove from your hand. Cleanse the head and start the process again, making contact with the client's skin.

8   Eye pads can be placed over the eyes if the client prefers – it does prevent any product getting into them.

9   Place the applicator head on to the neck and gently increase speed control until the desired action is achieved, ensuring client comfort.

10   Work upwards on the neck and face in straight lines (as in the diagram opposite) and avoid the delicate skin around the eyes.

11   Work over the area for 5–7 minutes.

12   Reduce speed control to a minimum, turn off the machine and remove the brush from the skin.

13   Remove any remaining product with damp sponges and continue the facial routine.

Risk assessment for brush cleansing equipment

Refer to Follow health and safety practice in the salon, pages 68–90, for a complete discussion of risk assessment.

Hazards: only look for hazards that you could reasonably expect to result in significant harm under the conditions in your workplace. Use the following examples as a guide.

- **Fire** (e.g. from electrical flex or lead)
- **Burning of equipment** (through motor running too fast)
- **Moving parts of machinery** (e.g. dropping heads on to client's face when removing them)
- **Ejection of materials** (spitting products into client's eyes)
- **Spillage** (e.g. from too much product applied to heads)
- **Electricity** (e.g. poor wiring)
- **Manual handling** (lifting machine)
- **Loose heads** (if not inserted into handle firmly enough)

Steaming with a brush cleanse

If a steam treatment is indicated for the type of skin being treated, it should be given either before brushing (to soften dead cells and open pores) or in conjunction with brushing – this ensures the area is also kept moist throughout the treatment. It will depend upon the skin texture – too much stimulation will not be good for a delicate skin type. Be guided by your particular manufacturer's instructions.

Care and maintenance of brush heads

After use, clean the brush head thoroughly in hot, soapy water. Rinse and dry. Place in a sanitiser between clients to avoid the risk of cross-infection. Be guided by your particular manufacturer's instructions.

Product exfoliators

If the client is restricted for time, steaming and brush cleansing may be too time-consuming. Exfoliators are now very popular in salons. In this situation the use of a product exfoliator is very effective: it can be applied easily, and is quickly removed after priming the skin to be receptive for massage and mask therapy.

The exfoliator may take the form of granules in a dry form, which you mix into a paste with warm water and massage into the skin. Product houses also make exfoliants which are pre-mixed in tubes and are so gentle some of them can be used daily. Dead skin cells are removed by abrasive powders, such as finely ground olive stones, nuts, oatmeal, corn-cob powder or synthetic micro-beads, buffing the skin. (Refer back to the product information on exfoliant use, page 286.)

There is a difference between exfoliants professionally applied in the salon and those sold to clients for use at home. Professional exfoliants have slightly stronger ingredients and require training for application; they also have activators and accelerators which need to be mixed in proportions suitable for each skin type.

The only drawback with using exfoliating products is that they can get a bit messy! Make sure the client's turban is protected with an extra layer of tissue, and put a double thickness of couch roll under the client's neck and shoulders to catch any fallen product. This can then be removed prior to the massage starting. It would be very uncomfortable for the client to be lying on granules throughout the rest of the treatment. Your fingers will also tend to pick them up, especially if you are using an oil medium, and you will drag them over the face – which will be scratchy.

The client may prefer to use eye pads to avoid getting any granules in the eye. Remember also to check the client's ears – and chest area (and in the bra!) – when removing the product, and certainly before she leaves the salon, as granules tend to fall in and look unsightly. The more you have to work with, the harder it is to remove and the messier it seems to get. Practice makes perfect, and in time you will be able to judge the amount of product needed quite effectively.

Using and adapting massage techniques

Facial massage

All massage is extremely therapeutic, whether of the face, scalp or body. It is very relaxing both to give a facial massage and to receive one. A good therapist knows her massage movements so well that she doesn't have to think about where her hands go next, and she can also enjoy the experience.

Massage movements can also be incorporated into a cleansing routine, and most other facial and cleansing treatments.

To be truly relaxing, a good massage has continuity, rhythm and the correct depth, appropriate to the area and the needs of the client.

Facial massage has several benefits.

- It helps dead surface cells to loosen and be shed. This helps the natural exfoliation process and produces a clean-looking, fresh complexion.
- Facial muscles are relaxed, and they receive more blood supply because of the stimulation to the circulation. This improves the tone and strength of the muscles, giving a firmer facial appearance.
- As the blood circulation is improved the face area is warmed. This is very relaxing if muscles are clenched and tense in the jaw and forehead.
- An increase in lymphatic drainage to the face (massage always flows in the direction of the lymph nodes) produces an increase in cellular activity and the removal of toxins. The sebaceous glands are stimulated to increase sebum production, and this keeps the skin protected and supple.

To make the treatment doubly effective, and help the massage medium penetrate deeper into the skin, try the application of heat on to the skin with either hot towels, steaming or exfoliation by brush cleansing.

Psychologically, massage is very beneficial. It is so relaxing that some clients drift off to sleep! The gentle rhythm is soothing and calming. The atmosphere in your working area should enhance this; relaxing music helps the process along and encourages the client to let go of conscious thought and drift away.

Your massage movements may need adapting for the different skin types, conditions and mediums, as well as muscular tension present and the client choice of medium. You should ask the client if she prefers oil or cream. Oily skin is best massaged with cream to avoid adding oil to the skin. Dry skin soaks up oil (although the client may prefer cream) – make sure you have enough medium on at the beginning so the massage is not disturbed by you breaking contact to apply more.

Minor contra-indications, such as a bruise, can be avoided and muscular tension in the upper back will require firmer movements. Check with the client if she prefers a firm massage or more gentle massage – ideally, facial massage will relax the client to such an extent that she goes to sleep, so avoid vigorous movements.

Massage mediums

Some product houses supply their own massage medium in their treatment range which has the same active ingredients as their face masks and cleansers. Some mediums have aromatherapy oils already added – such as Decleor products. Always follow the manufacturer's instructions and remember to check if your client has a nut allergy before using almond oil or any other nut-based oil.

Facial massage movements

Massage movements are performed with the hands over the neck, shoulders and chest, as well as the facial area. The movements require practice in order to perfect the skills and outcomes required.

Movements are adapted according to the client's needs and relate directly to the facial analysis or the consultation. It may be that your client has specific areas of tension, or that her skin is particularly dry and therefore needs an oil, rather than a cream.

The basic massage movements are classified by their names (in French) and their particular effects and benefits to the skin. These are:

- effleurage
- tapotement
- petrissage
- frictions
- vibrations.

There are two types of effleurage: superficial and deep.

Superficial effleurage

This is a light, flowing pressure used at the beginning and the end of most treatments. It introduces your hands on to the client, spreads the massage medium and can be a great linking movement to help the massage flow.

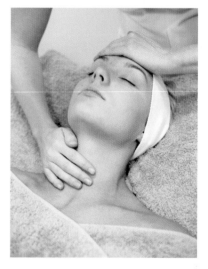

A facial massage can be very relaxing

Provide facial skincare

Think about it

How you approach massage also affects your client and the mood of the treatment. If you are rushed and hurried, no benefit will be gained by your client. Be calm, fully prepared and collect your thoughts before you begin. Giving a massage should be a little like meditation for the therapist – a quiet, soothing time for you both.

Use the entire palmar surface of the hands, keeping the fingers together and the thumb either close into the side of the hand, or open and out of the way. The area being massaged is covered by all or part of the palmar surface. Pressure should be light and even, with good contact with the skin, and the hands should be warm and relaxed.

Superficial effleurage does not normally affect the circulation as it is not a deep movement, so it can be used in any direction.

The benefits of superficial effleurage are:

- relaxation of tense muscle fibres
- a general feeling of relaxation
- stimulation of sensory nerve endings and a feeling of pleasure
- introduction of the massage medium and cream on to the skin
- a soothing and calming sensation.

Deep effleurage

This is the same type of movement as superficial effleurage but with more pressure applied – not too much to make the sensation uncomfortable, but enough to encourage muscular relaxation and for you to feel the tension knots.

Maintaining contact with the skin helps avoid overstimulation of the nerve endings. This is because when contact is broken and then re-established, it sets up a reflex response in the nerve endings, which prevents the muscles from relaxing.

The benefits of deep effleurage are that it aids:

- venous return
- arterial circulation by removal of congestion from veins
- desquamation.

Petrissage

There are four different categories:

- kneading
- wringing – mostly used on body
- picking up
- rolling – mostly used on body.

Think about it

Always use effleurage to link petrissage movements.

Petrissage always follows effleurage. It is a compression movement performed using intermittent pressure with either one or both hands, using the hands in different positions. Most petrissage movements work on all or part of a muscle and it is important that, as a muscle is slowly released from application, pressure is reduced.

Petrissage movements must be applied rhythmically and not in a hurried way. Too much pressure may result in damage to the skin – adaptation to the client's needs is vital.

Petrissage has several benefits.

- Aching, hard muscles are relaxed, helping to prevent the formation of tension modules.
- Skin regeneration is stimulated.
- It has a toning effect on muscle tissue.
- It helps eliminate muscular fatigue by aiding in the removal of lactic acid.

- It helps the removal of waste products and lymphatic flow.

Frictions

Frictions are classified within the petrissage group, but their purpose differs. Friction movements will loosen adherent skin, loosen scars, and aid in absorption of fluid around the joints. The pressure is firm and the movement is usually applied in circular directions on the face. Fingertips or thumbs are mostly used in small areas.

Frictions have two main benefits.

- Adhesions and loose skin are freed.
- Scar tissue can be stretched and loosened.

Tapotement

Tapotement is a percussion movement and involves what its name implies – tapping. The tips of the fingers are used over the face to create very light tapping movements, which stimulate the skin.

It is very important that sufficient adipose tissue is present to perform the treatment. It is not used on sensitive skin to avoid possible overreaction and skin damage.

Tapotement has two main benefits.

- It increases localised blood supply.
- It increases nervous response due to stimulation.

Vibrations

Vibrations are fine, trembling movements performed on or along a nerve path by the fingers. The muscles of the operator's forearm are continually contracted and relaxed to produce a fine tremble or vibration, which runs to the fingertips. It is used at the occipital region in facial massage.

The benefits of vibrations are:

- it can relieve pain
- it can relax the client due to its sedative effect.

> **Think about it**
>
> Make sure you have enough of the massage medium on the skin. If you have too little, the hands become sticky and the movements will not flow. If you have too much, it will run down the client's face! If in the first application you can judge that the client's skin is dry and is soaking up the cream or oil, then apply a little more at the beginning of the second application, rather than having to stop the massage to apply more.

> **Think about it**
>
> Different product houses have different massage routines and you will be taught various movements when you do your training for them. Over time and with lots of experience, you will find your massage routine grows and evolves – you will leave out some movements and put in others. Remember, movements for your assessments need to be recognisable to your assessor – so stick with the routine in the book until you have passed this unit and then you can adapt your massage to suit you and your client.

Provide facial skincare

My story

Salon life

My name is Candice and I was having trouble remembering all the information about products, massage movements and skin types for facials at Level 2. I have written out my procedures on to small postcard size reminder cards in step-by-steps and I have been using them on my trolley as I work.

I asked my mum and sisters to have facials at home for me to practise my skills and then they started coming into college to model too. It has really made a difference to my confidence – I can now complete my massage without having to refer to my sheet. I would say to anyone just starting that you need to keep practising your skills – it really does make you perfect!

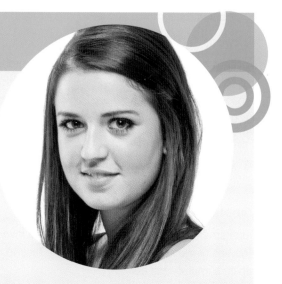

Effects of facials

Benefits of a facial for the client:

- Professional skin analysis for correct diagnosis of skin type

- Healthier looking skin and general health benefits due to better circulation of lymph and blood

- Mental and physical relaxation

- Aftercare advice and product recommendations

Benefits of a facial for the therapist:

- Excellent retail opportunities in recommending products

- Diversity of treatments and clients keeps the day interesting

- Good recommendations and treatments can improve client's confidence as well as their skin – this can be very rewarding

Ask the experts

Q *What is the most important part of a facial?*

A The consultation. You need to understand the client's needs before you begin so you can choose the right products and give the correct aftercare advice.

Q *What if a man wants a facial? What should I do?*

A Male skin is slightly thicker but you can follow the basic routine, just as you would for a female client. You will have no make-up to remove but cleansing is still important. For comfort, ensure your movements go downwards with the hair growth pattern rather than against it. Use clean sponges when removing products as cotton wool may get stuck in beard hair.

Top tips

- Practise, practise, practise until facials are routine to you. This allows you to concentrate on the client and their needs rather than focusing on what you are doing.

- Don't be afraid to try new products – the more knowledge you have, the more you can offer your clients.

- Be flexible. Product houses have different methods and procedures and your massage movements will evolve and develop as your confidence grows. When you have qualified you may change and adapt your massage routines according to who you are working with – sharing good practice and picking up tips from more experienced therapists is a great way to learn.

Step-by-step facial massage routine

Female client

All movements should be carried out six times. The massage should last for 20 minutes.

1 Apply massage medium all over the face, neck and shoulders and spread evenly. With both hands together, start at chin, and move down either side of neck towards shoulders.

2 Apply pressure over the chest and go over the shoulders, working along the upper back towards the spine.

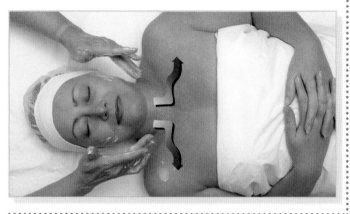

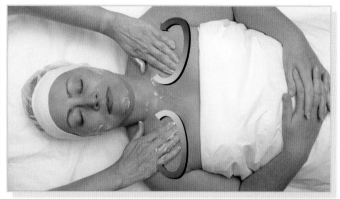

3 When your hands reach either side of the spine, work upwards and gently stretch the neck, lifting the head slightly off the couch.

4 Face brace: with hands in an upside-down prayer position, begin under the chin, with heels of the hands resting lightly on the chin. Work upwards, over the cheeks, lifting quite firmly. The cheeks will move slightly, as the client is relaxed.

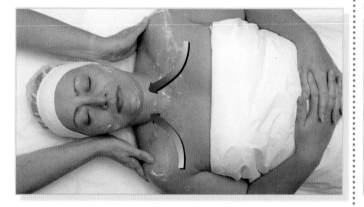

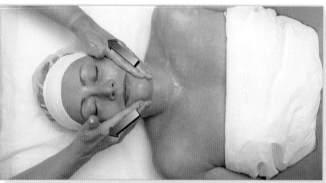

5 Finish with a firm, lifting movement on the forehead.

6 From the forehead, gently slide the hands back to the jawline.

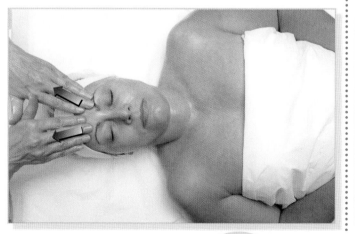

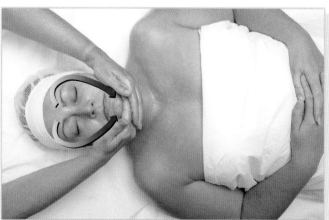

Provide facial skincare

7 Perform rotaries of petrissage, starting from the chin and moving down either side of the neck towards the shoulders and beyond, paying special attention to the arm and deltoid muscle. Use small circular motions across all of the chest area. You may only be able to use your fingertips if the client is small — no long nails!

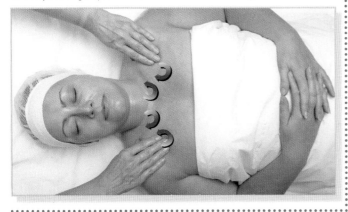

8 Continue your circular massage up the sides of the neck, ready to begin another movement.

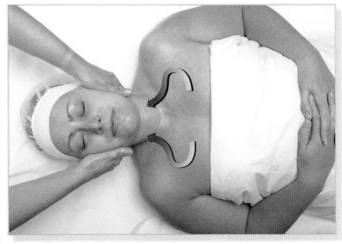

9 Turn your hands into loose fists and rotate your fingers to form knuckling. Come down from the neck and across the chest, over shoulders and back to the occipital cavity.

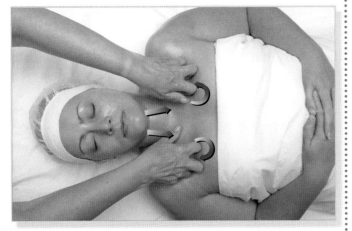

10 Finish the movement at the jawline ready to begin alternate triangular sweeping.

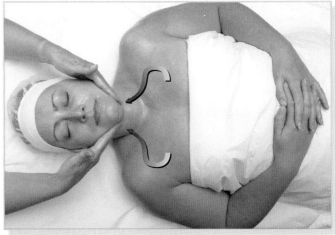

11 Support the jaw with your left hand; with the right hand, stroke down the right side, to the shoulder. Stroke across the chest to the other shoulder.

12 Take your right hand behind the shoulder.

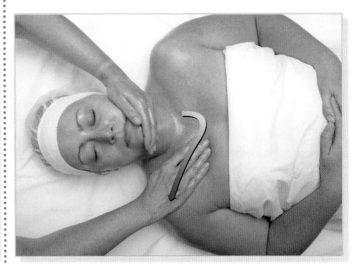

13 Stroke your left hand across the chest to meet the right hand at the right shoulder.

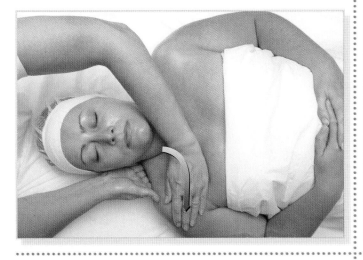

14 Bring the right hand back up to the jaw and left hand back across the chest.

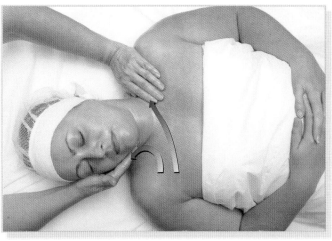

15 Bring the left hand back up to meet at the jaw.

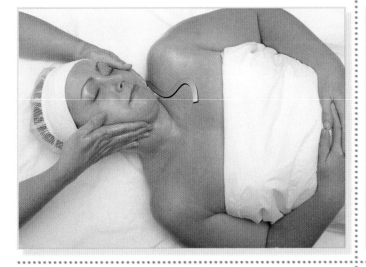

16 Bring the right hand back down at the shoulder.

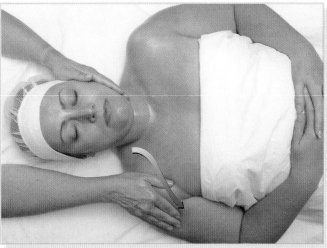

17 Perform trapezius rolling – work hands together on one side, then the other.

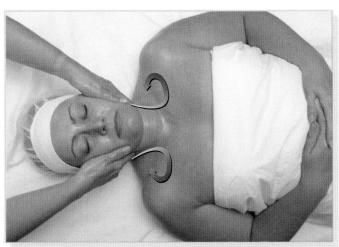

18 Cheek lift – index finger to little finger – turn and twist off.

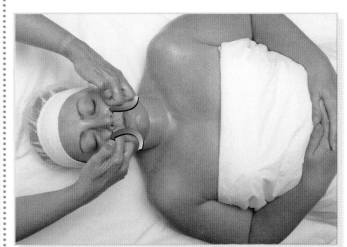

19 Tap along the jawline.

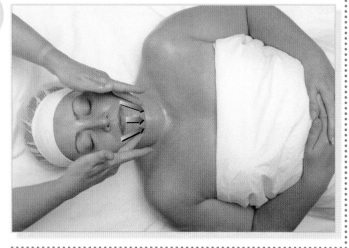

20 Perform rotaries along jawline — thumbs abducted — centre outwards.

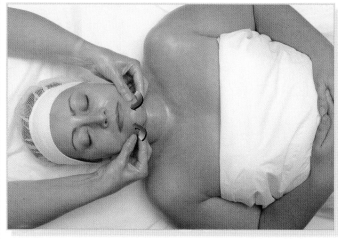

21 Knuckle over chin and cheeks.

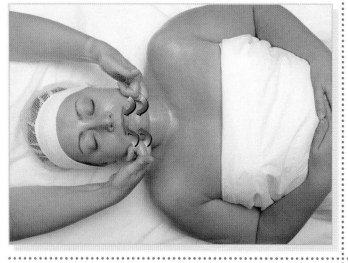

22 Facial lift — work hands along each side of the face — lift and join hands together over the forehead, then divide off.

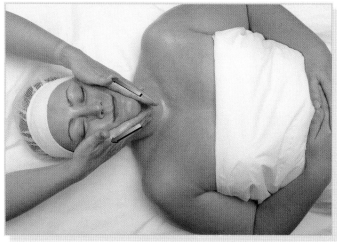

23 Forehead brace — both hands lift up the eyebrows to the hairline.

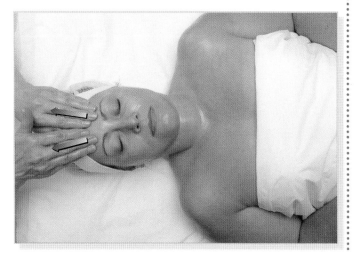

24 Turn hands sideways and gently pull the forehead from the centre, smoothing out the temples.

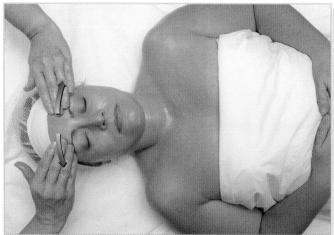

25 Finish with slight finger rotation pressure at the temples.

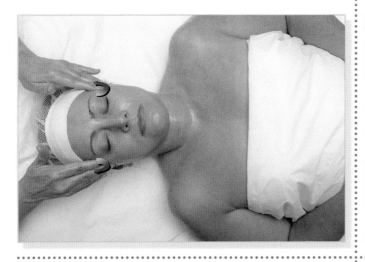

26 Slide hands down to the jaw. Pinch along the jawline, using thumb and forefinger.

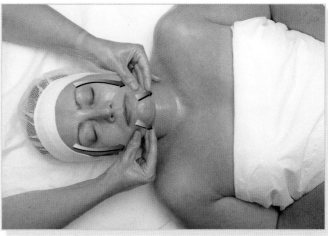

27 Using alternate hand movements, begin roll patting over cheeks and forehead. Repeat this movement over both sides of the face.

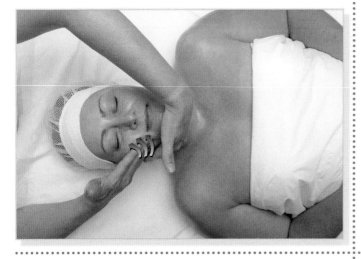

28 Tap over cheeks, using light pressure – fingertips only.

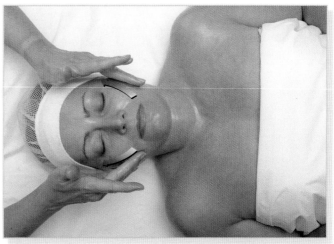

29 Apply frictions, using index fingers, around mouth and chin.

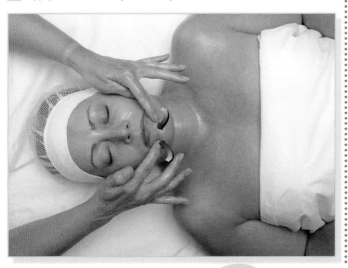

30 Apply frictions, using index fingers, around nostrils.

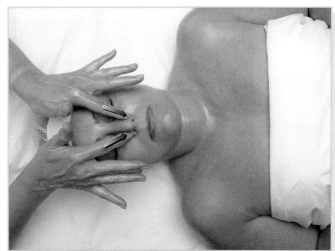

Provide facial skincare

31 Work upwards along nose with index fingers.

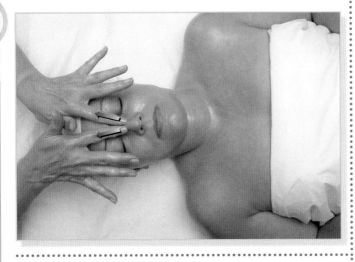

32 Zigzag with middle fingers going into a V created by the other hand over forehead.

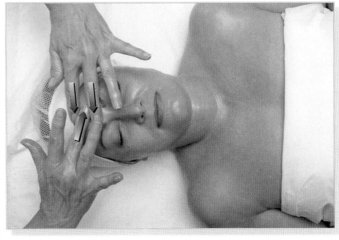

33 Working right across and down the forehead, cover all areas – this movement is especially appreciated by clients who suffer from headaches.

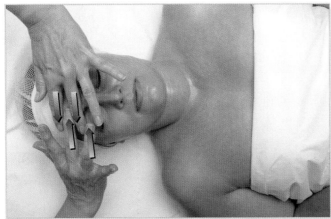

34 Do small circular pinching movements along the length of the eyebrows.

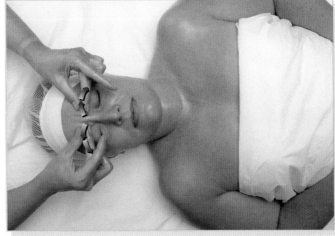

35 Piano playing across brow: circle eyes and bring all fingers across the brow. Start with little finger and finish with index finger.

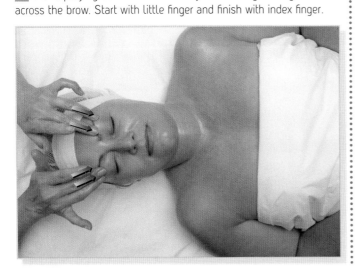

36 Pinch brows – centre to sides. Slide back and repeat.

37 Come back to jawline and begin superficial effleurage down either side of the neck.

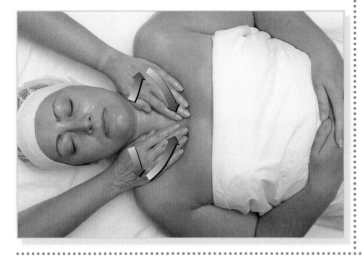

38 Perform superficial effleurage over shoulder area, gradually slowing down as you finish the massage.

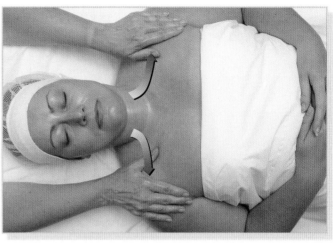

Male client

1 Cleanse as per a female client, making sure to treat the entire forehead. Long hair may still require a headband.

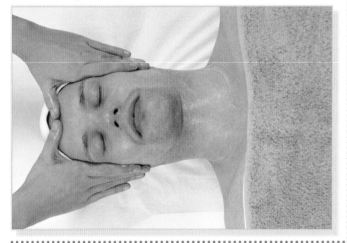

2 Use sponges and warm water to remove cleanser rather than cotton wool, which tends to break up over facial hair causing fluff.

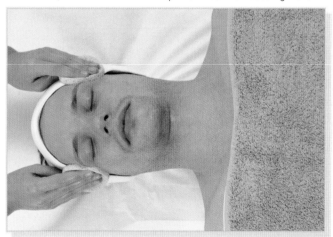

3 A facial scrub or mask will exfoliate and deep cleanse the pores, especially if the client isn't shaving.

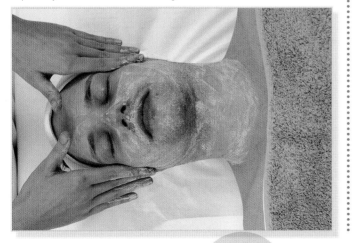

4 Remove scrub or mask with warm water and sponges. Pat dry, tone and moisturise.

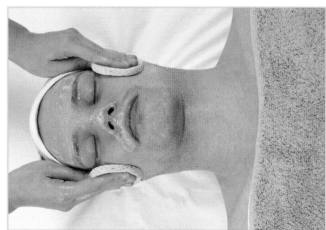

Applying mask treatments evenly and neatly

A large variety of face masks are available, both over the counter and in salons. Face masks can be made out of many different natural ingredients, and there is a huge choice of prepared or ready-mixed masks. They can be divided into two categories.

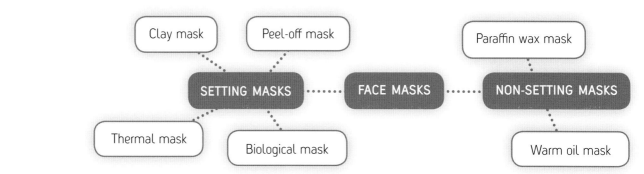

Types of face mask

Masks can have different actions depending upon their formulation.

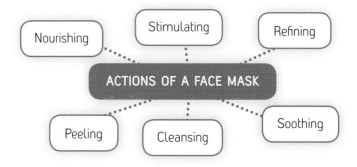

Actions of a face mask

The choice of mask depends on accurate skin analysis and knowledge of the effects of the basic mask ingredients.

Some masks come already mixed and some need mixing – generally the pre-prepared types tend to be more expensive. The ones that need mixing require more skill and knowledge of the ingredients and proportions, but the basic ingredients can be purchased in bulk and stored.

Natural ingredients can also be used as a face mask and provide great variety and fun!

Properties of face masks

- They should be smooth and free from gritty particles and unpleasant odours. In powder form, they should be easily dispersed in water to produce a paste.
- They should be easily removed from the face after use without causing discomfort.
- They must be harmless to the skin and non-toxic.

Contra-indications to the application of face masks include:

- skin disorders and diseases
- excessively dry or sensitive skin
- loose, crepey skin
- cuts and abrasions
- recent scar tissue.

Note: Clients who suffer from claustrophobia may prefer a non-setting mask.

Materials required for a face mask treatment include:

- bowls
- spatulas
- mask brush — flat and sanitised
- damp cotton wool
- headband
- tissues
- skin tonic
- moisturiser
- couch roll
- client record card
- scissors for eye pads.

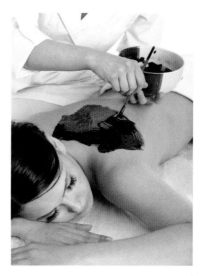

Masks can be used on the body too

Clay masks

Clays can be classed as natural ingredients because they are found in the earth. They are good at drawing out impurities and deep cleansing. Some can be quite stimulating and are good for improving the circulation; others are mild and soothing on the skin. The key is to know which ingredients are suitable for which skin type.

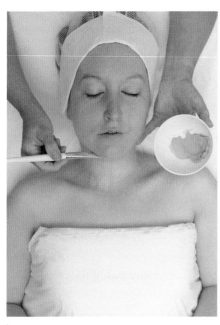

Fuller's earth face mask application

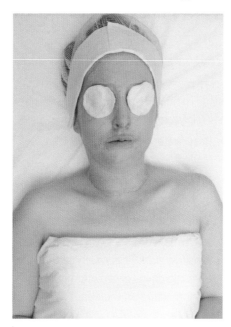

Fuller's earth face mask

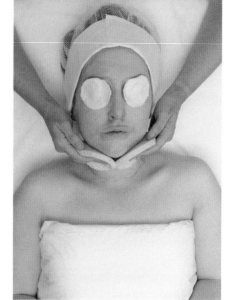

Removing a Fuller's earth face mask

Provide facial skincare

Skin type	Clay powder	Benefits	Mixed with
Dry	Calamine (a pink powder)	Contains zinc carbonate to soothe the skin and calm down a high colour	Rose water, orange flower water (or distilled water for sensitive skin)
	Magnesium carbonate (a white powder)	Refines and softens the skin, mildly astringent	A couple of drops of vegetable oil, almond oil or glycerol can be added
Greasy	Fuller's earth (a grey/green powder)	Deep cleansing	Distilled water with a drop of witch hazel if required. Witch hazel is not suitable for a sensitive, greasy skin as it can be quite stimulating
	Sulphur (a pale yellow powder)	Drying action so can be used on individual blemishes	Distilled water with a drop of witch hazel if required
Normal (balanced)	Magnesium carbonate (a white powder)	Refines and softens the skin, mildly astringent	Mix with equal proportions of rose water, orange flower water or witch hazel
	Calamine (a pink powder)	Contains zinc carbonate to soothe the skin and calm down a high colour	Mix with equal proportions of rose water, orange flower water or witch hazel
	Fuller's earth (a grey/green powder)	Deep cleansing; not suitable for sensitive skin as it can be quite stimulating	Mix with equal proportions of rose water, orange flower water or witch hazel
Combination	Follow the dry/normal skin for cheek areas and greasy skin for T-zone skin, depending upon the severity of each area		

Active ingredients

A clay mask needs to be mixed with active ingredients to turn the powder into a liquid paste. The liquids are selected to complement the skin type and mask to be used – they reinforce the action of the mask.

- **Rose water** gives a mild toning effect, which increases the toning action of a mask. Made from rose petals. Recommended for dry, normal and mature skin types.
- **Orange flower water** gives a stimulating, tonic effect. This is natural plant extract from the fruit of the tree.
- **Citrus dulcis** is very fragrant. Recommended for normal, dry and mature skin types.
- **Witch hazel** has a drying, stimulating effect, so is contra-indicated on fine sensitive skins; it is much better suited to greasy or combination skins. It is made from the dried leaves and bark of the hamamelis virginiana tree. It has a tissue-firming action on the skin.
- **Almond oil** can be used on dehydrated or neglected younger skins or on the more mature skin. A natural oil obtained from the kernels of the seeds of whole almonds, it improves the condition of the skin.
- **Distilled water** is ordinary water that has had the chemicals, such as magnesium bicarbonate or calcium carbonate, removed from it. These can be removed by boiling the water or chemically removed by water softeners.
- **Calamine lotion** is a liquid which contains zinc carbonate to soothe and heal the skin. Iron oxide produces the pink colouring.

Think about it

Always check your own posture and position for both mask application and massage techniques – your position should minimise fatigue and the risk of injury. If you have been sitting when giving the massage, you may wish to get up and apply the mask from the front, facing the client, instead of stretching over and getting backache.

Skin type	Recipe	Time on face
Normal	1 part kaolin 1 part Fuller's earth Mix with water and a few drops of witch hazel to form a smooth, thin paste	8–12 minutes
Dry	1 part kaolin 1 part magnesium carbonate Mix with rose water or orange flower water to form a smooth, thin paste	10–15 minutes
Oily	Fuller's earth Mix with witch hazel to form a smooth paste	5–15 minutes
Sensitive	1 part calamine 1 part magnesium carbonate Mix with rose water to form a smooth paste	5–10 minutes

Mask type	Recipe	Time on face
Sulphur mask (for acne)	$\frac{1}{2}$ tsp Epsom salts 1 tsp oatmeal 1 tsp magnesium carbonate 1 tsp precipitated sulphur Mix with hot water to form a paste	Apply over gauze, leave for 15 minutes, keeping warm with infrared lamp
Stimulating mask (for open pores, capillaries and contracting the tissues)	6 parts magnesium carbonate 2 parts fuller's earth Mix with rose water or almond oil according to the moisture content of the skin	5–15 minutes
Astringent mask (to dry an oily skin)	6 parts magnesium carbonate 1 part calamine Pinch of alum Mix with witch hazel	Apply over gauze Apply one coat until almost dry, then apply second coat and leave for 10 minutes

Peel-off masks

Peel-off masks are gel or latex based. (Paraffin wax masks also come into the peel-off category, although they are classed as non-setting.) Because perspiration cannot escape from the skin's surface, moisture is forced back into the epidermis. Some peel-off masks also create heat, so could come under the thermal category.

Gel masks are purchased as a ready-made suspension containing starches, gums or gelatine, to allow the correct consistency. Synthetic non-biological resins are commonly used as well. The mask is applied over the skin. When it makes contact it immediately begins to dry. It can be peeled off over the face as a whole facial mould when sufficient technique has been mastered. The gel mask can be used on most skin types, depending on the ingredients used, so check with individual manufacturer's instructions.

A latex mask is an emulsion of latex and water. The water evaporates leaving a rubber film to form the mask. Alternatives are synthetic PVC resins. These have a firming, tightening effect on the skin and can be used on a dry or mature skin.

Think about it

The setting times for all types of masks, including paraffin wax, are to be used as a general guide only, and you should go by the client response and how the skin reacts to the mask ingredients – this is why it is important never to leave the client unattended. Mask setting depends upon many variable factors: how active the ingredients are, how warm the room is, how hot the client is, what skin type the client has, if the skin is particularly sensitive and even hormone fluctuations (which often affect body temperature). Always judge by looking at the skin, asking the client and remove the mask immediately if you think the skin is reacting.

Think about it

A gel mask does adhere to the facial hair and can be painful during removal, rather like a plaster coming off! If the client has a lot of facial hair, offer an alternative mask.

Provide facial skincare

Biological and natural masks

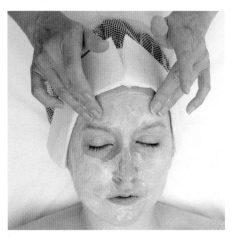

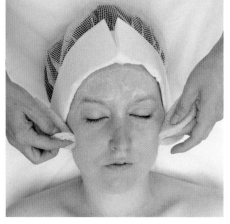

Work the exfoliant mask into the skin using small circular motions

Remove mask thoroughly with warm water and sponges

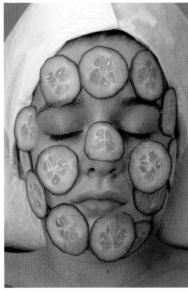

A natural cucumber mask

These include the following:

- **Fruit extracts**, e.g. avocado mashed to a smooth paste. Action: helps stabilise the skin's pH and acid mantle.

- **Herbal and vegetable**, e.g. cucumber sliced and placed over the skin. Action: calming or astringent effect.

- **Biological**, e.g. natural yoghurt applied in bought state. Action: refines the skin's texture, helps rid skin of waste, counteracts possible infection.
  Egg mask – with almond oil for dry skin or lemon for oily skin.
  Honey mask – has a softening effect on dehydrated or mature skin.

Warm oil masks

The skin is cleansed, and a piece of gauze is soaked in warm olive or almond oil. Eye pads are placed over the eyes, and the gauze is carefully put on to the face. An infrared lamp is placed in position for 10–20 minutes. The distance of the lamp is determined prior to application to suit the client's skin type.

The time of the treatment will depend upon the client's skin tolerance and how hot they get, whether the skin starts to show erythema and client preference.

Indications for use

- Crepey, finely lined skin
- Premature ageing
- Dehydration or dry skin
- Younger skin as a preventative measure

It is important to prepare the client and couch adequately to protect all areas.

Effects

- It cleanses and aids desquamation.
- It increases smoothness, softness and elasticity.
- As the mask works on heat penetration, the skin will absorb cosmetic preparations more easily, so make-up should be avoided.

Massage oil into the skin after application for maximum benefit. Ensure toning and moisturising is thorough without overstretching or over touching the skin.

The client should be advised that the skin might have an uneven appearance directly after application for 3–4 hours.

Risk assessment for warm oil equipment

Refer to Follow health and safety practice in the salon, pages 68–90, for a complete discussion of risk assessment.

Hazards: only look for hazards that you could reasonably expect to result in significant harm under the conditions in your workplace. Use the following examples as a guide.

- **Fire** (e.g. from electrical flex or lead)
- **Burning of equipment** (through light bulb burning out)
- **Burns to skin** (lamp too close to skin, left on too long, treatment not timed)
- **Ejection of bulb** (hot bulb falling on to skin, not screwed in properly, lamp should not be directly over skin)
- **Electricity** (e.g. poor wiring)
- **Manual handling** (outer casing is hot and will burn if towel is not used for protection)
- **Falling machinery** (if supporting arm is not screwed in properly)
- **Contamination** (from brushes and equipment not sufficiently sterilised)
- **Cross-infection** (if possible contra-indications are ignored)

Paraffin wax mask treatments

Preparation

A small amount of sterilised paraffin wax should be poured into a small, clean bowl lined with foil. (Wax heaters may be too large to be mobile.) The working temperature is 49°C.

The wax treatment may be applied within the facial routine in place of a setting mask. Disposable paper should cover towels for protection.

Application

Eye pads are put in place. Wax should be applied in a firm build-up over the neck, cheeks, chin, nose and forehead, using a small brush. The client should have complete confidence in the treatment and your presence so she can relax.

- Wax must be applied to a clean skin that is free from oil, cream, etc.
- The protective band should be checked to avoid soiling.
- The mask is applied as a thin, even film over the face and neck with a brush or spatula.
- Eyes, nostrils and mouth areas must be avoided.

The application must be accomplished quickly and neatly.

Note: A combination skin condition may require the application of two or more masks to suit the different areas.

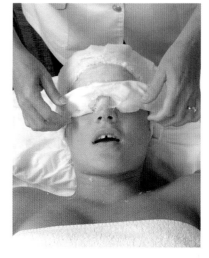

Removing a paraffin wax mask

Depending upon the skin type, time may vary between 10 and 20 minutes. This will depend upon the skin's reaction and client tolerance to the ingredients – do not let the mask dry on for too long as it will be very difficult to remove.

Remove the eye pads, gently slide the fingers under the edges of the mask, place the hands under the mask at the throat, pulling the mask up a little at a time and taking care that any bits of mask are stuck to the main bulk. Pressure toning with water may be suitable, but usually it is best to leave this.

Risk assessment for paraffin wax equipment

Refer to Follow health and safety practice in the salon, pages 68–90, for a complete discussion of risk assessment.

Hazards: only look for hazards that you could reasonably expect to result in significant harm under the conditions in your workplace. Use the following examples as a guide.

- **Fire** (e.g. from electrical flex or lead)
- **Burning of equipment** (through low wax level in the tank)
- **Burns to skin** (from not testing wax temperature first on self)
- **Ejection of materials** (spitting hot wax)
- **Electricity** (e.g. poor wiring)
- **Manual handling** (spillage possible if moving when in liquid form)
- **Falling machinery** (if not securely positioned on a trolley)

Effects

- Natural perspiration cleans the skin.
- Circulation is improved.
- Dead cells are removed and desquamation is improved.
- Elasticity, smoothness and softness of texture are increased.
- Removes cellular matter.
- Moisturises the skin.
- There is a local increase in temperature.

Indications

- Dry, dehydrated skin
- Mature skin, where regeneration is needed without overstimulation
- Crepey, finely lined skin
- Uneven-textured skin (unstable pH) to promote desquamation and refine texture
- Seborrhoea conditions, to remove oily blockages and surface adhesions

Contra-indications

- Highly nervous, tense clients, or those suffering from claustrophobia
- Extreme vascular conditions
- Sepsis, skin infection and irritation

Client preparation

- The client should be prepared as for cleansing.
- Hair and clothing should be well protected.
- The face should then be cleansed to remove all make-up.
- After deciding on the formula, the powder ingredients are placed in a bowl and mixed to a smooth paste by gradually adding the liquid.

Basic mask formulation

As every facial diagnosis differs slightly, no formulation can be assumed to be suitable for all skin conditions. No rules can apply in mask therapy due to the variety of mask products and the different actions they are capable of producing. Observation and client discussion regarding tolerance to the mask will increase your knowledge of the skin's reaction to certain ingredients.

Final tips for face masks

- Follow the manufacturer's instructions.
- Always use the mask that complements the products being used, e.g. René Guinot or Clarins or whichever range the salon is using.
- Always do a thorough facial analysis to be able to decide the correct mask for the client.

Provide aftercare advice

After a facial it is important to recognise that the immediate aftercare is as important as the long-term aftercare if maximum benefit is to be gained from the salon treatment. Much of this information can be found in Display stock to promote sales in a salon. Read that unit for tips on how to promote additional services and give accurate information.

Think about it

When you have finished the client's treatments always check that the client is satisfied with the results and that they meet the agreed treatment plan. Provide a hand mirror so the client can see just how clean and fresh the skin has become.

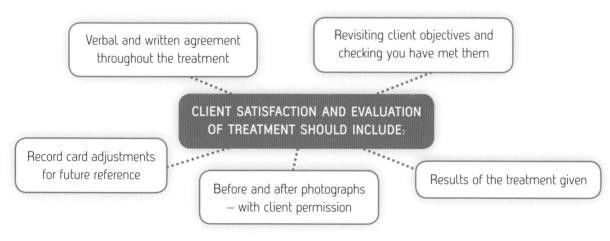

Verbal and written agreement throughout the treatment

Revisiting client objectives and checking you have met them

CLIENT SATISFACTION AND EVALUATION OF TREATMENT SHOULD INCLUDE:

Record card adjustments for future reference

Before and after photographs – with client permission

Results of the treatment given

Provide facial skincare

Giving suitable advice and recommendations

Always talk through the aftercare with your client. The client should leave the salon knowing exactly what to do to help the skin and to reinforce the benefits of the salon treatment.

Immediate aftercare to avoid contra-actions

The skin has been deep cleansed, stimulated and nourished. No aftercare is needed except to leave it alone. Avoid picking, squeezing pimples or touching the area.

◉ Avoid the temptation to apply make-up for 12 hours, where possible.

◉ Evening cleansing is not necessary, but if the client prefers, a light cleanse, tone and moisture may be recommended.

◉ Suitable and compatible home care products should be recommended. These will complement the work of the therapist in the salon.

◉ Explain to clients that while it is unlikely that contra-actions will develop after a facial, they should avoid any overstimulation and further heat treatments. If a reaction is going to occur, it will usually be a reaction to a cream used while the facial is going on, not afterwards.

◉ Highly perfumed products should be avoided.

◉ No depilation (hair removal) should take place after a facial.

◉ If any rash, irritation or itching occurs, suggest putting a cool flannel to the area. Remove the offending product from the skin with damp cotton wool, and apply a light calamine lotion to soothe the skin.

Long-term and home care advice

◉ Regular use of home care products will help the skin.

◉ Regular facials will help to regulate a problem skin; timings and intervals are a personal decision between the therapist and client and may depend on cost.

◉ Future treatments may be discussed with a view to specialist help for specific problems, such as facial steaming for comedone extraction, or regular paraffin wax mask application for a dry skin condition.

◉ Targeting a problem and then giving intensive treatments to help that condition is very rewarding. The client is pleased and the therapist has job satisfaction.

◉ A treatment plan should make allowances for timing intervals, the cost involved and how convenient it is for the client to get to the salon.

◉ Give the client a price list and all relevant information for present and future treatments with you.

◉ Give your client accurate information about additional products and services. Refer to Display stock and promote products and services to clients in a salon, pages 117–33.

A client leaving the salon in a relaxed and satisfied state is very rewarding, but your work is not yet over. There are important details to complete, which are as much a part of your job role as everything else that you do. These include completing client records accurately. Take time to fill out all parts of the record card:

◉ Were there any reactions during the treatment that will affect the future treatment plan?

Think about it

Your workstation may be shared by other therapists. Most salons have a waxing area, a facial area and a body treatment section, so if your next client is in the waxing room, you have to leave your facial station clean for another therapist to use. Would you like to inherit a messy work area from another therapist?

- Did the client express any preferences or dislikes for massage movements, products or mask?
- Would you leave something out next time?
- Did the client feel claustrophobic with eye pads on?
- Were products purchased?

Finally, you must leave the work area and equipment ready for further treatments.

Frequently asked questions

Q What instructions should I give to a male client booking in for a facial?

A All treatments are private and confidential whether the client is male or female. Facial massage includes the upper back and shoulders, so upper clothing will be removed but the chest will be covered with a towel to keep the client warm. Advise the client to have as close a shave as possible on the morning of the treatment, to avoid dragging on the facial hair. He should wear loose clothing to aid relaxation, such as a tracksuit or casual clothing rather than a formal suit.

Q What action should I take if I discover the client has a contra-indication to a facial treatment?

A If the contra-indication is an infection or inflammation, stop the treatment immediately, and suggest that the client sees their GP. You must not make a diagnosis, only a recommendation that the client seek medical attention. If the contra-indication is of a minor nature, simply avoid the area and adapt the treatment accordingly.

Q How would I recognise the signs or symptoms of skin damage?

A The skin ages prematurely causing breakdown of collagen and elastin, which supports the skin, and uneven pigmentation can also occur. There may be contamination of the skin, clogged and blocked pores, irritation and a tendency to comedones and allergic reactions. Skin damage causes dehydration and overactivity of the sebaceous glands resulting in problems. The skin may be overstretched. Inappropriate products can cause comedones to form or an oversensitive skin.

Q Why is it important to complete client records accurately?

A To record relevant details to be able to contact the client if necessary; to provide full and accurate information which will ensure client safety; to ensure consistency of treatment regardless of who performs the treatment; to record the number of treatments in a course and the date of each one; to record changes to the treatment programme or contra-actions if they occur; to record the progress of the condition or treatment success; to safeguard the salon and the therapists against clients taking legal action for damages or negligence.

Provide facial skincare

Check your knowledge

1 Dehydrated skin has the appearance of:
a) shiny nose and forehead
b) blackheads and papules
c) tightness and flaky patches
d) redness and irritation.

2 Skin ages faster due to:
a) Stress, smoking and exposure to ultraviolet light
b) Too hot bath water
c) Too many beauty treatments
d) Poor choice of products.

3 The skin type which has oily and dry areas is known as:
a) unusual skin
b) problem skin
c) combination skin
d) sensitive skin.

4 Restrictions for a facial treatment would include:
a) Bruising
b) Impetigo
c) Herpes
d) Scabies.

5 Massage is good for the skin because:
a) it helps bring oxygen to the skin surface
b) it cleanses the skin
c) it smoothes out wrinkles
d) it makes you thinner in the face.

6 The most suitable cleanser for dry skin is:
a) cream cleanser
b) milk cleanser
c) wash-off cleanser
d) baby lotion.

7 A contra-action to a face mask would be:
a) Milia
b) A rash or itching
c) Blackheads
d) Keloid tissue.

8 Erythema is when the skin becomes:
a) rehydrated with moisture
b) flushed with blood
c) cleansed with a face mask
d) darker as in a tan.

9 An example of a bacterial infection would be:
a) Conjunctivitis
b) Herpes simplex
c) Bruising
d) Chloasma.

10 A sensitive skin would show as:
a) Dry and tight to the touch
b) Flaky and peeling
c) Blackheads and pustules
d) Red and flushed with broken capillaries.

Getting ready for assessment

Simulation is not allowed for any performance evidence within this unit.

Your assessor will observe your performance on **at least three occasions**, **each involving a different client**. As there are considerable ranges to cover for this unit, it is likely that you will be doing facial assessments for some time and you must practically demonstrate in your everyday work that you have met the standard for improving and maintaining facial skin condition.

Remember also that some clients will cover more than one range, for example, a sensitive skin may also be mature and dehydrated, so you can cover several ranges in one go!

Over a period of time, you must practically demonstrate that you:

- have used all consultation techniques
- have carried out at least one of the necessary actions
- have carried out treatments on two of the three skin conditions
- have used all types of facial products, massage mediums, massage techniques, masks and provided all types of advice
- have used all types of equipment.

The best source of evidence is during a realistic practical workshop where you carry out the required treatments encompassing the skin types mentioned in the ranges. However, if you do not have a client with a specific range – for example, you may never have a client requiring a cold compress – then written papers, projects or a case study of home treatments (ideally with photographic evidence) are also acceptable forms of supporting evidence. If you get to the end of your assessments and a range is still outstanding, you may be able to show understanding through full oral questioning depending on your assessor and the demands of the Awarding Organisation.

Provide eyelash and brow treatments

What you will learn

- Prepare for eyelash and brow treatments
- Provide eyelash and brow treatments

Introduction

This unit focuses on ways to enhance the appearance of eyebrows and lashes by carrying out a range of treatments. As well as eyebrow shaping, and eyebrow and eyelash tinting, this unit will cover how to carry out an eyelash perming treatment. This is a very popular treatment and so it is useful to know how to carry it out.

Each of the treatments can be either combined or carried out independently to meet the requirements of the client.

Some therapists view this section as 'small treatments', but it should not be undervalued. Clients can instantly see an improvement with an eyebrow shape, eyelash tint or application of artificial lashes. Eye treatments can be easily slotted into other treatments: for example, added into the facial while the tint is processing. Remember to include these 'extras' in the cost.

My story

The value of small treatments

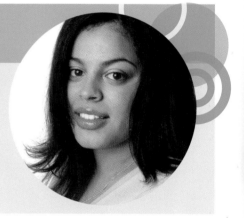

My name is Holly. When I first started working in a salon I did not like having only the small eye treatments in my column, especially as my colleagues had larger treatments and could earn more commission from the sale of additional products, for example after a facial. However, my manager encouraged me to use the time with the clients to discuss and introduce other treatments that the salon offered. I found from this that a number of clients booked in not only for further lash and brow maintenance treatments but also for treatments we had discussed. I now value these small treatments as a time to discuss other services with clients.

Benefits of eye treatments for the therapist:

- easy service to fit into salon day
- clients find immediate result pleasing
- excellent opportunity to promote other services
- enhances wedding, prom and seasonal promotions.

Prepare for eyelash and brow treatments

In this outcome you will learn about:

- preparing yourself, the client and work area for eyelash and eyebrow treatments
- using suitable consultation techniques to identify treatment objectives
- interpreting and accurately recording the results of tests carried out prior to treatments
- providing clear recommendations to the client
- selecting products, tools and equipment to suit client treatment needs.

For advice on safe and effective methods of working practice, refer to individual treatments:

Shape eyebrows — page 338

Tint eyebrows and lashes — page 340

Eyelash perming — page 349

Refer also to Professional skills, Follow health and safety practice in the salon and Provide facial skincare.

Leaving the work area suitable for further treatments

Always leave your working area as you would wish to find it. Restock tissues or cotton wool, if you have used the last of them, or at least inform the person whose job it is to restock the workstations. Put lids back on pots to prevent products drying out, or oxidising.

Remember that your next client may not be at that couch — you may have to go into the waxing area, or the massage room, and it is not professional to leave a mess for another therapist to tidy up.

Ensuring the client's records are up to date and accurate

While waiting for the tint to develop or the perm to process, you can sit with your client and update her client record card. Although she will have her eyes closed, you can talk to her about aftercare, product use, and caring for her lashes at home, as well as filling in the details of the day's treatments. Now is a good time to check that her address and other personal details are correct, and add any purchases she will be taking home with her.

Using consultation techniques

As with all treatments, you will need to carry out a consultation, to check for any contra-indications that may prevent the treatment taking place and to discuss the client's requirements. These contra-indications apply to all eye treatments. (For information on consultation techniques and contra-indications, refer to Professional skills, pages 1 and 3 and to Follow health and safety practice in the salon.)

You will need to ensure that the consultation process does not discriminate against clients from different cultures, religious backgrounds or who have disabilities or illness unless any of these areas would deem the treatment unsafe or inappropriate. For example, you should avoid discussing religious topics with clients. You may also need to research illnesses and disabilities to ensure that your client receives the best possible treatment and service.

As with any treatment, if the client is under 16 years of age, signed parental or guardian consent needs to be obtained before treatment can commence and the parent or guardian must be present during the treatment. Every other client would be required to sign to confirm that contra-indications have been checked and that they confirm the treatment plan.

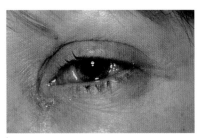

Conjunctivitis

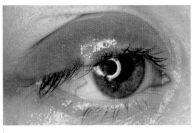

Stye

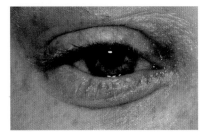

Eczema

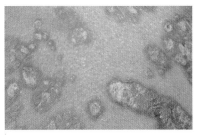

Psoriasis

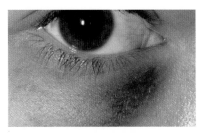

Bruising to the eye area

If the client is having a treatment for the first time it is important to highlight the benefits of the treatment to them, especially if they are apprehensive.

Benefits for the client could include:

- fairly quick treatment (depending on the service)
- immediate result and effect
- excellent treatment for clients who wear glasses
- minimum pain from shaping.

Identifying contra-indications to treatment

During the consultation, you will need to find out if your client has any contra-indications to the treatment by asking her questions and doing a visual check of the area to be treated. Remember to record your client's response to the questions asked. You should also look out for a range of conditions that will contra-indicate treatment. These are the main conditions to look out for:

- Conjunctivitis – this is a nasty eye condition. The eyelids are red and sore, with itching. Mainly caused by bacteria present. It can be irritated by a virus or an allergy.
- Stye – this is a small boil at the base of the eyelash follicle. It is raised, sore and red, and there may be considerable swelling in the area.
- **Blepharitis** – an infection of the lid causing inflammation of the eye, which will look red and sore. Depending on the severity of the condition, you may need to advise the client to see their GP before eye treatments are undertaken.
- Viral infections – this could include a cold.
- Bruising to the area.
- Reaction to a sensitivity test for tinting or perm products.

You should also be aware of some other conditions:

- Hypersensitivity – if a client has hypersensitive eyes, it is very important to use hypoallergenic products when cleansing the eyes and ensure a sensitivity test is carried out before the products are used.
- Active eczema or psoriasis – the area should not be treated, especially if the skin is open or weeping when it is vulnerable to infection and the condition can be spread.
- Common cold – easily recognised: runny or blocked nose, dry skin around the nose, sneezing, watery eyes, headache.
- Hay fever – an irritation of the nasal membrane resulting in watery eyes, runny nose and sneezing.
- Watery eyes – an irritating condition, in which the eye area becomes moist, which may make it difficult for the client to have eye treatments.
- Recent operations – a general rule of thumb is to wait six months before treating an area with scar tissue. However, if it is a minor operation, and you have your client's and her GP's approval, go ahead, but avoid the area itself.
- Bruising to eye – easy to recognise, a bruise shows as blue/black and yellow skin colouring. Do not treat a bruised eye.
- Facial piercing – care should be taken if a client has a piercing on the brow area. The piercing should be removed or covered with a suitable dressing before treatments commence. The therapist should only go ahead if she thinks that it is safe to do so or if the end result will not be compromised.

• **Contact dermatitis** – this condition can affect both the client and the therapist. You will need to check whether the client is allergic to **latex** as gloves are worn in all eye treatments. If the client has an allergy, then **powder-free** vinyl or **nitrile** gloves should be worn. A sensitivity test should be carried out prior to tinting to ensure that allergic reactions and dermatitis do not occur. If therapists have skin contact with tint and peroxide, it is possible that they could develop contact dermatitis, so safe working practices should be adopted.

Remember that it is not your place as a therapist to mention specific conditions to your client as you are not medically trained. You can recommend that your client see their GP over a condition, but do not name the condition, or offer any diagnosis or cure. Ensure advice is given without causing undue alarm or concern to the client.

Providing recommendations to clients

During the consultation you will gather the information you need to recommend the most appropriate treatment plan for your client. Do make sure that you agree all aspects of the treatment plan with the client before you begin, and encourage them to ask questions to clarify any points they do not fully understand. The use of a mirror for the client as a visual aid will ensure that you clarify the result the client wishes to achieve, especially when shaping the brows.

Planning the eyebrow shape

Eyebrow shaping is the removal of superfluous hair to enhance the shape of the natural brow. Superfluous hair is the term used if hair growth is normal but the client feels it is unattractive. When shaping the eyebrows you need to plan the treatment carefully, because it cannot be undone. Discuss the needs with your client before commencing the treatment. You may have very different ideas.

Important tools for shaping are a mirror and an eyebrow brush. If the brows are very fair or a sparse grey, you can identify the hairs that are to be removed by using a light application of eyebrow powder or an eyebrow pencil.

Facts about eyebrows

Every natural eyebrow is different in shape, hair type and colour. As well as this, to achieve the most flattering effect, you need to consider both facial and eye types.

Most hairs on the brows are **terminal hairs** (refer to Related anatomy and physiology, page 252). The terminal hairs of the brows, unlike other terminal hairs, are usually short in length but are still there for protection. The reason we have hairs on the brows and surrounding the eyes is to stop debris entering the eyes and to keep germs out. The hairs are also there to protect the eyes from excessive light damage.

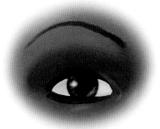
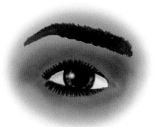

Eyebrows differ in shape, hair type and colour

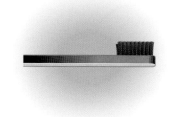

An eyebrow brush

Provide eyelash and brow treatments

Eyebrow shapes

It is recommended that the normal eyebrow should look like the wings of a bird in flight: thicker at the inner corner of the eye, tapering to an arch and narrowing at the end of the brow. As the eyebrows frame the face, they should be in balance with the rest of the facial features.

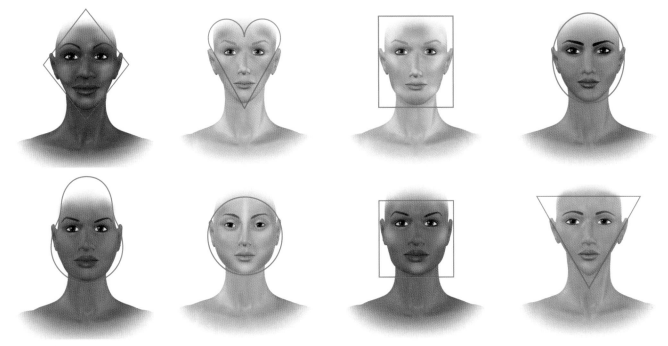

The following indicate the effect of shapes.

Angular shape

This shape can define a round face. Enhance this shape with shading and contouring of the eye make-up for elegance.

Rounded shape

Suitable for clients with large eyes or a wide forehead, a rounded shape can enhance the client's eyes. The eyebrow line should follow the frontal bone and be shaped to
a taper.

Arched shape

Sometimes referred to as 'sweeping', this shape is very flattering on most clients. It gives width and expression to the eye. It opens the eye and can help to balance a prominent nose or a large mouth. An arched shape can also be used to detract from a high forehead.

Low arched shape

This shape works well for a client with a low or small forehead by giving the illusion of more length. It is sometimes referred to as a straight shape.

Wide-set eyes

If a client has wide-set eyes, extend the eyebrow to inside the corner of the eye.

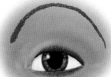

Angular shape

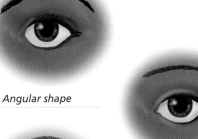

Rounded shape

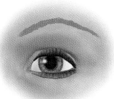

Arched shape

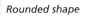

Low arched shape

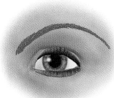

Wide-set eyes

Other factors that may influence the shape of the brows.

- The natural shape of the brows. If the client has been shaping her own brows, it may be necessary to let them grow for a short time before shaping them professionally; in the meantime, stray hairs can be removed to keep them neat.

- Client age. More mature clients might have some coarse hairs, which can be long, white or discoloured. These can be removed, provided that doing so does not alter the brow line or leave bald patches. Ideally, the brow should be of medium thickness. Too thick, and it can give an older appearance. Thin eyebrows give a severe appearance.

- Fashion trends. Each season sees new fashion trends, which have an effect on eyebrow shapes and eye make-up. This should also be considered before shaping the brows.

Other approaches which may be suitable for the client

- Semi-permanent make-up. This should be applied only by professionals. Pigment is applied to add colour to the brows, e.g. to disguise a bald area.

- Hair transplants. These are already available in the USA for clients with sparse brows.

- Artificial individual eyebrow hairs. These are applied in the same way as individual eyelashes and are not permanent.

- Eyelash perming can be used to create a curl on the lashes and is a salon treatment that lasts approximately 4–6 weeks.

- Waxing, epilation (sometimes called electrolysis), threading and laser (IPL) treatments can all be used to remove unwanted hair. Further information about these treatments can be found in Remove hair using waxing techniques, page 405.

Measuring the eyebrows to decide length

Once you have carried out the consultation and discussed the client's needs, you need to measure the length of the brows. Here are some points to help you when deciding the correct length and shape for your client. (If the brows are unruly or very light you may need to use a brush to shape the brows or eyebrow powder to enhance the colour of the brows. This will help you measure correctly.)

- Place an orange stick in a straight line from the side of the nose to the inner corner of the eye. This is where the eyebrow should begin.

- Place an orange stick from the side of the nose to the outer corner of the eye. This is where the eyebrow should end.

- Ask the client to look straight ahead. Hold the stick vertically so that it runs through the lateral edge of the eyes. This is where the highest point of the arch should be.

- Hold the stick horizontally and it should more or less connect the beginning and end of the eyebrow.

These are useful guidelines. With practice you will learn to train your eye.

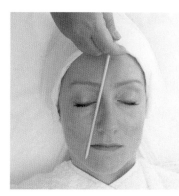

Line up the orange stick with the corner of the mouth and the edge of the nose: the beginning of the eyebrow should start where the orange stick rests on the skin

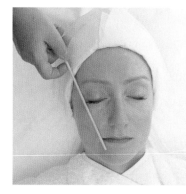

Line up the orange stick with the edge of the mouth and the outer corner of the eye: the end of the eyebrow should be where the orange stick rests on the skin

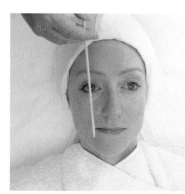

The arch of the eyebrow should match the middle of the pupil. This is your shape guideline; any stray hairs outside the shape can be plucked out

Think about it

You can only work with the eyebrow's natural shape so you may need to discourage your client from expecting unrealistic outcomes.

Provide eyelash and brow treatments

Selecting suitable products, tools and equipment

This will depend upon the results of the sensitivity test, consultation and the treatment being undertaken.

Equipment required for eyebrow shaping

- Tweezers (rounded, slanted, pointed, claw or automatic)
- Damp cotton wool
- Orange stick
- Antiseptic solution
- Aftercare solution or ice pack
- Disposable gloves (refer to your professional body for guidance or visit the Habia website)
- Tissues
- Bin and bin liner
- Sterilising dish
- Mirror
- Eyebrow brush
- Headband
- Eyebrow pencil or eyebrow powder
- Skin warming products, e.g. hot cotton wool or heated towels

Tweezers

There are two types of tweezers used for eyebrow shaping.

Automatic tweezers

These are designed to remove the bulk of excess hair. They have a spring-loaded action.

Manual

These are used to remove stray hairs and accentuate the shape of the brow. Various ends are available – slanted ends are generally considered to be the best for eyebrow shaping.

For equipment and materials for eyelash and eyebrow tinting, see page 343.

Protecting the client: personal protective equipment for eyebrow and eyelash treatments

It is advisable when carrying out treatments around the eye that you wear gloves, so as to protect you and your client from infection and contamination. Blood spots may be produced when shaping – this is a normal reaction to tweezing or waxing of the brows.

There are several different types of protective gloves available. Traditionally, gloves are made of latex, but a number of people have developed allergies to latex. If you or a client show signs of redness or irritation when in contact with latex gloves, an alternative made of either vinyl or nitrile that are powder-free should be used.

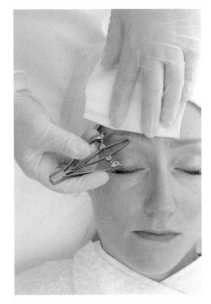

Using spring-loaded automatic tweezers

Think about it

It is important that all tweezers are ready for use, and they should be sterilised between clients, either in an autoclave or in a sterilising solution. It is important that this is carried out as blood and tissue fluids can be drawn during treatment, and these could cause contamination. Any tissue fluid drawn should be disposed of, in accordance with health and safety regulations, to prevent contamination.

Care should be taken when putting on and removing gloves to avoid cross-contamination. Gloves should be removed by turning inside out and disposed of in the contaminated waste bin.

Preparing the client

After completing the consultation:

- Secure client's hair with headband or turban.
- Place towel or tissue or cape over the client's chest.
- Position client comfortably; couch or chair should be slightly elevated.
- Remove all accessories, e.g. earrings or facial piercings. Clients who wear contact lenses may find treatment more comfortable if they remove them prior to treatment.

Risk assessment for eye treatments

Refer to Follow health and safety practice in the salon, pages 68–90, and Professional skills for a complete discussion of risk assessment.

Hazards: only look for hazards that you could reasonably expect to result in significant harm under the conditions in your workplace. Use the following examples as a guide.

- **Chemicals** (e.g. eye damage from glue in the eye)
- **Allergies** (allergic reaction to glue, tint or latex)
- **Cross-infection** (blood spotting from the eyebrow shape)
- **Contact dermatitis** (continued use of products without the protection of suitable gloves can cause a reaction to the therapist's hands which can be spread to other areas of the body if extreme sensitivity occurs)

Provide eyelash and brow treatments

In this outcome you will learn about:

- communicating and behaving in a professional manner
- following health and safety working practices
- positioning yourself and the client correctly throughout the treatment
- using products, tools, equipment and techniques to suit client's treatment needs
- completing the treatment to the satisfaction of the client
- recording the results of the treatment
- providing suitable aftercare advice.

Disposing of waste materials safely and correctly

Remember to dispose of all waste materials in the correct bin — if you have drawn blood when eyebrow shaping, the tissue and cotton wool are classed as contaminated material and should be put into a bin liner, which then goes into the yellow bin, to be taken away by your local contractor. Refer to Professional skills, You, your client and the

Think about it

If the treatment requires that you use gloves, check with the client before treatment starts whether she has a latex allergy. Any allergy should be recorded on the client record card.

Think about it

Be sure to clarify the shape required with the client before commencing any treatment. If the client is nervous, explain the procedure and reassure her as you progress.

Details of shape, thickness, texture and required shape should all be added to the client record card.

Think about it

All tinting and adhesive products that are used on the eyes are controlled by the Control of Substances Harmful to Health regulations (refer to Professional skills, page 49). All therapists should refer to the Manufacturers Directives Schedule (MDS) on how to use the products and COSHH data. These regulations govern the correct use, storage and disposal of products.

Provide eyelash and brow treatments

law, page 54 and Follow health and safety practice in the salon, for the legal aspects of your actions. Tint brushes, dishes, etc. can be cleaned and made ready for use, if reusable. If the tinting brush is a disposable one, put it in a bin with a liner — tint will stain anything it comes into contact with that is porous, including hands and overalls.

Shaping eyebrows

It is important that the client understands the treatment procedure and the shape is discussed before the treatment commences. The therapist should check the shape at regular intervals. The procedure for shaping eyebrows is as follows.

1 Remove all traces of make-up and clean the area with an appropriate cleanser. Wipe with sanitising solution and prepare the area.

2 Inspect the treatment area to assess the amount of work required. Measure shape (see page 335) and consult the client. A magnifying lamp can be used to give maximum visibility.

3 Brush the brows into shape before you begin.

4 Open pores — it is often suggested that before you begin shaping, you should place warm, damp cotton wool pads over the area. This relaxes hair follicles and softens the eyebrow tissue, making hair removal easier.

5 To remove hairs, gently stretch the skin between your fingers and pluck out the hairs in the direction in which they grow. Begin by removing the stray hairs between the eyes. Hairs below the natural brow shape can then be tackled. The few odd hairs that grow unevenly above the brow may also be removed, provided they do not form part of the main eyebrow growth. If there are any tough, spiky or white hairs, these can sometimes be removed without spoiling the overall shape.

6 Consult the client as you work; ensure she has a hand mirror and consults with you as you proceed.

7 Place the removed hairs on a tissue placed at the side of the client, or held wrapped around your fingers.

8 Periodically soothe the client's brow with antiseptic, as this helps to remove any stray hairs.

9 When all the shaping is complete, place a dampened cotton wool soaked in witch hazel, ice pack or soothing antiseptic solution over the area to soothe, cool and remove excess erythema (for information on erythema, see page 339).

10 Give aftercare advice and book the client's next appointment.

If blood or tissue fluid is accidentally drawn during the treatment, the following steps should be taken.

1 Apply pressure to the area with clean cotton wool soaked in sanitising solution.

2 Do not panic. Keep calm, and explain to the client so she is aware of the problem.

3 Apply soothing solution to the area.

4 Dispose of waste carefully in accordance with health and safety regulations and local by-laws.

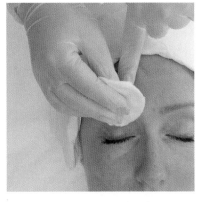

Placing hot cotton wool pads on the brow opens the pores (step 4)

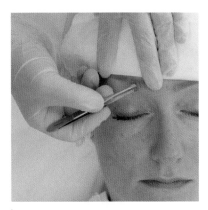

Stretching skin and tweezing near to the root will minimise discomfort

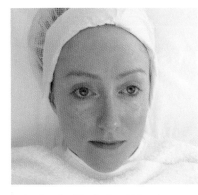

The finished look should be clean and tidy and open up the whole face

An eyebrow re-shape may take up to half an hour although the service time for a regular treatment is 15 minutes. In all cases it would depend on the density of the hairs, shape required, hair growth and the client requirements. Clients who visit the salon regularly often have an eyebrow tidy as an integral part of their treatment plan. On average, an eyebrow tidy would be carried out every 4–6 weeks.

Aftercare

Clients should be given the following aftercare advice when they have had an eyebrow shape or tidy.

- Cooling mild antiseptic products, e.g. witch hazel, should be applied.
- No make-up should be applied to the area for 12 hours, as the follicles are open and infection may occur.
- Stray regrowth hairs can be removed at intervals to prolong the effect.

Think about it

A nervous client may require eye pads or be advised to keep eyes shut. Heavy brows should be gradually reduced over two or three visits to minimise discomfort and allow the client to become accustomed to her new image.

Trouble-shooting eyebrow problems

Bare sparse brows

Fill in with pencil, using short strokes in the direction of the hair growth, and blend with a brow brush. Ensure that the pencil is sharpened as you move from one eye to the other, to prevent cross-infection.

Stray hairs

Remove any stray hairs with tweezers.

Thin brows

Instead of a pencil, try a shade of powder that matches the brow colour. Apply with a stiff brush, following the natural line, and ensure that you blend in well to prevent the line looking harsh. This will create the illusion of doubling the thickness.

Unruly or thick brows

Long, unruly hairs should be trimmed. Hold the brows straight with a brow comb and trim to the required length. To help the hairs to lie flat, use either a little hair gel or a small amount of hairspray on a comb. Never spray directly on to the face.

Think about it

Contra-actions usually take the form of erythema to the area, but in some cases blood spots occur and sometimes swelling. You should try to reduce the swelling before the client leaves the salon, by applying a soothing antiseptic. In extreme cases, a cold compress or ice should be applied. All contra-actions should be recorded on the client record card.

Ensure all equipment is sterilised and accessible

↓

Carry out consultation

↓

Check for contra-indications

↓

Discuss client requirements

↓

Remove contact lenses if necessary

↓

Cleanse area

↓

Measure brows

↓

Pre-warm area

↓

Shape as required

↓

Soothe area with suitable solution

↓

Give aftercare advice

↓

Show client finished result

↓

Record details of treatment on client

Eyebrow shaping

Think about it

Your posture is important when carrying out a shape. Ensure that the client is at the correct height so that you can clearly see the hairs. You may need to use a magnifier to help you if the hairs are fair or white.

Provide eyelash and brow treatments

Tint eyebrows and lashes

Tinting has several benefits to the client.

- Eyebrows help to emphasise facial expression and eyelashes frame the eyes.
- Tinting may be carried out on clients with light-coloured brows and lashes to define their appearance.
- Brows and lashes can be tinted to complement hair colour.
- Tinting can mean that coloured mascara need not be applied, which is good for those who are allergic to it, or in the summer months when mascara is likely to smudge if it is very hot.
- Tinting is also ideal for clients who wear glasses or contact lenses.

Key terms

Contra-action – an adverse physical reaction during or after the treatment. This should be recorded on the record card.

My story

No more smudges

My name is Zaida, and I'm a chef in a busy hotel. Although my working environment is hot and steamy, I like to wear a little make-up. I was finding that whichever brand of mascara I used, by the end of the day it had run. My friend suggested I had my eyelashes tinted. I went to the local salon and I had a tint test to ensure that I was not allergic to the products. Two days later I had my lashes tinted – I was delighted with the results. That was over two years ago. Since then I have had my lashes and brows tinted regularly and for my sister's wedding I had an artificial lash application. I no longer have to put up with smudged mascara!

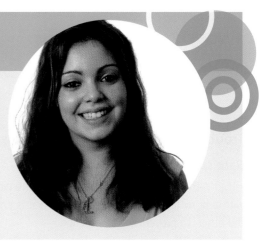

Performing a sensitivity test

A sensitivity test should be carried out prior to tinting or the application of perm products with the product that you plan to use. A suitable area should be selected, usually behind the ear or the crook of the elbow. An area nearest to the eye would be the most suitable for a more accurate result.

Many professional associations now recommend that this test be carried out 24–48 hours prior to each treatment, even on a client who regularly has the treatment at the salon. The client may have become sensitive to the product, or the salon may have changed products and therefore the ingredients may be slightly different from the ones used previously.

All tests should be recorded on the client record card with the date the test was carried out and the results of the test. An allergic reaction would show as a red, itchy, sore area. Treat with a cold compress and soothing cream. This reaction would mean that the client is unsuitable for the treatment.

If the test is not carried out and a problem does occur, it is possible you could invalidate your insurance policy. A test only takes a few minutes and can easily be performed by the receptionist.

Method

- Cleanse the area of the skin to be tested (behind the ear or the crook of the arm).
- Mix the same make and colour of tint to be used with the manufacturer's recommended quantity of 10 per cent volume peroxide.
- Apply the tint to the area selected with a brush, about the size of a ten pence coin.
- Allow to dry.
- Ensure the client is aware that the tint should be left on the skin for 24 hours. If no reaction occurs, then wash off.
- If a reaction occurs, the tint should be removed immediately with water and a soothing lotion applied to the area.
- A reaction will be recognised by an itching, red-hot inflamed area. This should be treated with a soothing substance.

Precautions for lash and brow tinting

- Discuss the client's requirements with her prior to beginning the treatment.
- Ensure all equipment is clean and sterilised.
- Ensure all eye make-up is removed with a non-oily product.
- Check for contra-indications.
- Ensure client has removed contact lenses.
- Ensure area is thoroughly cleansed.
- Apply barrier cream to the skin around the eyes only and not to the hair to be tinted, as the tint will not act. The barrier cream is used to prevent the tint spreading beyond the area being treated.
- Ensure the client keeps her eyes closed at all times when the tint is on the lashes to prevent tint from entering the eyes and causing irritation. As a therapist, you are responsible for giving your client full instructions. This is vital, especially when treating nervous clients.
- Do not leave the client while the tint is processing.
- Complete details of the tint on the record card.
- Ensure that the eyebrows are tinted prior to shaping, to avoid tint seeping into the follicles, resulting in a reaction.

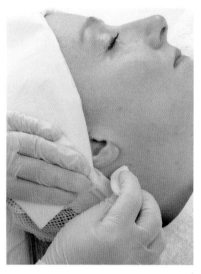

Patch test: cleansing the area first

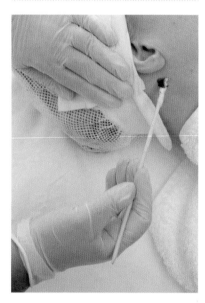

Patch test: applying the product

Provide eyelash and brow treatments

For your portfolio

Carry out a skin sensitivity test for tint and the application of eyelash adhesive. Record the date on your client record card and note the result in 24 hours. Make a note of the make of product that you have used.

Think about it

Always note the date and the results of the patch test on the client record card. The details on the card should include:

- date of patch test
- products used
- development time of the treatment
- areas treated
- contra-actions
- aftercare.

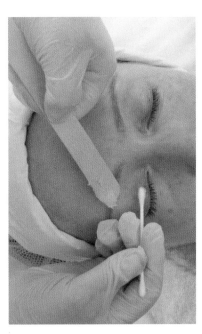

Decant the barrier cream onto a spatula and paint onto the skin surrounding the eyebrow to prevent accidental staining

Key terms

Oxidation – chemical reaction that occurs when peroxide and dye are mixed together.

Think about it

Although you will not be in contact with blood or tissue fluids during tinting, it may be advisable to wear protective gloves to prevent contact with the tint, which may cause dermatitis. This will also prevent accidental staining of the fingers when applying the tint.

How colour works

The selected dye and hydrogen peroxide are mixed together to produce a chemical reaction. When first applied to the hair, they enter the middle of the hair as small particles, but, because of the chemical reaction, they swell. This swelling prevents the colour from coming out when washed and so becomes permanent. This process is known as **oxidation**. The colour of the hair changes and this will remain until the hair grows or falls out.

Never mix the ingredients until you are ready to use them. Oxidation starts to occur and the tint starts to work as soon as it is mixed, so if you prepare them too early the product will not be able to enter the hair properly, resulting in poor colour.

Always replace caps on the tint and hydrogen peroxide as they will oxidise and future results will be unsuccessful. When using two colours of tint, mix them together and then add peroxide.

Choosing a tint

The skin around the eye is very thin and sensitive, therefore dyes designed for eyelash and brow tinting have been specially formulated to avoid any eye or tissue reactions. Any other type of dye or any hydrogen peroxide solution stronger than 10 per cent dilution should not be used in this area. It is dangerous and may even cause blindness.

The products used for eyelash and brow tinting are usually available as creams or gels in basic colours of black, blue, brown and grey. These colours are mixed to form variations in tone: for example, blue/black provides a darker colour.

The choice is a matter of personal preference and depends on:

- the client's overall skin type and hair colouring
- the type of eye make-up usually worn
- the age of the client.

As clients grow more mature, they lose a lot of natural colour from their hair and eyes. Brown or grey tints are preferable to black for producing a softer, more natural effect. This is an example of when you need to be aware of the fact that the client's expectations may not be realistic. The client may expect a very dark finish or longer eyelashes, where this may not be possible. It is therefore your responsibility to explain to the client that certain expectations cannot or should not be achieved, due to suitability. It is important to provide the client with sufficient professional advice and emphasise that lash and brow treatments are designed to enhance the natural features.

This applies to shaping and eyelash perming too. Expectations are realistic when they can be achieved with success and when the treatment is suitable for the client. The effect of tinting depends on the natural colour of the hair: for example, blond hair colour develops rapidly, usually in 5 minutes; red hair is more resistant and development will take longer, perhaps 10 minutes; white hair will take slightly longer to process, due to the lack of the pigment melanin. Make sure the colour you choose gives a realistic natural effect.

Preparing the client for tinting lashes and brows

◉ Help the client into a comfortable, semi-reclined position and protect hair and clothing.

◉ Clean and tone the area to ensure that all grease and make-up is removed from lashes and brows. If grease is left on the skin, a barrier will be created and the tint will not take properly.

◉ Protect the skin above the eyes with a barrier cream. Take care not to get any barrier product on the lashes or brows that require tinting. Use a tipped orange stick or cotton bud to apply the barrier cream to the skin above the eyes.

◉ When applying the cream below the eyes, either stroke it directly onto the skin and position the **eye shields** on top, close to the base of the lashes, or coat the underneath surface of the shields with barrier cream and slide them into position.

Key terms

Eye shield – used to protect the eyes during a treatment; may be made of paper or cotton wool.

Applying lash tint

Precautions should be taken to ensure that neither the tint nor the applicator penetrates the eye. There should not be any problems provided:

◉ the eye is well supported by gently holding the area

◉ the tint is applied carefully

◉ the lashes are not overloaded with tint

◉ the client's eyes are kept still and closed.

Tinting – what you will need

- Tinting equipment
- Protective headband and towel
- Couch roll to protect the work area
- Small non-metallic bowl for mixing tint (a metal one would react with the hydrogen peroxide)
- Lined container for waste
- Sterile spatula
- Sterile applicator or tipped orange stick
- Clean water in the event of eye irrigation becoming necessary
- Hand mirror
- Client record card
- Materials
- Damp cotton wool and tissues
- Eye shields made from cotton wool or paper
- Selection of coloured tints
- Hydrogen peroxide (usual 10 per cent volume, but always check the manufacturer's instructions)
- Eye make-up remover (non-oily)
- Cleanser and toner
- Gloves
- Barrier cream
- Tint stain remover

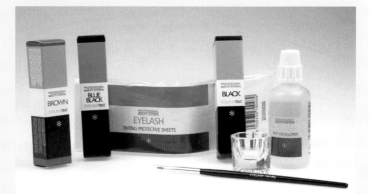

Provide eyelash and brow treatments

Step-by-step eyelash tinting

1 After placing shields under the eyes, begin to apply tint to lower lashes, made up to manufacturer's instructions. Ask the client to close her eyes, and apply tint to the top lashes. Cover the eyes

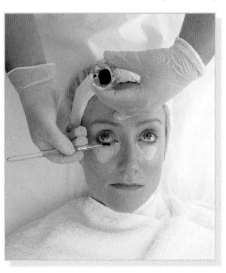

2 While the lash tint is developing you can tint the eyebrows if required

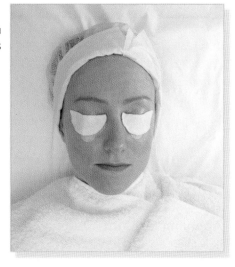

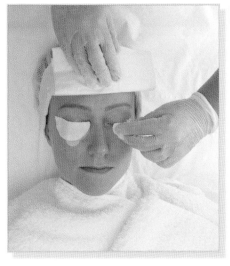

3 When processing time has elapsed, remove all traces of the tint

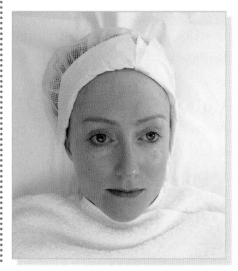

4 The finished eyelash tint defines the lashes and enhances the eyes

1   Once the client has been correctly positioned and the make-up removed, mix the correct colour of tint according to the manufacturer's directives. Measure out approximately a 5 mm length of tint with 2–3 drops of hydrogen peroxide, mixed in a tinting bowl with a disposable brush or an orange stick to a smooth paste.

2   Remember, before applying the tint a barrier cream should be applied to prevent staining.

3   Ask the client to look upwards and cover the lower lashes with tint (if the client has watery eyes, the lower lashes can be covered with the upper lashes when the eyes are closed, but the result is often not so effective). (See photo 1.) Make sure you do not ask the client to look up into the overhead light as this will over-sensitise the eyes and make them water.

4   Ask the client to close the eyes and apply the tint to the upper lashes.

5   Gently lift the skin to the eyebrows, so the tint can be applied right down to the base of the lashes and include shorter hairs which grow near the inside corner of the eyes.

6   If the client complains of discomfort or the eyes begin to water, remove the tint immediately using damp cotton wool pads, and irrigate the eye.

7   Note the time and allow for the tint to work according to the manufacturer's instructions. The colour should be checked at intervals and the tint reapplied if necessary. As a guide, allow 5–10 minutes, depending on the colour characteristics of the client.

Removal of eyelash tint

If the client experiences irritation, stinging or burning, the tint should be removed immediately before the end of the processing time. Even if a client has not had a negative reaction to a sensitivity test, some clients may find that the process irritates the delicate skin around the eye. The same would apply for the application of eyelash glue.

1   Place a pad of damp cotton wool on each eye. Hold the eye shield and pad of cotton wool together at the base and swiftly remove, enclosing any excess tint.

2   Remove any remaining tint with slightly damp cotton wool, using a gentle downward motion, and remove excess with a cotton bud. (See photo 3.)

3   When both eyes have been cleaned, ask the client to carefully open the eyes.

4   Support the eye and work quickly on the lower lashes with damp cotton wool and a cotton bud.

5   Stand in front of the client to check that all the tint has been removed.

6   Finally, wipe the area over with damp cotton wool to remove traces of the barrier cream.

7   Offer a hand mirror to view the final results.

8   Inform the client of possible contra-actions and aftercare. If irritation occurs, apply a damp cotton wool compress to the area.

9   Enter details on to the client record card. This should include the colour selected and the processing time for the tint, and any contra-actions and other information relevant to the treatment.

The process of eyelash tinting should take about 20 minutes.

Applying eyebrow tint

Step-by-step eyebrow tint

This can be performed after lash tinting, prior to shaping. Many salons and therapists perform this treatment while the lash tint is processing, to ensure they are cost-effective with their time. If shaping is carried out first, the tint will seep into the open pores, causing irritation.

1   Prepare the skin and brows the same way as for treating the lashes. Apply barrier cream around the eyebrows taking care to avoid the hairs.

2   Apply the tint against the hair growth using an orange stick or a fine brush, working gradually from the outer and underneath hairs towards the centre.

3   After one minute, remove a little tint from the inner corners of the eyebrow and check how the colour is developing. Apply more tint and repeat colour checks at one-minute intervals until the desired effect has been achieved. The developing time for tinting brows is much shorter than for lashes, usually 1–3 minutes. Always refer

Ensure all equipment is hygienic and close to hand

⬇

Carry out a consultation (ensure a patch test has been carried out). Check for contra-indications

⬇

Remove contact lenses if required

⬇

If shaping is to be carried out always tint first and shape after

⬇

Cleanse area with non-oily product

⬇

Apply barrier cream and preformed shapes if tinting lashes

⬇

Mix tint and apply (never pre-mix the tint). Note processing time on client record card

⬇

Remove tint after the required processing time

⬇

Show client results. Give aftercare advice

⬇

Record details on client record card

Eyebrow and lash tinting

Provide eyelash and brow treatments

to the manufacturer's directives for product guidance. Care must be taken to prevent the brows from becoming too dark as this can create an unattractive harsh effect.

4   Remove tint with clean, damp cotton wool.

5   Wipe over the area to remove all traces of barrier cream.

6   Discuss the final effect, possible contra-actions and aftercare with the client.

7   Enter details of the treatment on the client record card.

The process of eyebrow tinting should take approximately 15 minutes.

How to irrigate the eye

If tint accidentally enters the eye, do not panic; the client may be feeling discomfort and a slight burning sensation. Calm the client and explain the procedure you are going to follow.

1   Tilt the client's head slightly to one side. Carefully trickle some tepid water into the corner of the eye and allow the eye to be rinsed of the foreign body. In your first aid kit you may already have an eye irrigation bottle that contains sterilised water for this purpose.

2   Hold some tissue or a small kidney dish to collect the excess water.

3   Apply a damp cotton wool compress to cool and soothe the eye.

It is not acceptable to use an eyebath because of the risk of cross-infection.

Possible causes of eye irritation include:

◉ very sensitive eyes

◉ too much or incorrect strength of hydrogen peroxide

◉ something in the eye

◉ inadvertently poking the eye.

Assessing the results

It is important that the client is shown the results of the treatment to ensure satisfaction before she leaves the treatment room.

◉ A successful tinting treatment produces the required colour changes to the lashes and brows without staining the skin.

◉ Even the shortest eyelashes should be coloured from the base.

◉ The appearance of blond roots after the eyelash tint shows that not enough care was taken. The skin fold of the eyelid was probably not lifted away from the base of the hairs when applying tint.

◉ The tint will not have covered the brows successfully if:
  – there was grease or make-up on the hairs
  – old tint was used
  – the hydrogen peroxide had lost strength
  – the tint and peroxide were incorrectly mixed
  – the tint was removed too soon.

Aftercare

As with all treatments, the client should be advised against touching or rubbing the areas immediately after the treatment. If redness or irritation occur, apply a damp cotton wool compress.

The client should be aware that the effects will last approximately 4–6 weeks as the hairs grow out. Strong sunlight will make the results fade faster.

Product safety data

Product	Description	Ingredients	Hazards	Flammability	First aid procedures	Spillage	Handling and storage
Eye make-up remover	Prepared from mild cleaning agents in a cosmetic base	All ingredients commonly used in cosmetic products and meet accepted standards of purity	Non-hazardous under normal conditions of use	✗	Ingestion: drink milk or water Eye contact: wash well with water; if irritation persists, seek medical advice	Clean using absorbent material, followed by washing with detergent and water to avoid slippery floors	No special precautions
Eyelash tint	Oil/water-emulsion (cream)	Water/cetearyl alcohol/PEG-sorbitan lanolate/sodium cetearyl sulfate/diaminotoluene/aminophenols/dyest. CI 77499 and/or 77007/no preservatives	Non-hazardous on its own; becomes hazardous when mixed with hydrogen peroxide	✗	Ingestion: drink a lot of water; seek medical attention Skin contact: remove with water; if irritation occurs, seek medical attention Eye contact: avoid by careful observation of the instructions for use; if contact occurs, rinse immediately with warm water	Clean area immediately to prevent staining Always wear gloves and avoid contact with skin and eyes	At least three years, when kept under normal stocking conditions

Product	Description	Ingredients	Hazards	Flammability	First aid procedures	Spillage	Handling and storage
Eyelash tinting peroxide	Mixture of oxidising agents, wetting agents, pH adjusters, fragrance and water Contents: hydrogen peroxide	All ingredients commonly used in cosmetic products and meet accepted standards of purity	Hazardous if precautions are ignored	✗ Note: Hydrogen peroxide may react with other chemicals to form explosive mixtures; combustion may occur if hydrogen peroxide is allowed to dry on paper, wood, hair, etc.	Ingestion: seek medical attention immediately Skin contact: avoid; always wear rubber gloves when using product; if skin contact occurs, wash well with soap and water; if irritation persists, seek medical attention Eye contact: avoid; wash well with water and seek medical attention	Clean area with plenty of water and dispose down drain; do not absorb into flammable material such as tissue or couch roll	Always wear gloves and avoid contact with skin Store in a cool place away from direct sunlight; store in the original container only and keep closures tightly sealed Contamination of solutions containing hydrogen peroxide can result in instability with liberation of heat and oxygen
Eyelash tint stain remover	Mixture of ethanol and fragrance oils in solution	All ingredients commonly used in cosmetic products and meet accepted standards of purity	Hazardous unless normal safety precautions followed	✓ Ethanol content: 50 per cent w/w Note: In event of a fire, evacuate areas known to contain products and inform fire service of their presence	Ingestion: avoid, drink plenty of milk or water Inhalation: avoid, may cause dizziness, remove to fresh air Skin contact: avoid prolonged contact with skin; if irritation persists, seek medical attention	Clean contaminated area with plenty of water, wash with detergent and water to avoid slippery floors; do not absorb on to combustible material such as tissue or couch roll	Store in a cool place away from direct sunlight; large quantities should be stored in fire-resistant store

Eyelash perming

This treatment is a semi-permanent way of curling the upper lashes and the result will last from 4–6 weeks: as the old hairs are lost and replaced with new hairs the curl diminishes. The use of perming solutions, although chemical-based, are far less damaging than regular use of eyelash curlers.

Eyelash perming is recommended:

- to emphasise the eyelashes, making the eye look larger and to give more definition
- for clients who wear contact lenses or glasses
- for mature clients with sagging eyelids
- for clients who do not wish to wear mascara
- for sportswomen
- for clients living or working in a hot environment
- for clients who have short, straight lashes
- for special occasions or holidays.

There are a variety of eyelash perming products available and most companies offer training sessions. It is always important to follow the manufacturer's directives when using any product, but special care should be taken when working with chemicals around the sensitive eye area. Refer to COSHH regulations.

How perming works on the eyelashes

When perming, the lashes are curled and stretched over small rods and curled into shape using a chemical product. Today most of these products are referred to as cold wave gels or lotions. This term is used to distinguish the products from heat perms, which require heat to activate the chemical process. This would be unsuitable for the delicate eye area.

The gel breaks down the structure of the hair, and once broken the hair can then take on the shape of the curling rod. When this curl has taken place, a second gel is applied to fix the eyelash into the new shape. The gel is often referred to as a neutraliser or oxidising agent.

Consultation

It is important with all treatments to carry out a thorough consultation and to establish what a client requires from the treatment. The same contra-indications checks apply to perming as for other eye treatments. It is vital that no skin infections or open wounds are present, as a chemical is being applied to the skin. Ensure no reaction has occurred during the sensitivity test. A reaction would show itself as itching, redness and swelling. Treat with a suitable product.

Preparation of the client

- Ensure the client is in a semi-reclined position.
- Remove jewellery — remember piercing around the eyebrow area.
- Remove contact lenses if required.
- Secure hair away from the face.
- Protect the client's clothing.
- Ensure all products and basic trolley equipment are close to hand. Remove all eye make-up by using non-oily eye make-up remover.
- Have water ready to irrigate the eye if required.

> **Think about it**
>
> The products to be tested are adhesive perm solution and neutraliser. They should be tested as with tinting in the crook of the client's elbow or behind the ear.

Provide eyelash and brow treatments

Step-by-step eyelash perming

1 A full consultation follows a skin sensitivity test which should be carried out at least 24 hours previously. Thoroughly cleanse the eye and lashes removing all traces of make-up.

2 Blot the eyes to ensure they are grease free and dry. A non-oily remover should be used to avoid any grease forming a barrier.

3 Use a cotton bud to thoroughly check the lashes are clean and dry.

4 Choose a suitable-sized rod, depending on the lashes and the curl required.

5 Apply a small amount of adhesive to the main body of the rod. Check no lashes are caught underneath. Bend and shape the rod to sit tightly in the eye shape.

6 Curl lashes over the rod with no bends or kinks. Use a cotton bud to apply the solution to the lashes. Follow manufacturer's directives for development and neutralising times.

7 The finished result should be curly but natural looking with not too tight a curl. Tinting can be carried out during the procedure, but check recommended instructions.

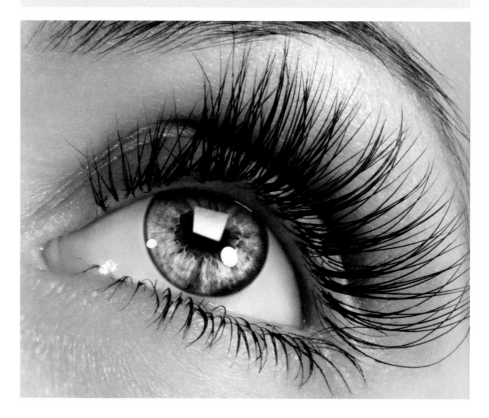

Eyelash perming can produce stunning results

Problems with eyelash perming

Problem	Cause	Solution
Too curled	Rod too small	Re-perm using a larger rod, half the time
No result	Too large a rod Insufficient processing Incorrect neutralising Oil barrier on the lashes	Re-perm
Uneven curl	Incorrect position of rod Uneven application of gel/lotion Not curling all the lashes over the rod	Re-position rod
Buckled or hook ends	Failure to wrap hair correctly around the rod	Trim ends of lashes carefully

Provide aftercare advice

It is important that you ensure the client receives the correct aftercare advice for the treatment that has been undertaken. You could provide an aftercare leaflet that covers eye treatments highlighting the relevant points for the client to take away.

Frequently asked questions

Q	Why is it important to carry out a sensitivity test?
A	To ensure that the client is not allergic to any of the products used in the treatment. This should be done prior to the first tint or application of lashes.
Q	Why should a sensitivity test be carried out each time the client comes for a treatment?
A	To ensure the client has not become sensitive to the product causing irritation. As a salon you may have changed products. You could invalidate your insurance if a problem arises and this procedure has not been carried out.
Q	Do I have to pre-warm the area prior to shaping?
A	You do not have to pre-warm the area, but this procedure helps to minimise discomfort as the heat opens the hair follicles – making removal easier and less painful for the client.
Q	Why is it important to use a non-oily, eye make-up remover prior to treatment?
A	Oil-based products will form a barrier over the lashes, making the application of artificial lashes or tint non-effective.
Q	Why should a barrier cream be applied prior to tinting lashes and brows?
A	This barrier cream prevents tint seeping onto the surrounding skin, causing unsightly staining of the area.

Provide eyelash and brow treatments

Check your knowledge

1. What type of condition is blepharitis?
   a) Fungal
   b) Viral
   c) Bacterial

2. How would you minimise discomfort when shaping the brows?

3. What facial features would you use to aid measuring the shape of brows?

4. Name two types of eyebrow tweezers.

5. Why is it important to carry out a sensitivity test before carrying out a tint or a perm?

6. How often should you carry out a sensitivity test for tint and adhesive products?

7. Why is it important to mix the tint just before you use it, and not in advance?

8. How long would you leave a tint on the brows?
   a) As long as the client wants
   b) According to the hair type
   c) According to the manufacturer's directives

9. Why should you tint before carrying out a shape on the client?

10. Which three activities should be avoided after having a brow shape?

11. What is the suggested brow shape for a client?

12. What action would you take if blood spotting occurred when brow shaping?

13. Why should you carry out a sensitivity test for adhesives before perming lashes?

14. What percentage of peroxide is used when carrying out an eyelash or brow tint?
    a) 5 per cent
    b) 15 per cent
    c) 10 per cent

15. Name the solutions that are required when perming lashes.

16. State three reasons why a client may require permed lashes.

Getting ready for assessment

Your assessor will require you to show competency in the skill areas of shaping, tinting and eyelash perming. However, your assessor will determine whether you need to show competency three times for each skill area, or just show one treatment for each skill area on three different clients. Evidence to support your work may be in the form of photographs or video, employer's or client statements, written papers or project work.

Remember that a client may wish to have all three treatments on the same salon visit. You may also carry out a treatment while the client is having another treatment. An eyelash tint can be performed while the client has a facial mask. These combined treatments maximise salon revenue and save precious salon and client time.

When tinting and applying perm products it is important to remember that the client must have a sensitivity test for the products you are using.

When tinting you only need to show that you have practically covered two colour characteristics (light and dark being more common that white and red). However, your assessor will need you to show that you would be able to treat all colours in the range effectively and will require supporting evidence to prove this. These outstanding ranges may be covered by written work or oral questioning.

You must show that you can carry out a total brow re-shape as well as general brow maintenance, and that you can apply both types of artificial lashes and have used adhesive and solvent products.

You must also show that you can carry out a thorough consultation for each treatment, prepare the working area as necessary, give suitable aftercare advice for whichever treatment you have performed, and deal with a contra-action if it arises. This could be irrigating the eye or identifying a reaction to a sensitivity test or a contra-indication to the treatment.

Provide eyelash and brow treatments

Apply make-up and instruct on make-up application

What you will learn

- Prepare for make-up
- Apply make-up
- Prepare for make-up instruction
- Instruct on make-up application

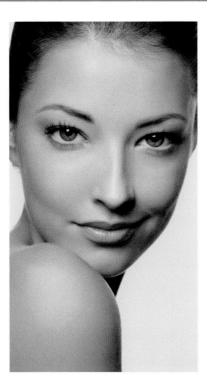

Introduction

These units are presented together as there are many aspects of providing a make-up service where you must also provide the client with valuable skincare information to ensure they gain the most from the service. You may also promote further treatments that can enhance the client's skin and overall appearance.

The subject of make-up application is one that most of you will associate with becoming a beauty therapist. The combined unit focuses on the use of make-up to enhance the appearance, for day, evening and special occasions with the added component of how to instruct clients on the most suitable skincare and selection of products to suit their skin type. This is an important skill if you wish to become a make-up artist, a trainer or pursue a career as a make-up consultant for one of the large cosmetic houses. Most women have used make-up to enhance their appearance and have been pleased with the results — whether it was for hiding a blemish, for a special occasion or just a night out with friends. However, few people know how to use make-up to their best advantage, so it is very rewarding for a therapist to accentuate a client's best features and to enable her to disguise or minimise areas that she is not as happy with. Applying make-up correctly and selecting suitable skincare products can help you do all this: providing the correct base to work on and understanding how to apply make-up to enhance features can boost confidence and self-esteem.

To help with make-up application and selection of skincare products, refer to You and the skin, and Provide facial skincare, for more information on skin types and how to recognise them, skin conditions that are treatable, and contra-indications that will prevent the treatment or require the therapist to adapt the treatment plan. Although techniques are the same regardless of skin type, a good knowledge of the client's skin is vital if you are going to do the best for the client.

It is also important to ensure that you understand the client's needs, including the time she may have available to spend on applying products and her budget.

Benefits of skincare and make-up session for the client:

- one-to-one, non-intimidating personalised service to suit individual requirements
- individual demonstration and trial
- tailored skincare/make-up planning.

Benefits of skincare and make-up instructional sessions for the therapist:

- one-to-one, personalised service to the client
- opportunity to promote salon products and treatments
- increase in clientele and commission for the therapist
- promotes salon or own business.

Benefits of group demonstration for the client:

- fun activity to do with friends
- informative without the focus just on you — good for people who don't know what to expect!

Benefits of a group demonstration for the therapist:

- targets a larger audience
- as well as all of the above.

Prepare for make-up and prepare for make-up instruction

In this outcome you will learn about:

- preparing yourself, your client and your work area for make-up
- using suitable consultation techniques to identify treatment objectives
- carrying out a skin analysis
- providing clear recommendations to the client
- selecting products, tools and equipment to suit client treatment needs, skin types and conditions.

Ensuring all tools and equipment are cleaned

As with all salon treatments, hygiene is paramount and make-up services are no exception. The equipment and products should be cleaned after each treatment and the **cut-out method**, where products are **decanted**, should be used, to prevent contamination of the product and cross-contamination from client to client.

Brushes and sponges

These need to be cleaned in hot, soapy water, which should be worked into the fibres before rinsing under running water. Brushes should then be given a final clean in an alcohol solution or suitable brush cleaner before drying naturally – this will prevent the bristles from becoming misshapen. Sponges require soaking for at least one hour in a suitable disinfectant, and should then be rinsed thoroughly.

Palettes

These should be scrubbed to remove waxy deposits, then dried thoroughly.

Maintaining industry hygiene and safety practices

There is little risk of products becoming infected if good hygiene procedures are followed. However, to prevent infection by products which are normally applied directly to the face, these simple rules should be followed.

- ◉ Eye and lip pencils – sharpen before use to expose a new surface.
- ◉ Lipsticks – transfer a small amount on to a spatula before applying. Use a disposable lip brush.
- ◉ Pressed powders (eyeshadow and blushers) – either transfer products on to a palette or have a good supply of clean brushes.
- ◉ Mascara – use a disposable mascara wand for each eye.
- ◉ Wash and disinfect hands before you begin the service. If you are carrying out a demonstration in a hall or similar venue a sanitising hand gel may be used.

For information on facial treatments refer to Provide facial skincare, pages 267–325, and for the difference between sanitation and sterilisation refer to Professional skills, page 38.

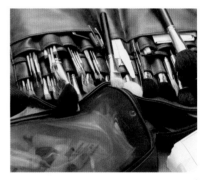

Always ensure your make-up brushes are clean before you put them away

Key terms

Cut-out method – decanting a product from a larger container onto a spatula or into a bowl for use during a treatment.

Decant – removing a product from a larger container to a smaller container.

For your portfolio

Investigate the type of brushes that are available on the market.

Apply make-up and instruct on make-up application

Leaving the work area in a condition suitable for further services

It is important to leave the working area clean and tidy. Ensure that all products are put away and that brushes and sponges are cleaned ready for use – clean brushes in warm, soapy water and rinse well. Allow the brushes to dry naturally if possible, so that the shape of the brush is not distorted.

Disposing of waste materials

Contaminated waste should be disposed of according to legislative requirements. Any other waste products can be put with the normal rubbish, but remember to abide by COSHH guidelines for safe disposal of all products used within the salon. If carrying out a make-up service and applying false lashes, read the manufacturers' guidelines for disposal of adhesive or solvent products.

If you are carrying out a demonstration outside the salon, ensure that all waste is disposed of in accordance with the law.

Preparing for a skincare or make-up service

The working area should be clean, tidy and well organised. Ensure you adhere to a professional standard regarding your appearance and that your working area complies with the health, safety and hygiene regulations. Consult your professional body for guidelines to prevent cross-infection. The main sources of infection during make-up are usually contaminated products, dirty tools and equipment, and applying make-up and skincare products over infected areas.

Make-up and skincare activities can be carried out individually or you may be asked to do a promotion or presentation to a group. Whichever method you are using it is important that you act in a professional manner. Whether you are in a cubicle with a client in a one-to-one setting or giving a presentation in a community centre, you should maintain the same high standards.

Identify the client's treatment objectives

Before a make-up application/instruction or skincare lesson can take place, a full consultation should be undertaken so that an accurate assessment of the client and her needs can be made. This should be both by visual assessment of the skin and by asking a series of questions.

Visual assessment

This should be carried out on a cleansed and toned dry face with the hair secured away from the face. The skin should not be moisturised at this stage because this will make the skin slightly greasy. A suitable moisturiser for the skin should be applied before the application of make-up. Refer to Provide facial skincare, pages 271–92, for information on facial analysis, cleansing and toning routines.

You should analyse the client's skin type, facial features and bone structure in an upright position.

Think about it

For every client, you will need their signed, written, informed consent before carrying out the service. Anyone under the age of 16 will require parent/guardian informed and signed consent for these services to go ahead, and the parent/guardian must be present throughout the service.

When carrying out an analysis for make-up the light should be falling directly onto the client's face. The light should be a combination of natural daylight and warm white fluorescent light.

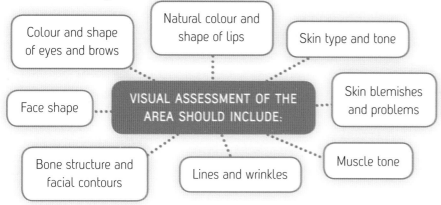

Colour and shape of eyes and brows

Natural colour and shape of lips

Skin type and tone

Face shape

VISUAL ASSESSMENT OF THE AREA SHOULD INCLUDE:

Skin blemishes and problems

Bone structure and facial contours

Lines and wrinkles

Muscle tone

Questioning the client

As well as the visual assessment, you should ask the client a few simple questions to help you both agree on a realistic service plan. Some useful questions to help you assess the client are listed below.

- How much make-up do you usually wear?
- What do you think are your best/worst features?
- Do you have any allergies or sensitivity to make-up or other related products?
- Is the make-up for a special occasion?
- Are there any colours you like/dislike?
- Are you trying to create a special look?
- What skincare regime do you use at present?
- Do you have any areas of particular concern/outcomes you would like to address/ achieve? (This will encourage the client to ask any questions that she may have.)

It is important to ask the client open questions so that you can gain maximum information. Always be positive, even if the client has no skincare regime.

When you have gathered all the information you can agree a suitable plan for your make-up and skincare instructional session or make-up application. You may have differing views from your client, so it is important to agree on a suitable and realistic plan. Remember, too, that the plan should reflect the client's level of ability. If she is a novice at applying skincare products and make-up, there is no point in giving her a complicated routine to follow.

Apply make-up and instruct on make-up application

Key terms

Sensitivity – the ability to react to a stimulus. This could be caused by an allergy such as hayfever or as a result of improper use of products over a period of time.

Allergic reaction – unpleasant reaction of the body when coming into contact with a particular ingredient, product, chemical or substance; symptoms may include sneezing, redness of the skin, skin rash, inflamed eyes and mucus membranes.

Hypoallergenic – designed to cause fewer allergic reactions.

Identifying if clients have contra-indications to make-up

Allergic reactions and sensitivity testing

European Union (EU) and US legislation requires that cosmetic companies conduct very strict safety tests on materials they use to formulate products. Nevertheless, there will always be some people who are allergic to a substance which other people can tolerate without a problem. It is therefore essential that you complete a **sensitivity** test if you are concerned that the client may react to a product. This can be done by testing a small sample of the product behind the client's ear or in the crook of the elbow. If a reaction occurs within 24 hours the product should not be used. A reaction could include:

- redness (erythema)
- swelling
- irritation to the area.

Treat with calamine lotion and a cold compress as necessary.

In some instances, medication can affect the condition of the skin and cause sensitivity to occur. Always carry out a thorough consultation and contra-indication check. If the client has an unidentified condition, recommend that she visits her GP for a diagnosis and treatment. Never diagnose yourself.

If the client has had **allergic reactions** to skincare products or make-up in the past, ensure that the products you select are **hypoallergenic**.

How long do cosmetics last?

The European Union Cosmetics Directive 1993 states that products which contain no preservatives and natural ingredients with a shelf life of less than six months have to be stamped with an expiry date. Cosmetics that have been tested and meet the European safety requirements are not required to be date stamped. The EU gives a shelf life for cosmetics that is approximately 30 months from the time of manufacture, although this may vary depending on the product, so you could calculate how long you have had a product from the day that you opened it. The time after opening is denoted by a special symbol that looks like an open jar; inside the symbol will be a number that will reflect the number in months that the product can safely be used without harm.

The product should also state its function, have a batch number on it just in case there is a problem during manufacture and the product needs to be recalled and, finally, any precautions for use.

Risk assessment for make-up application

When carrying out any treatment a therapist should conduct a risk assessment to identify any problems that may occur when carrying out the treatment or service.

Hazards: only look for hazards that you could reasonably expect to result in significant harm under the conditions in your workplace. Use the following examples as a guide.

- **Allergies** (allergic reaction to make-up)
- **Cross-infection** (infections spread from tools)
- **Irritation** (caused by scratchy tools)
- **Contamination** (caused by ignoring contra-indications to service)

Even though as a therapist you have carried out a thorough consultation, a client may still react to a product and you need to remove it quickly. It is always worth having an eye irrigation bottle that contains sterilised water just in case a client reacts to an eye make-up product. This is for future reference and for insurance purposes.

Many of the topics relating to both the application of skincare products and the application of make-up are covered in more depth in Provide facial skincare, pages 267–327 and Professional skills.

Ensuring lighting is suitable for make-up application and instruction

It is important to work in good lighting when applying make-up to the client, carrying out make-up instruction and, where possible, for demonstrations. Always try to face natural light. Natural daylight is pure white light, but this light does not just fall on the face from above — it is reflected from any light coloured surface it hits. Natural daylight is the only light that shows true colours, but it is also the harshest form of light as it shows up imperfections. To achieve the best from your make-up, a combination of natural light and warm white fluorescent lighting gives the best effect.

Artificial lighting

Make-up colours tested in the wrong light can give the wrong effect when applied. It is therefore important to be aware of the differing effects of various types of lighting.

Standard light bulbs

These produce a yellowish colour which dulls blue tones and makes red tones appear darker. A light bulb cover with a shade directs the light down, creating unnatural shadows.

Fluorescent tubes

White tubes give out a harsh, blue-white light which makes colours appear cold. If the fluorescent tube is covered by a diffuser, this will soften the effect and create very little shadow. Warm white tubes with a diffuser will therefore be the best type of artificial light for matching make-up colours.

Skin analysis

The knowledge you require to prepare the client for treatment is the same as that required for a full facial treatment as covered in Provide facial skincare, pages 293–323. Whatever the environment you are working in and whatever the treatment you are undertaking, you will need to carry out a skin analysis in order to ensure the correct products are selected. This will cover:

- facial examination
- skin types, e.g. normal, dry, oily or combination (you need to be able to identify these skin types and mature, sensitive and dehydrated skin conditions, so you can recommend suitable skincare and make-up products to suit these skin types for your assessment)
- record cards.

Think about it

In some instances allergic reactions can be severe and will require medical intervention. In the event of a client being allergic to a certain product or substance, ensure that you always read the ingredients and refer to the manufacturer's instructions. Always record details on the client record card.

Think about it

Warm, white fluorescent light is the best substitute for natural lighting and the best for matching make-up colours.

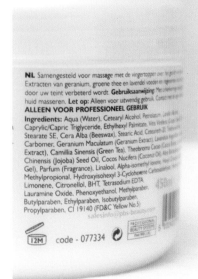

List of ingredients and shelf life of product

Apply make-up and instruct on make-up application

Refer to You and the skin, pages 183–206, for further detailed information on skin types and conditions.

Before carrying out any make-up services, you need to ensure that you establish the client's skin type, age range and condition and select suitable skincare and make-up products for both the client's personal use and instruction. (Refer to Provide facial skincare, pages 271–92, for more information on how to undertake a facial analysis and select appropriate products.)

Normal skin	Dry skin	Oily skin	Combination skin	Sensitive skin	Dehydrated skin	Mature skin
Eye make-up remover – lotion Light cleansing lotion Facial wash if preferred 10–20 per cent alcohol toner Light moisturising lotion/cream Eye lotion/gel Gentle exfoliant Non-setting mask	Eye make-up remover – oil or cream based Cream cleanser 0 per cent alcohol toner Cream moisturiser Gentle exfoliant Eye cream Neck cream Non-setting mask	Eye make-up remover – lotion based Cleansing lotion or milk Facial wash or gel 25–50 per cent alcohol toner Cleansing grain or peel Moisturising milk Light eye gel Clay-based masks	Products to suit the variation in skin types – however, if the client has sensitive skin in the combinations, this should always take priority over other types of product	Treat as dry skin – consider using hypoallergenic products	As dry – recommend gentle exfoliation and facial treatments such as a galvanic facial to push moisture into the skin	Cream-based products that are suitable for drier skin and alcohol-free toners that prevent the skin from drying out, night, eye and neck creams should be recommended. Additional treatments such as non-surgical face lifts could also be discussed

At a glance – suitable skincare products for different skin types

Providing recommendations to the client

The client should be shown how to use each of the recommended products; it is important for the therapist to let the client know the frequency of application, methods of application and any special equipment that should be used. This should be done by the use of demonstration and client application as a trial, diagrams, written home care leaflets as well as verbal instruction.

Think about it

If a product starts to smell, change colour or separate, it should be thrown away. Always refer to the manufacturer's instructions for use and storage and look at the symbol denoting the number of months the product can be used for once opened. If products are used incorrectly or not stored properly, then they will deteriorate more quickly than indicated on the symbol.

Think about it

You should have available a variety of products and equipment to suit all skin types and effects that you wish to create suitable for a varied range of clientele.

Selecting appropriate products, tools and equipment to suit the needs of your client

Basic trolley set-up for a skincare instructional session

- Variety of cleansers, toners and moisturisers for each skin type
- Exfoliants
- Facial washes/scrubs
- Eye creams
- Neck creams
- Lip balms
- Masks
- Magnifying lamp
- Headband
- Cotton wool/facial sponges
- Tissues
- Spatulas
- Facial consultation charts

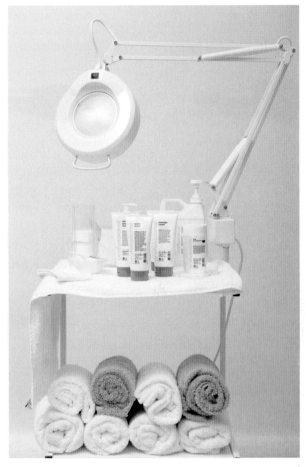

Trolley prepared for skincare instructional session

Basic trolley equipment for a make-up procedure

- Towels or gown
- Headband
- Make-up sponges
- Make-up brushes
- Make-up products
- Spatulas
- Palette
- Sharpener
- Cotton buds
- Mirror
- Brush and comb

All brushes should preferably be disposable to prevent cross-infection.

Apply make-up and instruct on make-up application

Make-up brushes

A good set of brushes is essential in the application of any make-up. There are individual brushes available for each stage of make-up application. For maximum benefit it is important to understand their usage.

Face-powder brush

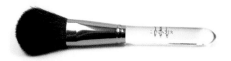

This is the largest brush as it covers the largest area. It is not restricted to defining shape, its primary purpose being to blend loosened face powder into the skin.

Blusher brush

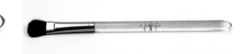

Used to apply blusher to the cheekbones. It looks similar to the powder brush but is slightly smaller in order to work on the cheekbone area.

Contour brush

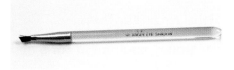

This brush has several uses: to apply contour powder under the cheekbones, to shade and highlight the face.

Eyebrow brush

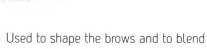

Used to shape the brows and to blend colour. It has short nylon bristles and may have a small comb on the other side to separate lashes.

Eyeliner brush

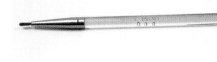

For the application of eyeliner or to blend in kohl pencils along the rim of the eye, a very thin, pointed brush is required.

Angled eyeshadow brush

To apply and blend powder eyeshadow. The angle of the brush is important, it allows you to follow and blend into the socket area.

Eyeshadow brush

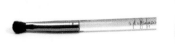

Used for general shading purposes. It is similar to the angle brush but with a straight edge.

Fluff brush

This brush is used to finish off the blending of eye make-up. It is the largest of the eye brushes and needs to be very soft, as it is used to soften the edges without disturbing the shape of the make-up.

Sponge applicator

The sponge is good for applying both loose and powder eyeshadow. It is also used for blending and softening harsh pencil lines.

Lip brush

To apply lipstick, the brush must have short thin bristles to make it flat. This helps to give a clean outline to the lips.

One-to-one make-up and skincare sessions

The criteria for this qualification will allow you to deliver make-up and skincare sessions to individual clients and groups (the group may be two or more people or you may make a presentation to a large number of people). Your assessor and training establishment will discuss with you the requirements you need to complete your assessments successfully.

A one-to-one make-up or skincare session usually takes place in a salon, in a well-lit cubicle or working area, and takes little organisation, except for clean tools, a good selection of products and the necessary accessories of tissues, cotton wool and cotton buds, as well as a large mirror. (Refer to basic trolley set-up on page 363.)

When the client books in for a lesson, it is a good idea to suggest she brings her existing make-up — it might simply be that the client has excellent products and colours, but she just does not know how or where to use them, or she might be concerned about overusing them — or the range of skincare products she currently uses.

When using instructional techniques, whether for skincare products or the application of make-up, you are teaching the correct use and application in order for the client to gain the best results. With make-up application the best way to do this is to ask the client to follow your lead. You do one side of the face, and she matches the technique on the other.

For an individual skincare or make-up lesson you should:

- seat the client in an upright or slightly reclined position in good light
- discuss the client's requirements including any concerns
- remove any accessories, and make sure hair is secured off the face
- ask the client to remove her contact lenses if she has sensitive eyes
- protect the client's clothing
- check for contra-indications (refer to You and the skin, pages 208–213, for further information on contra-indications)
- carry out a thorough skin analysis on cleansed skin.

Make-up consultation should include:

- client preference
- face shape
- areas to be highlighted/shaded
- any areas requiring corrective make-up
- bone structure
- shape of head
- hair colour and texture
- skin colour and tone
- skin sensitivity
- cultural and religious considerations.

Think about it

Make-up is a very personal thing. While it is important to be sensitive to cultural differences, whatever your perceptions of your client's background might be, do not make assumptions about how she would like to look.

Key terms

Enhance – make something look better or more attractive.

Cultural and religious considerations

For some Asian women, facial adornment has religious significance that has its roots steeped in history. The application of facial and body adornment is a specialised art. If you treat people from several different cultures within your salon, it would be worth spending time researching this area. This would show excellent customer care to existing and prospective clients. You should also be aware of the ingredients in the make-up products and skincare range you use – some cultures and religions forbid the use of animal-based products.

- Agree a plan incorporating the above, taking into account the type of make-up required, the occasion, the colour of clothing to be worn, the client's clothing, and the client's skin type and tone, which should include both colour and muscle tone, condition and age group.
- Agree products with client.
- Apply the make-up and explain the procedure to the client.
- Assess the results with the client, entering the colours/products used on the record card.
- Recommend products for home care use.
- Check client satisfaction.

Face shapes

It is useful to consider some general descriptions of face shapes and some hair styles that can **enhance** make-up application. This will help when you are analysing the client's face shape at the consultation stage. Remember when applying make-up to clients from different ethnic origins that characteristic facial features can differ.

Any corrective work on black or Asian clients should be approached in exactly the same way as for white Caucasian clients, using contouring products to enhance or reduce areas. Refer to skin characteristics in You and the skin, page 199.

Refer also to You and the skin, page 207, for more information on face shapes.

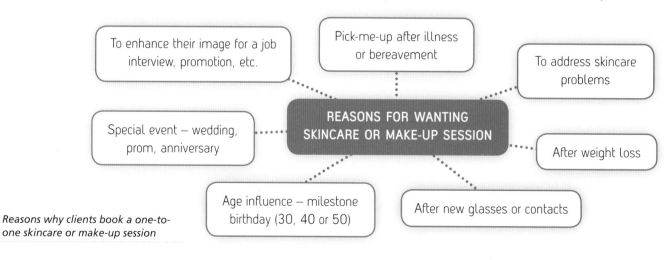

To enhance their image for a job interview, promotion, etc.

Pick-me-up after illness or bereavement

To address skincare problems

Special event – wedding, prom, anniversary

REASONS FOR WANTING SKINCARE OR MAKE-UP SESSION

After weight loss

Age influence – milestone birthday (30, 40 or 50)

After new glasses or contacts

Reasons why clients book a one-to-one skincare or make-up session

Group demonstrations

Local clubs and societies are often looking for opportunities to engage interesting speakers. You could offer to give a talk to the local Women's Institute (WI), mother and toddler group, slimming group or women's group, or your salon might be approached by one of these groups asking for a make-up or skincare demonstration. This is your opportunity to talk about the various treatments your salon offers or, if you are a mobile or independent home-based therapist, an opportunity for you to promote your business.

All of these groups are potential customers, so a professional, yet friendly, approach is essential. Your aim is to encourage them to come to you for the treatments and services you are demonstrating!

My story

Salon promotions

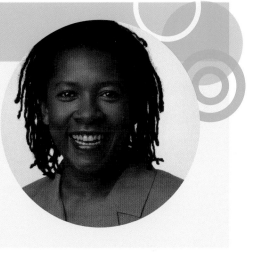

Hi, my name is Sam. I am manager of a large salon in Kent. Until recently, my therapists were all reluctant to take part in promotional events, so I devised an in-house training session to get them used to public speaking and doing demonstrations to larger groups. We invited family and friends along so that it was not so intimidating, and presented some of our latest treatments. We also did skin mapping. The session was a huge success, and it gave the therapists real confidence. We now do seasonal promotion evenings, and all the therapists enjoy taking part. It has increased our clientele and retail sales. It's also worth remembering that some product companies will provide a small amount of money for the organisation of a promotional event.

Meeting individual needs and interests

When organising a demonstration, you will need to consider:

◉ the age group of the audience — this will impact on the type of skincare or make-up you focus on

◉ the size of the group

◉ the type of demonstration — for example face painting would interest a mother and toddler group but may not interest the WI

◉ the time of day when the event is to be held — day, evening or special interest, e.g. prom/ball/bridal

◉ different product types, for example emphasis on products with sunscreens and protection from the environment — this could include:
  – moisturisers and age-defying hand creams
  – products designed for sensitive skins/hypoallergenic products
  – suitable cosmetic make-up for treating skin disorders, port wine stains, etc.

If you are carrying out a group demonstration/instructional demonstration, there are a number of factors that you should consider to ensure that your audience is engaged.

Venue and format

Some points to bear in mind:

● Where the event is to be held is very important. The venue can be anywhere, from the local village hall to a hotel (most commonly used for bridal fairs) to someone's home. Find out where and when, and then consider both the risk assessment aspect and health and safety implications, along with the general ambience, warmth and suitable lighting for undertaking a make-up and skin care demonstration. Remember natural daylight is the best lighting for make-up. Does the room smell pleasant? Some halls can smell musty so you may need to think about room fragrances.

● You will need to check whether your insurance will cover you to do the demonstration. You should not assume that your public liability and indemnity insurances are valid when you are working away from your own premises (see Professional skills, pages 60–61). You also need to consider your car insurance: are you covered by business insurance and are your products insured when stored in and transported in your vehicle?

● Accidents happen, and it is your responsibility to ensure that both you and your audience are adequately protected; both externally, for problems with the building, fire regulations, etc., for internal areas, such as safe seating and non-slip flooring.

● Ask the group's organiser if the premises have an up-to-date fire certificate, if there has been a recent risk assessment of the building and what access and exit facilities are available. Are there fire exits?

● Will a first aider be present at the demonstration? What happens if a member of the group has an accident or is taken ill? This needs to be considered before the event so that contingency plans can be put in place — after the event is too late and may leave you and the organiser with serious issues of compensation or neglect charges.

● If the demonstration is for people who have disabilities, then responsibility should be taken by the organisers to ensure that sufficient carers are present to support the audience. It should not be your responsibility to take guests to the toilet or deal with a medical emergency — you are not trained to do so. Find out if there are facilities for people with disabilities such as ramps and toilets.

● For your own safety, ask the organiser about parking and how to get in to the building. A dark parking area may leave you vulnerable, and carrying your demonstration materials, make-up and stand up several flights of stairs because the lift is not working may not be very practical. Ideally, easy access on the ground floor is preferred, with well-lit parking available. You may need to enlist some help in setting up.

● If you are giving a presentation to a large group, make sure that they will be able to hear you. You may need to see if the venue has appropriate sound appliances that you can use.

Budget and cost

The other important aspect of the group demonstration is who pays and for what. The issues of budget and cost should be sorted out at the planning stage. If your salon is approached by an organisation, the organiser will usually ask how much you charge for a make-up demonstration. Some salons would consider this an ideal opportunity to enhance their client base and a means of advertising, and would therefore agree to the demonstration for free. Other salons would look at the time involved, the wages of the member of staff to be covered and the cost of materials, and then calculate a set fee to cover their overheads. This is up to the individual salon — there is no right answer.

The timing of the demonstration may affect the issue of cost. If the therapist goes in her own time after work to an evening event, then she may expect to be paid for it. Often, bridal fairs are held over a weekend to allow people who work during the week to attend. This may mean the therapist is working on her only day off, Sunday, and she may wish to be paid. If she attends on Saturday, who will cover her clients in the salon? This could become expensive if a relief therapist has to be brought in or clients cancelled to allow the therapist time to attend a demonstration she is giving, with no charge.

However, often it is worth the investment for the publicity generated, and the profile of the salon can be raised enormously. Lots of business comes out of demonstrations, and further treatments and services can be linked into the make-up demonstration — facials, top-to-toe bridal treatments, skin improvement, and so on.

All of this needs discussing with the organisers and your line manager within the salon before you agree to the demonstration.

Products

The number of people attending the demonstration will affect how many products, testers and display materials you will need. This will also depend upon the type of demonstration you do. If it is a complete make-over, using one model who you have brought along to display your skills and entice people into the salon for treatments, then you will only need products for one. If you will be selecting a model from the audience, you will need one set of everything for each skin type.

If you are doing a demonstration en masse, where the audience actively participates, following your lead, applying their make-up as you go along, then many more products are required, unless everyone brings their own. As you are applying make-up to a clean skin, which has a make-up base or moisturiser on it, skincare products are essential, as well as a selection of make-up.

Active participation is a good idea, and encourages the audience to have the confidence to apply their own make-up. Make sure that everyone has a clear view of you and the step-by-step application.

Timing

It is important that you know how long you are expected to speak for and the length of time your full demonstration will take. If you are expected to take the whole meeting time, which may be several hours, you should have some activities which the audience can participate in, like a draw for a free treatment, to keep the interest high.

Have a dress rehearsal with a model before the day of the demonstration, so that you know how long the actual make-up application takes, and then add time for an introduction, and a question and answer session afterwards. This will allow you at the planning stage to tell the organiser that you will need a minimum of, say, an hour and a half, in which to work.

Setting up the room

The key to a successful demonstration is visibility. The audience needs to be able to see what you are doing, or they will lose interest and potential clients will have been lost. For good communication to take place, you also need to be heard, and a microphone may be needed for larger venues. A raised platform or stage is good for larger audiences, but it does not create an intimate, friendly feel, so it will depend upon the number of people and the facilities the venue has.

The best room set-up is a horse-shoe shape, with you and your model at the open end, with an eye-catching display behind you and all materials close at hand. This ensures everyone has a good view, you have command of the room and are able to make lots of eye contact to check that the audience understands your techniques and remains interested.

Try to be organised, so once you start and get into the swing of things, you do not have to return to your car for tissues, or stop the demonstration for any reason. This will break the attention span of your audience, and you will not appear to be professional.

Think through what you will need beforehand, and work logically so that nothing is missed.

Apply make-up and instruct on make-up application

In this outcome you will learn about:

- communicating and behaving in a professional manner
- following health and safety working practices
- positioning yourself and your client correctly throughout the treatment
- using products, tools, equipment and techniques to suit clients' treatment needs, skin types and conditions
- instructing the client on make-up application to promote understanding
- providing the client with written make-up instructions
- evaluating the effectiveness of the make-up instruction with the client
- completing the treatment to the satisfaction of the client
- recording the results of the treatment
- providing suitable aftercare advice.

For advice on safe and effective methods of working practice, refer to Individual services. Refer also to Provide facial skincare, pages 268–70, and Professional skills.

Introducing the demonstration

Once you have fully prepared your working area and the room is set up in a user-friendly manner so that everyone can see and hear you, you may begin.

It is important to consult with your model prior to starting — have a quiet word with her to ensure that your objectives marry up with her needs, and that she has no contra-indications present.

An introduction is always a good ice breaker, rather than just starting and hoping everyone will pay attention. It is a good idea to begin with something along the lines of 'Good afternoon, everyone — my name is Janine from Tranquillity salon, and I'd like to welcome you to Fern Hall for this demonstration.' Then tell the audience exactly what is going to happen and at what point they can ask questions. For example, 'I am going to give a make-up/skincare demonstration for about half an hour, talking you through the various stages, with some professional tips, and then there will be a question and answer session. After the tea break, we can talk about products and treatments.'

Using instructional techniques

For tips on general communication skills, refer to The workplace environment, pages 100–103. Below are some specific tools for a short presentation. Remember, these tips would also apply in a one-on-one session with a client:

- Pace your speech pattern — try to speak slowly and clearly, rather than very quickly, which is what often happens when you are nervous. Pace is literally the speed of the words. A calm, slow, measured speech reflects reassurance and confidence — the speaker is concentrating on getting across the message. Although interest and enthusiasm are important, these can sometimes lead to a more rapid delivery. Panic, anxiety and lack of confidence can produce fast, muddled speech.

- Do not be afraid of short pauses or silence while you are either allowing the information to sink in, or you are concentrating on applying the make-up. Break up the silence if you think it has gone on too long by commentary such as 'Always apply foundation after the skin has been moisturised. Allow the moisturiser to be absorbed for a few seconds before continuing with the foundation ...'

- Pauses can be either a comfortable silence, allowing reflection upon what has been said, or can be very awkward, even menacing. Judging a pause and knowing when to break it, takes a little patience and skill. Hesitation in speech patterns may indicate uncertainty or stress, or just tiredness, where the brain function is slowing down.

- Varying the tone of your voice enlivens speech and helps retain the listeners' attention. Flat, boring tones will not engage the audience and will not help them understand what is being said to them.

- Pitch is most noticeable when it is either high or low, and often reflects the emotional state of the person. Someone who is depressed often talks in a low, falling pitch, quite slowly, whereas a raised pitch conveys excitement, enthusiasm or anxiety. Voice coaches recommend to people in the public eye, who have to make a lot of speeches, to lower the pitch slightly and slow down their normal rate and rhythm of speech.

- The use of graphics, a PowerPoint® display (if you have the technology and the facilities are available) or pictures of make-up products and skincare products along with demonstration samples add interest. Visual aids always attract attention so always include these to enhance your demonstration/presentation.

- Make plenty of eye contact and try not to focus on one person as this may make them uncomfortable. Include everyone in your field of vision. Whether undertaking a group presentation or working with a client on a one-to-one basis, ensure that you give them your full attention. Focus on them when they are talking and be encouraging when they try out new techniques and products.

Apply make-up and instruct on make-up application

◉ Respond kindly when asked questions. Listen carefully to the query, rather than interrupting the person, and nod to show you have understood. If you answer one person well, it encourages others to ask questions, too.

As well as talking through your demonstration, remember not to stand in front of the model as you are working — the audience will not be able to see. You need to perfect the art of working at the side so that your actions are plain to see, and you can stop at each stage to show the audience or client the type of effect. For example, 'After foundation and powder application, the skin tone is even and blemishes are well covered, but the colour comes with the application of blusher, lipstick and eye products, so don't expect too much colour in the face at this time.' Then show the audience your 'blank canvas', with just foundation and powder on.

These are just a few pointers to help you prepare and carry out a presentation and these techniques can be used when working with smaller groups and one to one. You may need to adapt your methods of communication to meet the needs of the client and the size of your audience to make sure that they fully understand. To aid your explanation you should also explain the purpose of the tools and products — a thorough explanation could boost your retail sales.

Positioning your client

As a therapist, it is important to consider your posture as well as the client's when carrying out a service. When conducting a make-up application or demonstration you must be able to reach the client correctly. Positioning is important to prevent injury.

When working one-on-one with a client, allow them to look in a mirror as you work with the products so they can see exactly what you are doing, and if you are instructing, how the effect can be achieved.

Applying make-up products

Refer to Provide facial skincare for the correct skincare products to suit the skin type of the client. You will need to take into account the client's age, texture and skin tone. A suitable product will provide the correct canvas to ensure that the make-up lasts throughout the day.

To achieve a successful make-up application whatever the occasion, you need to understand how and when to apply make-up products. The following pages introduce you to the main kinds of make-up products before giving step-by-step guides to make-up application for various occasions and times of day.

My story

Salon life

My name is Yvette and I trained as a beauty therapist six years ago. I knew from the start that make-up would be my passion and since qualifying I have developed my own business promoting skincare and make-up to a variety of people. I find the work very rewarding and diverse especially when presenting to groups. I also undertake wedding, prom and special event make-up which is great fun. When I first started I decided to keep a notebook of my ideas and thoughts and I still use it to this day. It helps me with inspiration for new ideas – I cut out and keep clippings of pictures that have inspired me and pictures of work that I have done. It is also useful for jotting down ideas prior to using them on clients or you could collect together the ideas as a book for your clients.

Benefits to client and therapist

Benefits of make-up application for the client:

- Effect of treatment is immediately visible

- Sessions can be tailored to meet individual requirements offering a more personalised service

- Hands-on opportunities for client within a make-up and skincare lesson to ensure correct procedure is used at home

- Clients can try different products and ask questions

Benefits of make-up application for the therapist:

- Can be offered individually or to larger groups

- Group work allows the therapist to capture more potential client data, therefore increasing revenue

- Allows therapist to link sell products and other treatments

Ask the experts

Q *I sometimes struggle trying to find the correct shade of foundation. Do you have any tips that would help me?*

A Remember, if you can't find the correct shade of foundation then you can blend your own shades by mixing two or more colours together on a palette to obtain the right match. Use the colour wheel to help you remember which colours neutralise one another in order to get the right result.

Don't test foundation colour on the hand, as hands tend to be a completely different colour to the face. Test foundations on the jaw line for an accurate colour match. There is also nothing to stop you using different colour foundations for shading and highlighting purposes and to correct certain features.

Top tips

- For a flawless make-up application, a good base is essential and preparation is the key. A gentle daily exfoliant should be used after the cleanse to ensure the skin is smooth. This will prevent the foundation looking patchy.

- A great way to get the client to try a recommended product is to provide them with a small sample. This will allow them to try the product and see the results they get. Always write it on the client record so that you can follow up at the next visit.

- A small packet of shine paper is an excellent recommendation for a client who has an oily T-zone. Just press the paper over the oily area to remove excess grease and then finish with a pressed powder.

Apply make-up and instruct on make-up application

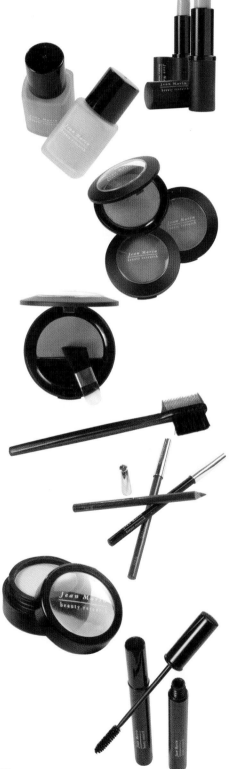

Key terms

Concealer – used to hide imperfections and to lighten and brighten areas. Available in many shades.

Sequence of make-up application

Concealer

This should be one or two shades lighter than the natural skin tone. Apply to the relevant area using a small brush or cotton bud. Press into the skin with a dry sponge. This applies both to the coverage of blemishes and to colour-corrective **concealer**. When using colour-corrective concealer (see page 376 for details) only apply to the areas that require it.

Foundation

The ideal shade will match the natural skin tone exactly – test the shade on the jawline. Work around the face using a damp sponge and fingertips, remembering to cover the eyelids and lips.

When you have finished, remove excess foundation from the hairline and eyebrows with some damp cotton wool.

Face powder

Tip a small amount of loose powder into a bowl. If using block powder, scrape a small amount off into a bowl and apply with dry cotton wool. Work downwards, covering the eyes and all of the face, and then blend with a powder brush.

Blusher and bronzing products

Remove a small amount of blusher or bronzer from the container and place on a make-up palette. Imagine a line from the centre of the eye to the cheekbones – blusher stops here. To apply, start at the hairline and follow the line to the cheekbones. Work down the face in the same direction as the facial hair. If corrective work needs to be carried out, apply according to the face shape. (See pages 381–83 for further information on contouring.)

Bronzers can be used to give the skin a sun-kissed look and can be applied to areas where the sun 'kisses' the face, such as the nose, chin and forehead.

Eyebrow pencil

Apply pencil if required. Brush brows to shape.

Eyeliner or kohl pencil

This can be applied to give definition to the eyes. A pencil creates a softer look, and can be used on the top and bottom lids. A liquid liner gives a more defined look, but is not always suitable for the more mature client (see page 386).

Eyeshadow

Place a folded tissue under the eyes – this will help to avoid shadow spillage on to the face. Apply individual eyeshadow colours. Blend on completion.

Mascara

Coat both sides of the lashes from base to tip using a disposable brush. Remove any specks with a cotton wool bud.

Lipliner

Apply to the outline of the lips. Ensure that colour is close to that of the lipstick, to avoid a harsh line.

Lipstick

Use a disposable lip brush. After the first coat, blot lightly and dust lips with face powder. Apply second coat.

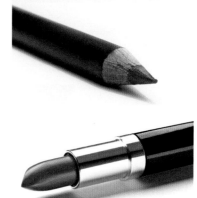

Moisturisers

These products come in many forms and your choice will depend on the skin type of the client. The purpose of a moisturiser when worn under make-up is to:

- even out the skin texture, and provide a smooth base for the foundation
- prolong the make-up by fixing it to the skin
- act as a barrier between the skin and the make-up by preventing pigmented products entering the pores, aiding cleansing.

Think about it

To minimise the risk of skin damage, you can use a moisturising product containing UVA and UVB sunscreens which protect against sunlight. These can be tinted to provide an alternative to foundation.

Concealing cosmetics

Concealer

Few people have a complexion without some imperfections or areas they wish to change – this can be done by using a concealer. Concealer should be applied on small areas where necessary before the application of foundation. Concealers come in various forms. They can be applied in a number of ways with a brush or sponge. You should only apply to the area where required. A stippling (or dotting) action may be best for coverage, especially to scars or blemished areas.

Cream concealer (camouflage)

Usually containing talc and kaolin, these creams have a thick consistency which completely covers all blemishes – including pigmentation marks, red birthmarks and dark shadows under the eyes. These creams come in a variety of colours that can be blended to match the skin.

Stick cover

These come in various shades to match the skin tone and are used to mask minor blemishes and imperfections (spots, dark circles under the eyes). They can be either oil-based or water-based.

Medicated sticks

These are available for applying to minor spots and blemishes, containing antiseptic and drying agents. Never apply directly onto the skin as contamination or cross-infection may occur.

Liquids

Liquid concealers are better for more mature skins where there are creases or wrinkles, as cream or stick concealers can clog in these areas, emphasising them. When covering crow's feet it may be best to use an anti-wrinkle product.

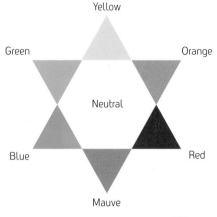

Yellow

Green

Orange

Neutral

Blue

Red

Mauve

Key terms

Colour star – also known as colour wheel; a chart showing the relationship of colours to each other.

Think about it

When using colour corrector cream, only apply to the area of the face where it is required.

Apply foundation over it, using a tapping action to prevent the corrector cream spreading and to ensure you achieve a smooth finish.

Correcting colour

Pigmentation creams can be used to help correct natural skin tone.

- Green is used to counteract high colour (redness).
- Lilac/pink brightens a sallow complexion.
- Peach is used to conceal blue veins and pigmentation.

The colour star

The **colour star** shows how opposite colours neutralise – for a basic corrective colour. So, for sallow or yellow complexions, rather than applying corrective cream all over the face a tinted moisturiser containing lavender, lilac or mauve could be used.

Primary colours	Secondary colours
Red	Green
Yellow	Orange
Blue	Mauve

The range of colours for both Asian and African skins is vast. However, the skin may contain primary colours so a product should be selected with the same primary colour. The range includes:

- pale olive
- yellow
- greeny olive
- warm russet
- warm brown/red
- brown
- grey brown
- blue black.

A tinted product could be used if required and may be a more suitable alternative than a heavier foundation. Imperfections on darker skin types are often less obvious than on white skin. Therefore the make-up that is applied should be mainly to enhance facial features rather than to conceal imperfections.

If loss of pigmentation is present (seen as lighter patches – vitiligo), a camouflage product may be required to disguise the pigmentation loss and to provide an even skin tone and base for the application of the other products.

Choosing a suitable foundation

A good foundation is probably the most important product when carrying out a make-up. The depth, tone and colour can affect all the products used. Foundations also provide a barrier to protect the skin and many now incorporate a sunscreen. A foundation is therefore used to:

- protect the skin
- conceal minor blemishes and imperfections
- provide a smooth finish
- enhance the natural skin colour.

Choosing a foundation for the client's skin colour and tone

The foundation should match the facial skin, but this is not always the case when the hair has been dyed and the colour and tone have been altered.

The therapist should be aware of various tones that occur naturally in the skin. The tone of the skin is created by pigmentation in the epidermis. Skin is therefore described as:

- light
- medium (containing neutral, pink, red or blue tones)
- dark.

You can match a foundation colour to any skin shade:

- neutral tones (match or add warmth: honey, gold, tan)
- pink/red tones (beige, olive)
- yellow/blue (rose, gold, bronze)
- dark tones (dark bronze, sun bronze, deep peach)
- medium tones (cool beige, soft beige, tan).

It is important to get a good colour match when selecting your foundation – you do not want your client to look fake with an orange face or have a ghostly appearance. It is worth remembering that there are many different variations in skin tone, so choose carefully. This may take you a little time or may require you to mix two or more colours together to achieve the desired shade and tone.

To test a foundation on your client for the first time, apply to the angle of the jawline. If the colour becomes darker or has an orange tone, you will need to choose a paler or cooler shade of foundation for your client.

Types of foundation

Foundations are available in many forms:

- cream
- liquid
- cake and pan cake
- gel
- medicated
- mousse
- mineral.

Most are oil-based or water-based with the addition of pigments for colouring and other ingredients to enhance and change their texture and aid the effectiveness of the product.

Cream foundations

This type of foundation blends easily on the skin because of the oil base, and contains wax, powder and a humectant (a product added to keep it moist), such as glycerol. This type of product gives medium coverage and is suitable for normal, dry, combination and mature skins. For a good finish this foundation should always be set with loose powder.

Liquid foundations

These foundations provide colour without being too heavy. They contain a higher proportion of water and give a light/medium coverage. In some products the oil is replaced with alcohol, which evaporates leaving only the powder and pigment. They are suitable for different skin types:

- oil-based – normal, dry and mature skin types
- water-based – combination greasy
- alcohol – greasy.

The base of the foundation should be marked on the container.

Cake foundations

These foundations are usually applied with a damp sponge, thinly or thickly as required by adjusting the amount of water used on the sponge. Cake foundations usually contain compressed creams with extra powder for good coverage. Cake foundations give medium/heavy coverage suitable for:

- normal skin
- combination skin
- blotchy, blemished, discoloured or scarred areas
- dry or mature (cream-based)
- greasy (powder-based).

Pan cake foundations

This product is used a lot in the Far East as it is suitable for humid climates. The colour that appears in the compact is the colour that will appear on the skin.

Gel foundations

A gel product will provide a thin, translucent colour that gives a natural look. Gels are produced like a liquid foundation but have an additional ingredient to produce a gel consistency, such as gum tragacanth. Gels produce a natural tanned effect and are very popular in the summer; many now contain sunscreens. They are suitable for:

- tanned skins
- smooth skin with no imperfections, requiring a natural effect.

Medicated foundations

This type of foundation is a liquid containing antiseptic ingredients, making it suitable for greasy, blemished skins. It can be used over mild acne, but care should be taken with hygiene. Remember that severe acne is a contra-indication to a make-up application.

Mousse foundations

This type of foundation is suitable for combination to normal skin. Most are made with mineral oils, although some are made with herbal extracts. If you do apply this foundation to oily skin, be aware that it can be streaky if not carefully applied.

Mineral foundations

These products are derived from natural sources and give long-lasting colour. They are excellent for oily skin types as they help prevent comedomes and blemishes.

For your portfolio

Look at one range of cosmetics available locally and see what types of foundation they offer. Are you able to buy suitable products for all skin types and skin colours?

Skin type	Recognition	Suitable foundation
Normal	Small pores, fine texture Soft supple, flexible healthy	Cream/powder
Dry/dehydrated	Matt, uneven texture Lacks suppleness Lines and wrinkles Dilated capillaries common on nose and cheeks	Cream
Oily	Shiny, thick blackheads, papules, pustules Open pores	Medicated liquid foundation Mineral foundation Non-oily block/cake
Combination	Any combination of skin types – most common: oily T-zone and dry cheeks	All-in-one fluid and powder combination Cream/powder combination
Sensitive/dry	Combination of dry cheeks and sensitivity Tight red appearance, broken capillaries	Hypoallergenic products
Sensitive/allergy prone	Reacts to products Skin flushes easily, which may appear as patches Dilated capillaries	Hypoallergenic products
Mature	Fine lines, crepey skin Poor muscle tone Broken capillaries Dry, thin and papery Pigmentation marks	Cream-based products

Summary of the most suitable foundations for the different skin types

Airbrush application

Many cosmetic houses and salons are now using airbrush applicators to apply foundation. The foundation is selected in the normal way to suit the client's skin colour and tones, and is then sprayed over the face. This form of application provides a flawless finish with no sponge or finger marks, and is excellent for bridal or photographic make-up.

Cautions when applying foundation

Apply with a clean sponge or flat brush — these help when applying to awkward areas such as nose or eyes. Thin coverage can be achieved by using a slightly damp, natural sponge. This type of sponge can, however, leave streaks because it is porous, so careful blending needs to take place. When a heavier coverage is required a latex sponge provides a smooth finish; a latex sponge is also less expensive. However, you should always check that your client does not have a latex allergy before using a latex sponge.

Blend from the centre of the face to the hairline; this prevents clogging foundation in the hairline.

You need to work quickly or the foundation will streak. Cover eyes and lips as this will provide a good base for eyeshadow and lipstick. When applying foundation to a more mature client, who may have crepey skin around the neck and eyes, add a little moisturiser — this thins out the foundation and helps to prevent creases.

Check the application around the nose, hairline and chin to ensure smooth application and no visible lines.

Apply make-up and instruct on make-up application

Face powder

For a really professional appearance, most cream-based make-up products should be set with powder. Loose powder should be used for all professional make-up applications and the correct shade of pressed powder supplied for retail purchase by the client. A powder is applied to:

- 'fix' the foundation
- absorb grease
- give a smooth, matt finish
- protect the skin
- reduce shine
- help conceal minor blemishes.

Loose powder

Loose powders come in two different textures: heavy and fine.

Heavy powders are often pigmented to complement the foundation and give a good cover; they contain a high proportion of kaolin and chalk.

Fine powders contain talc and a majority are translucent, which allows the colour of the skin or foundation to show through.

Some powders contain metallic particles for a pearlised effect, suitable for evening wear. If you decide to use a pearlised powder, remember that it will accentuate lines and blemishes, so it will not be suitable for mature or blemished skins.

Loose powder should always be applied in a salon in preference to pressed powder because of hygiene. If, however, you apply pressed powder it should be decanted on to a palette before being applied, to prevent contamination.

Pressed powder

This is a product in a block that fits into a compact. The binding agent is usually gum or wax, which joins the particles together. Pressed powder is used for touching up the make-up during the day; however, this powder is not fine enough to produce an even finish on freshly applied foundation.

Always avoid areas with excessive hair growth as powder will collect there and draw attention to the area. Also avoid applying to dry flaking areas, because the area will dry out further and it will be accentuated.

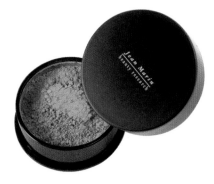

Loose powder should be used for all professional make-up applications

Cautions when applying powder

- Dispense a small amount on to a palette.
- Firmly screw up a cotton wool pad and press into the powder, shake off excess in rolling movements, gently press into the foundation, covering all areas including eyes and lips.
- Remove any excess with a brush — first against the hair growth and then down the face to smooth the facial hairs and produce an even finish.
- Use a clean brush to remove any powder that has settled on the lashes or eyebrows.

Contouring cosmetics

These are a range of products which are similar to foundations and powders, with the addition of coloured pigments. They come in powder, liquid, cream and gel. Contour cosmetics consist of:

- blushers
- **highlighters**
- shaders.

Blushers

Blushers add warmth to the make-up and give the skin a healthy glow to help define the facial features. They come in a wide range of colours. Pale colours can be used to soften and highlight areas. Bright colours can accentuate, and deep tawny colours and bronzes can shade areas. Blushers also come in a variety of forms, including mineral-based products, gels, creams and powders.

Gels

- Best on clear skins.
- Give cheeks a natural-looking, healthy glow.
- Good for the summer.
- Can be applied directly over moisturiser.

Creams

- Give skins a moist, dewy finish.
- Work best when applied over moisturisers and foundation.
- Good for normal or dry skin types.

Powders

- Matt or frosted finishes available.
- Applied for best results over powder with a large brush.
- Good on oily skins, but suitable for all skin types.

When choosing a blusher it should complement the foundation or natural skin tone. When applying a blusher it is best to build up the colour gradually to achieve the desired effect. It is the depth and tone of colour that needs to be selected carefully.

The use of blusher can help to alter the shape of the face. If you wish to reduce the width of the face, but give an illusion of length, keep the blusher to the side of the face, blending from just underneath the cheekbones to the temples. To create extra fullness, apply the blusher to the cheeks or blend from the angle of the cheekbones to the ears. If you do not wish to change the shape of the face, the blusher is usually placed on or near the cheekbones.

Key terms

Highlighter – used to lighten, brighten and accentuate an area.

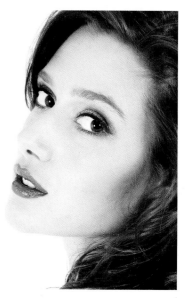

Blushers add warmth and give a healthy glow; highlighters emphasise features

Think about it

To check if the colour of the product is strong enough to show up effectively, take a small amount of the colour on to your finger – if the colour on your finger has the same depth as the compact, the colour is suitable.

Apply make-up and instruct on make-up application

Highlighters

Highlighters are used to emphasise features and to create the illusion of extra length and width. The pale colours of highlighters reflect light, brighten and accentuate an area. Use white, ivory and cream on pale skins for a subtle effect. When using a highlighter on a dark foundation it should belong to the same tone family:

- pale pink over rose shades
- pale peach over warm foundations.

Pearlised products are effective as highlighters, but avoid these on mature skins or hairy areas as they will draw attention to the areas.

Shaders

Shading is used to create artificial shadows or to reduce the size of areas. The colours suitable for shading contain brown pigments, which range from medium beige to dark brown. Beige is dark enough to shade when used over a pale base.

It is important to remember that the darker the foundation, the deeper the shade needs to be. Warm brown colours should be avoided as a shader as they tend to look orange when applied over foundation and then act as a blusher.

Cautions when applying contouring products

- Use soft, round-ended brushes that make blending easier.
- Tap any excess powder blusher on to a tissue or palette before applying, for a more subtle application. It is easier to build up colour in this way.
- When using a gel or cream apply with a damp sponge.
- Blusher application should start on the cheekbones level with the midpoint of the eye.
- Regularly check you are achieving a balanced effect.
- Keep blusher and highlighter away from the corners and the lines of the eye as they can accentuate fine lines.
- Ensure contouring is subtle for a natural day wear appearance.
- Use corrective techniques to try to achieve a balance in the facial features. This helps emphasise the best areas and takes attention away from problem areas.

Corrective make-up

Contouring products can be used effectively to emphasise and diminish areas to achieve the desired face shape. The oval face shape with almond-shaped eyes is often admired, although trends change with fashion and very few people truly fall into that category. When carrying out your consultation, ensure that both you and your client have realistic expectations about what you can achieve.

Key terms

Shader – used to reduce the size of an area and to change the shape of the face.

Think about it

Light colours define areas.

Dark colours make areas **recede**.

Key terms

Recede – disappear.

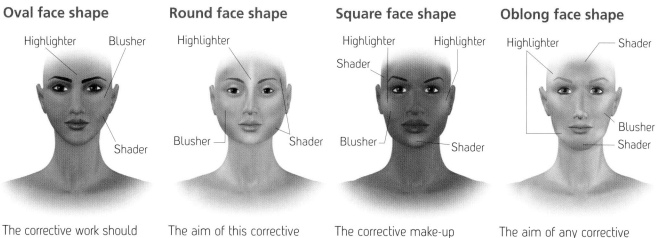

Oval face shape

The corrective work should create an illusion of length – to reduce the width from the sides of the face to the temples. To create length – subtle highlighter blended in a narrow strip down the centre of the face, apply blusher on the cheekbones up to the temples, shader over angles of the jaw and temple areas.

Round face shape

The aim of this corrective work is to soften the jawline and reduce the width of the forehead and lower half of the face. Shader should be blended over the angles of the lower jaw and forehead. Blusher should be applied upwards from under the cheeks towards the temples or along the fullness of the cheeks.

Square face shape

The corrective make-up should reduce the length of the face, and create width and fullness. This can be achieved by applying shader to the tip of the chin and the narrowest part of the forehead. Apply highlighter to the temples and lower jaw and blusher to the cheeks to add fullness.

Oblong face shape

The aim of any corrective make-up is to enhance bone structure and balance contours by blending blusher along the cheekbones towards the temples, applying shader below and highlighter above.

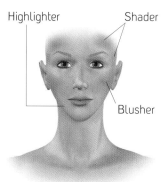

Heart face shape

The corrective work should aim to minimise the width of the forehead and widen the lower half of the face. This can be achieved by applying shader to the sides of the forehead and temples. Highlight the angles of the lower jaw. Apply blusher to the fullness of the cheeks.

Diamond face shape

The corrective work of this face shape is to reduce the length by applying shader to the tip of the chin and the narrowest part of the forehead. To give the illusion of width, apply highlighter to the sides of the temples and lower jaw. Apply blusher to the cheeks to create fullness in the centre of the face.

Pear face shape

The aim of this corrective make-up is to give width to the forehead by applying highlighter to the sides of the forehead and to reduce the width of the lower face through the application of shader on the side of the chin and angles of the lower jaw. Emphasise the cheekbones for a full appearance.

Triangular face shape

This corrective make-up is similar to that used on a heart-shaped face. The relatively wide forehead and narrow jawline need to be balanced to prevent the face from looking top heavy. Use shader to minimise the forehead width and create the illusion of width along the jawline by applying highlighter. Use blusher on the cheeks to balance the centre of the face and even up the whole shape.

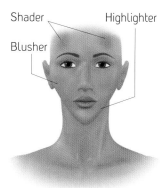

Apply make-up and instruct on make-up application

Eye cosmetics

The eyes are the focal point of the face. People often focus on the eye make-up as the eyes are used for communicating and expressing our feelings. The trick when applying make-up is to draw attention to the eyes and not to the make-up.

The use of colour can create illusions of depth, size and alter the shape. Always remember that lighter colours enhance, darker colours recede.

Care is always needed when working around the eyes, as the skin is very sensitive and thin and can be easily overstretched. The EC Cosmetics Directive of 1976 limits ingredients which may be contained in eye make-up products and only pigments which are known to be non-toxic and non-irritant are allowed.

Eyeshadow

Eyeshadows are used to emphasise the eyes and to coordinate the colour of the make-up and clothing. They are available as minerals, powder, liquid, gel and cream. Creamy, pressed powders are the most popular. Frosted products are available for highlighting and can be used to achieve a stunning effect when used for evening.

However, frosted and creamy products are not recommended for mature clients as they draw attention to lines and get trapped in crepey areas.

Powder shadows

These are talc-based with oil for a creamy texture, available in loose or pressed form.

Creams

Cream shadow contains wax and oil pigments, and is not so popular with mature clients as these products settle in the creases.

Gels

Gels give a natural appearance because they produce a translucent wash of colour.

Eyeshadow colours

- Dark, muted colours — use for defining and contouring. Effective on clients with dark hair and eyes. Applied with a fine brush, they can be used as a livening effect on people with light colouring.
- Pastel colours — produce soft effects, particularly on people with grey/blonde hair. They emphasise the colour of the eyes when applied in the same tone.
- Pale colours — have highlighting effects when contrasted with dark shadows. When applied near the brow makes the eyes appear bigger.
- Soft, muted shades — use when a more natural effect is required.
- Bright colours — use in young or fashion make-up. Some bright colours can be used as eyeliner to complement the eyeshadow, but be cautious when using bright colours on a mature client as they can give a hard and unattractive appearance.

Think about it

Foundation may also be used to change the shape of an area, minimise or make it less noticeable. To do this, use a foundation two or three shades darker than the natural skin colour and blend into the ordinary foundation with either a sponge or brush.

Applying eyeshadow to a range of eye shapes

Small eyes

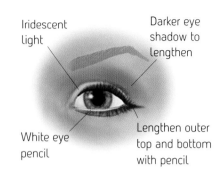

Iridescent light

Darker eye shadow to lengthen

White eye pencil

Lengthen outer top and bottom with pencil

Lengthen small eyes by applying a soft eye pencil to the outer third of the bottom lid extending outward. Use a short stroke to join this line to the upper lash line, then smudge.

- Use light colours and iridescent shadows on the lid for an eye-opening effect.
- Highlight with a frosted shadow under the brow for evening sparkle.
- Curl the lashes or have them permed before applying the mascara to open the eyes even more.
- Try lining the inside of the lower lid with a soft, white pencil – this will also give the appearance of the eye being more open.

Prominent eyes

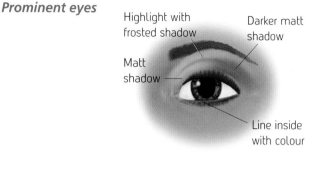

Highlight with frosted shadow

Darker matt shadow

Matt shadow

Line inside with colour

Use matt shadow on the lid and blend it into the crease. Apply a darker shade to the outer half of the lid, right over the first shade, and blend so the graduation looks natural and no harsh lines are visible. Highlight under the brow with a light or frosted shade.

If you wish to achieve a sultry look, which may be suitable for evening wear, line the inner rim of the eye with a soft eye pencil. Grey, navy, plum and black are excellent depending on the eye colour, but there are many more colours to choose from.

Round eyes

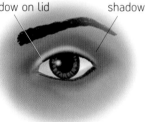

Matt shadow on lid

Darker matt shadow on outer 1/3 of eye

Line with pencil

Line outer 1/3 top and bottom with pencil to elongate

Elongate the eyes by using the deepest shades on the outer edge of the eye lid, and extend this to form a soft point. Lengthen the eyes even more by outlining the outer third of the top and bottom with a soft eye pencil, making sure that the outer point meets beyond the outer corner of the eye. Smudge for a softer effect. Narrow the eyes by lining the inner rim with a soft pencil.

Deep-set eyes

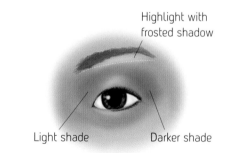

Light or frosted shadow on lid

Darker matt shadow

Use light or frosted shadows on the lid if it is appropriate for the client and occasion. Apply a darker shade above the crease to recess this area. Apply a little shadow or soft eye pencil on the outer half of the bottom lid to balance the depth of the eyes.

Oriental eyes

Highlight with frosted shadow

Light shade

Darker shade

Divide the area beneath the brow in half vertically. Use a lighter shade on the inner half and a darker shade on the outer half and blend well together. The application of a darker shadow creates a socket line. Apply a highlighter under the brow and blend together.

Almond eyes

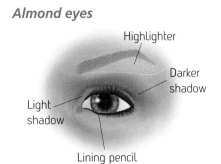

Highlighter

Darker
shadow

Light
shadow

Lining pencil

Close-set eyes

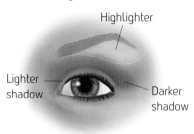

Highlighter

Lighter
shadow

Darker
shadow

Wide-set eyes

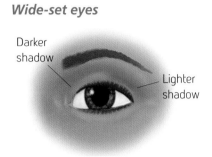

Darker
shadow

Lighter
shadow

Unless the eyes are set too close together or too far apart, you will not need to undertake corrective techniques. Choose colours that complement the iris, and ensure the brows are groomed to make application of shadows easy.

Keep all medium or dark colours on the outer half of the eye. This will draw attention outward and the eyes will seem further apart. Ensure that the brows have been correctly shaped to maximise the space between the eyes.

Extend the shadows to the inner corner of the eye and blend inwards to the bridge of the nose to minimise the space. Also ensure the brows are correctly shaped.

Cautions when applying eyeshadow

- Always use clean brushes and applicators. Do not overload the applicator with shadow as excess powder could fall into the eyes or on to the face – spoiling the other make-up. It is also not cost-effective to overload the applicator.

- Support the skin and protect the surrounding make-up with a tissue. Remember that the skin around the eye is very delicate, so do not be heavy handed and over-stretch the skin.

- Ensure your client keeps her eyes closed when applying the shadow and always keep the client informed of what you are about to do. Check the shadow is balanced on both eyes and evenly blended. If applying shadow beneath the eyes, ask the client to look away from the brush to prevent blinking or the eyes watering.

Eyeliner

This product is used for emphasising the shape of the eyelid and strengthening the colour of the lash line. It is good to use when strip lashes have been applied to give a more natural appearance. Liners are available in a number of colours and types. Like all make-up, eyeliner follows fashion trends. It was very popular in the 1950s and 1960s, and is currently enjoying a revival.

Cake eyeliner

This is the most versatile product but the most difficult to apply. It is applied with a fine brush that is dampened before applying to the eyes.

Liquid eyeliner

This is a gum solution containing pigments, which gives a heavier effect. It will provide a clearly defined line if correctly applied.

Pencils

These are available in a range of colours, usually soft enough to blend with the shadows because of their wax formulation, and should be used to complement the look that is required. Ensure they are sharpened between each eye to get an even application and to prevent cross-infection.

Kohl

This is a soft, waxy, black pencil which is applied to the inner rim of the lower eyelid to enhance the white of the eye. A kohl pencil is not recommended for use on a mature client as the effect can be harsh and can accentuate fine lines.

Cautions when applying eyeliner

- Gently lift the skin from beneath the brow so the line is drawn up to the base of the lashes.
- Ensure the client keeps the eyes shut when liner is applied to the upper lid.
- Always apply liner outwards towards the corner of the eye.
- Check that the thickness and angle of the eyeliner are the same for both eyes.

Mascara

Mascaras are available in a variety of colours – including clear mascara. Mascara is used to accentuate the eyes by darkening and thickening the lashes. Many now contain moisturisers and lash-building ingredients which include filaments of nylon and rayon. These fibres temporarily lengthen the lashes. Clear mascara enhances the natural features of darkened lashes and is especially useful after the lashes have been tinted.

When applying mascara with lash-building filaments be aware that the filaments can sometimes shed. If these enter the eye, they can cause irritation and this can especially aggravate the eyes of contact lens wearers.

Cake mascara

Cake mascara is made up of a mixture of waxes and pigments in a soap base, and is applied with a brush. This type of mascara is gaining popularity again in salons as the brush applicator can easily be cleaned and sterilised.

Liquid mascara

Applied with a brush or wand, this type of mascara is contained in a water or alcohol and water base with extra features: for example, waterproof, thickening, and protein enriched. Read the packaging to find out what the mascara contains. When applying this type of mascara to a client, disposable brushes should be used for each eye to prevent any contamination of the product.

Cautions when applying mascara

- Ensure that the client is relaxed as this makes the application of mascara easier – especially to the upper lashes.
- Apply mascara downwards on upper lashes and then upwards for maximum coverage.
- Place tissue under lower lashes, before applying, to prevent mascara marking the skin.
- Instruct the client to look away from the wand when applying the mascara to the lower lashes.
- Build up the mascara in fine coats to prevent clogging. Allow to dry between applications.

Think about it

Always check to see if your client wears contact lenses, even if they arrive at the salon wearing glasses. Lash tinting may be a preferred option for spectacle and contact lens wearers.

Apply make-up and instruct on make-up application

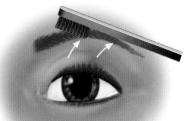

a Separate brow hairs

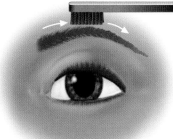

b Smooth them into shape

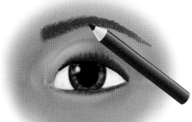

c Fill in the gaps and extend the length of the brow by using fine strokes that follow the natural hair growth

For your portfolio

Research one high street and one professional brand of cosmetics to compare the cost of the products and the variety of colour choice. Consider factors such as skin type and age range.

Eyebrow pencils

These pencils are used to strengthen the colour of the brows and define shape. They should be applied to the brow in light, feathery strokes for a natural look. The use of an eyebrow pencil is good for filling in bare areas if the brows are sparse. Use short strokes in the direction of the hair growth and blend into the natural brow shape with the aid of a brow brush.

Eyebrow pencils are produced in a limited range of colours to complement the natural brow colour. As with other pencils they should be sharpened after each eye to prevent cross-contamination occurring.

Cautions when using eyebrow pencils

- Brush brows into shape.
- Check the colour tone and shade of the pencil – this should look natural and complement the rest of the make-up.
- Ensure the pencils are sharpened after doing each brow, to prevent cross-contamination, and ensure feathery strokes are used rather than one harsh line for a natural look.

Lip cosmetics

There is a variety of cosmetics on the market for lips, in a range of colours and forms. There are lipsticks, glosses and pencils. These are used to define the mouth, by adding colour, and to protect the lips from the environment. Lip cosmetics can, as with other forms of make-up, be used as corrective make-up to enhance shape. All lip products contain the same ingredients of oils, fats and waxes, with the addition of safe pigments for colour.

Lipsticks

These contain a high wax content that makes them hard. Some products also contain sunscreens to protect the delicate skin of the lips from ultraviolet light. Lipstick should be applied with a brush to outline the mouth and spread colour over the lips evenly.

Lip gloss

This product can be used over lipstick or on its own for a natural look. It is usually of a gel consistency and is available in either lipstick form or as a gel.

Lip pencil

This is used for outlining the lips before applying lipstick and contains a high proportion of wax, which means it is less likely to smudge. It is useful to prevent lipstick colour from 'bleeding' into the fine lines around the mouth. It is also helpful for correcting lip shapes.

Lipstick sealer

Usually produced as a liquid, this is a colourless sealer, designed to prevent lipstick fading and to keep it in place. It should be applied with a brush.

Lip primer

This is used mainly for mature clients to prevent 'lipstick bleeding'.

Choosing a suitable lipstick

When selecting a lipstick it should be used to balance the colour scheme and coordinate with the clothing. Strong and vibrant colours draw attention to the mouth, so avoid them if you are trying to take the emphasis away from the mouth or jaw area. Strong colours look best with subtle and muted eye make-up colours.

Deep-colour lipstick or pencil should be used when outlining a corrective lip make-up. Pale, pearlised lipstick or lip gloss give lips a fuller appearance.

To reduce fullness, bronze, purplish pinks and blue-toned reds are useful.

Cautions when applying lip cosmetics

- Apply foundation and powder to the lips before applying lip cosmetics. This gives a good base and makes lip cosmetics last longer.
- Outline the mouth first and then fill in the colour.
- Blot the first application with a tissue as this helps to fix the colour.
- Apply a second coat for a final finish.
- Never apply lip cosmetics to any infected area or if the lips are excessively chapped or cracked.

Corrective lip make-up

Thin lips

The thickness of the lips can be increased by drawing a line slightly outside the natural lip shape.

Full or thick lips

Use dark colours to make the lips recede and create a new lip line inside the natural one by blotting out the natural line with foundation and powder.

Thin or straight upper lip

Create a new bow to the upper lip by pencilling just above the natural line to add fullness.

Thin lower lip

Create a new lower lip line slightly below the natural lip to give balance to the mouth.

Asymmetric lips

These lips are unbalanced so create a lip line where required to achieve balance.

Droopy mouth

Build up the corners of the lower lip, slightly extending upwards at the corners to meet the upper lip line.

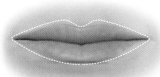

Thin lips

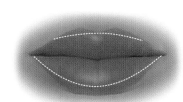

Full or thick lips

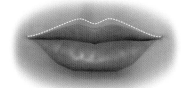

Thin or straight upper lip

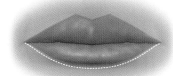

Thin lower lip

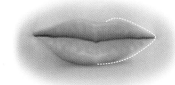

Asymmetric lips

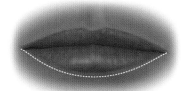

Droopy mouth

Apply make-up and instruct on make-up application

Facial problem areas

Jawline shapes

Broad jaw

A broad jaw can be minimised by the use of a darker shader, starting from the temple area down and over either side of the angle of the mandible (refer to Related anatomy and physiology, page 230), bringing the centre of the face into sharper focus and so creating a more balanced width.

Narrow jaw

Narrow jaws are highlighted to create an illusion of width.

Square jaws

These can be shaded with a darker foundation applied to the width, to appear more rounded.

Chin and neck shapes

Prominent chin

A dark foundation or shader should be used on the chin, and sometimes a touch of blusher can be just as effective.

Receding chin

A lighter foundation or a highlighter will make a receding chin appear more prominent.

Double chin

A double chin or loose skin should be shadowed, with a dark foundation or shader.

Thin neck

This should be highlighted to create the illusion of roundness and prominence.

Thick neck

This requires shading to make it appear smaller.

Nose shapes

Large or protruding nose

This is made smaller by applying a dark foundation or shader, blending it smoothly into a lighter foundation on the sides of the cheeks. Blusher should be kept away from the nose.

Short nose

This is made narrower by shading the sides of the nostrils.

Long, thin nose

This can be broadened by applying a highlighter foundation down its centre to above the tip, which is to be shaded.

Colour and skin pigmentation

Freckles and moles

These can be faded with the use of a good foundation or cream which is slightly thicker. It must be toned into the rest of the foundation, otherwise it will stand out.

Age lines

Creases round the mouth and crow's feet around the eyes can be softened by making the eyes appear fuller. This is achieved by the use of a lighter coloured foundation applied over the area. The crevices appear to be lifted out and less noticeable, but do not apply too heavily or you will make the areas more noticeable.

Clients with contact lenses or glasses

The effects that glasses have on the appearance of the face and make-up will vary according to the colour of frame, frame size and lenses.

Frames

- Heavy frames – can take strong lip colour and eye make-up to help balance the facial features.
- Lightweight frames – ensure the colours are soft, using liner or mascara. Eyebrow pencil to define the brows and lashes will look more subtle with this type of frame. Bold colours will make light frames recede.
- Coloured frames – make-up should complement them. Muted shades should be used if the frames are very bright.

Lenses

- Short-sighted – these make the eyes appear smaller.
- Long-sighted – these lenses make the eyes look larger.
- Tinted lenses – these lenses may change the colours of the make-up.

Contact lenses

Some clients are quite happy to have their lenses in place when the make-up takes place, but you should always take the following precautions to prevent irritating the eyes.

- Work gently.
- Avoid heavy creams that could smear the lenses.
- Avoid creating dust that could land on the contact lenses and irritate the eye, and always ensure the client keeps the eyes closed when applying powder shadow.
- Use eye make-up shadows with a creamy pressed texture.
- Use mascara without alcohol and added fibre filaments.

Make-up for day, evening and special occasions

Bridal make-up

Many brides have their make-up applied professionally so that they can be confident of looking their best. Therefore, to ensure you give the best advice, a preliminary consultation is essential. During the consultation you need to find out the following details.

- The date and time of the wedding. The final appointment must be scheduled within the overall preparations, as ideally make-up should be applied before the hair is dressed and the dress put on.
- Details of the dress – design, colour and material. Colours will look stronger if the dress is white. Lightweight fabrics need softer make-up than heavier fabrics.
- Hair style and headdress – this can affect the facial features.

Remember that lipstick and nail colours need to tone with the colour scheme of the dress and flowers. Pearlised products will emphasise flaws and defects and eye make-up will lose definition in photographs.

When carrying out bridal make-up, avoid stimulating the skin for 48 hours before the wedding. Shape eyebrows and apply individual lashes one or two days prior to the

> **Think about it**
>
> The bride wants to look beautiful and radiant, but she also wants to be recognised – it is not the time for a dramatic change.

wedding. Apply fake tan one or two days prior to the wedding if the dress is low cut and reveals paler areas of the body.

It is important to promote waxing, manicure and pedicure treatments before the wedding for a truly well-groomed appearance and for honeymoon preparation. Many salons include wedding packages in their price lists that include these treatments.

Photographic make-up

Many large photographic studios now employ a make-up artist to help clients get the best from their photographs. This service is included in the cost of the photographic package. You need to consider the following points.

- Lighting can be hot and make-up may melt, so do not apply a heavy make-up, and cool the skin if possible during application.
- Avoid greasy products and creamy, textured products as these emphasise shine, creases and open pores.
- Reapply translucent powder to achieve a matt finish.
- Pearlised products can cause glare and emphasise flaws.
- Ensure that all products are well blended. This is particularly important around the jaw and hair lines.
- Highlight under the eyes, chin and sides of the nostrils before applying foundation, to prevent discoloration and shadow created by skin folds.
- Use highlight and shadow techniques to create facial contours and define bone structure. Foundation should be as light as possible to enhance the contour cosmetics.

Creating mood

Colour can create the correct mood when taking photographs.

- Strong, rich colours create vibrant, active moods.
- Pale colours give a calming feel.
- Oranges and yellows give a feeling of warmth.
- Blues and greens have a cooling effect.

Contrasting colours

Red will bring the subject towards you or expand an area when taking a photograph. Blue allows the area to blend into the surroundings. Therefore, when selecting shades of make-up, it is important to look at the surroundings as well as the clothing or the effect you are trying to create may be lost. Using strongly contrasting primary colours could add emphasis to certain areas.

Lighting

If the photograph is to be taken outside, you need to be aware that the light will constantly change. It is for this reason that professional photographers use lighting when working outside to get controlled and better results. If, however, you have to work with natural light, remember:

- early mornings — when the sun is low, photographs will have more depth
- midday — natural light is flatter so little emphasis and depth are achieved
- strong sunlight — this will create hard outlines
- cloud — photographs taken when the light is diffused by light cloud gives a less harsh appearance of soft shadows and subtle highlighting.

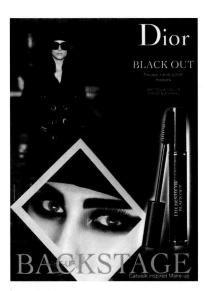

Photographic make-up can use dramatic effects

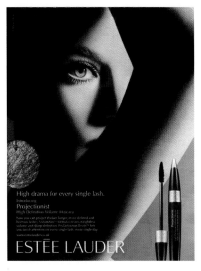

Lighting effects can have strong impact on the finished look

Step-by-step daytime make-up, converted to an evening look

Service time for day make-up = 30 minutes, evening make-up = 45 minutes

1 Prepare the client, in an upright position, fully covered and the skin lightly moisturised. Headband and tissues protect the hair. It is best to apply daytime make-up in natural daylight.

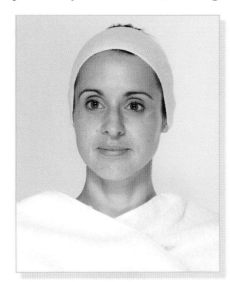

2 Apply concealer/colour corrector, if needed, followed by suitable foundation for the skin type.

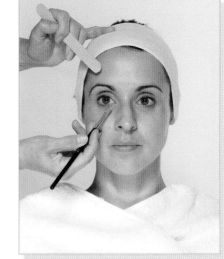

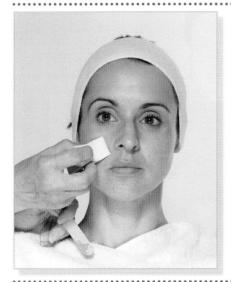

3 Apply foundation with a damp sponge or clean fingertips. Work from the centre of the face outwards using light movements.

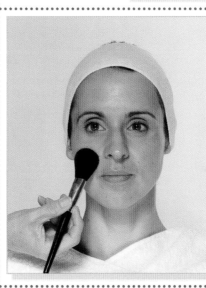

4 Using dry cotton wool, lightly pat on loose powder to set the foundation. Remember eyelids and lips. Using a large round brush, remove any excess powder, using downward strokes.

5 Shader, blusher and highlighter can now be applied to contour the face, as discussed in the treatment plan. Always decant products.

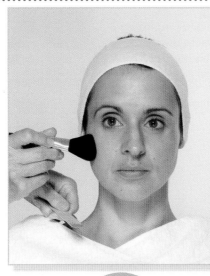

6 Apply eyeshadows, remembering to use disposable applicators and to decant the colours on to a palette, to avoid contaminating the remaining eyeshadow.

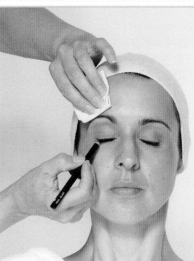

Apply make-up and instruct on make-up application

7 Apply eyeliner or pencil, without dragging on the eye, and remember to sharpen the pencil between clients for hygiene reasons.

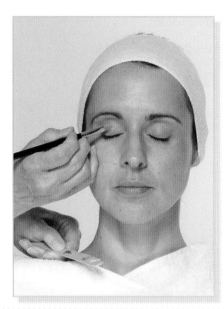

8 When applying mascara, remember to support the eye with a tissue, ask the client to look down, and stroke upwards, with the eyelash growth. A disposable wand is always used.

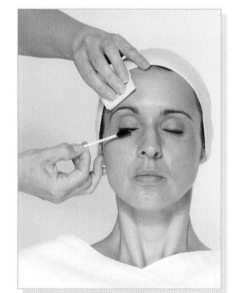

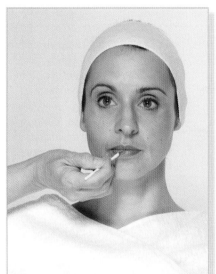

9 Lip liner and lipstick are next. Remember to sharpen the lip pencil, and to decant the lipstick onto a palette, applying it with a clean brush.

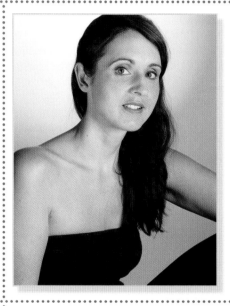

10 Show the client the finished result with all covering removed. Her own hair and clothes will give a natural look. Hold the mirror upwards for a flattering result. Ensure that the make-up effects combine and complement the client's look to create the image that she desires, and check that she is pleased with the result.

11 To convert the make-up for an evening look select complementary colours. These may contain a shimmer.

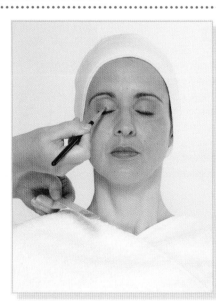

12 Additional eyeliner and mascara can be used to enhance the eyes and give lashes a more defined appearance.

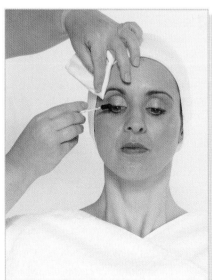

13 Apply blusher or bronzer to the cheekbones. These products may contain luminescent particles to enhance the cheeks.

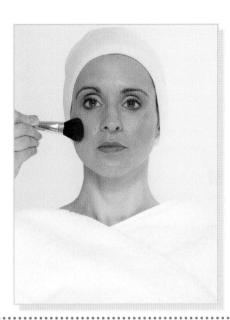

14 Lip products are usually darker for evening wear. A gloss may be applied over the lipstick for added sheen.

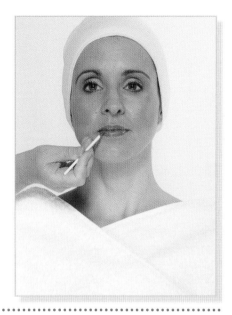

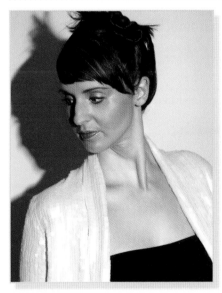

15 Evening make-up is more dramatic so false lashes could be applied to add impact. These should be applied prior to additional eye make-up.

Think about it

Application time should be approximately 45 minutes for a make-over. A lesson in skincare or make-up application should take 75 minutes. If you are demonstrating to a larger group, your time may be adjusted according to the service that you are presenting.

Think about it

To carry out an effective make-up service, you need to be able to identify and treat the client's individual skin type. Therefore, it is essential to have prior knowledge to ensure the best results.

Apply make-up and instruct on make-up application

Step-by-step special occasion make-up

Service time = 45 minutes

Special occasion make-up can be a little more individual than day make-up, but not quite as heavy as evening make-up. The key to making the whole look glamorous but not overdone is to coordinate the make-up colours with the outfit and add a touch of sparkle, with a lip gloss or shiny eyeshadow. Ask the client what she will be wearing; see the outfit, if possible, and definitely have a trial run before the event.

1 Study the client's natural skin and hair colouring, to avoid choosing make-up colours that clash. Research the type of special occasion and what the client will be wearing.

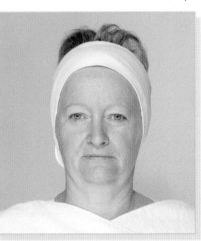

2 Decant and apply concealer/ colour corrector, if required. Take into account that your client may or may not be used to wearing much make-up. Keep application and colour light, particularly when applying make-up to mature skin.

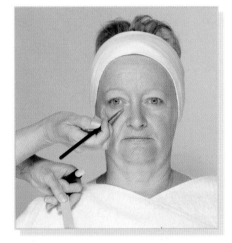

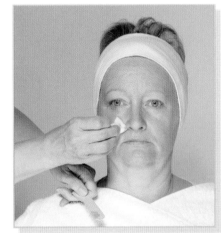

3 Apply foundation with a sponge or clean fingertips, blending from the centre of the face, outwards. Ensure foundation chosen is suitable for skin type — foundation for mature skin should be light in texture and colour.

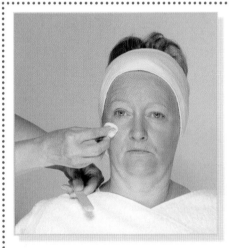

4 With a dry piece of cotton wool, pat loose powder all over the face, remembering eyelids and lips. Translucent powder is suitable for mature skin.

5 A light stroke with a large blusher brush will remove any excess powder. Stroke the brush all over the face, in a downward motion, to avoid a powdery look to the face.

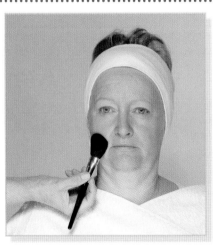

6 Eyeshadow is decanted and applied lightly over the lids. If the client wears glasses, or has quite lined eyelids, make the colour and application fairly light.

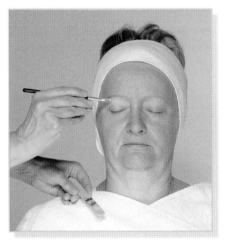

7 Apply a light application of mascara using a disposable wand. Soft shades of navy, grey or brown mascara are less harsh than black on mature skin.

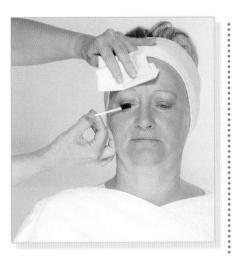

8 Decant the blusher on to the wooden spatula and apply lightly to the cheeks. Soft corals, peaches or pinks usually suit mature skin.

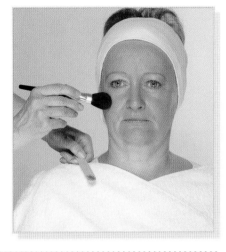

9 Sharpen the pencil and apply a light lip liner, which prevents the lipstick bleeding into the lines around the mouth.

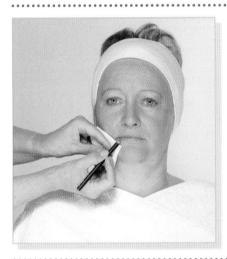

10 Choose a complementary lipstick and decant, then apply.

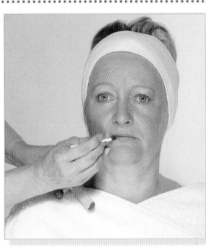

11 You gain the whole effect for special occasion make-up if you have a complete dress rehearsal – including the hat!

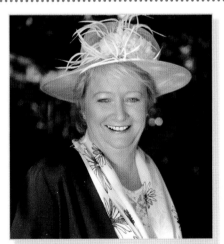

Children's face painting

Although not strictly a salon treatment, from time to time clients may request children's face painting for parties and birthday treats. No special skill is required – you just need some water-based face paints (child friendly for easy removal) and a flair for invention.

Apply make-up and instruct on make-up application

Recording the results of the treatment

Ensure that all records are kept up to date. For a make-up service this should include all products and shades used; any recommendations you have made; and products that have been purchased, so that you can follow up this information on subsequent visits. Skincare products should be recorded in the same way — remember that it would be worth making a note on the record card of any samples that you have given to the client. This will allow you to follow up their success at the next client visit.

TREATMENT SHEET (make-up) | Date: 18/5/2010 Client ref no. 789

Any factors which need to be considered today: Client going to wedding in June (mother of the bride). Outfit – gold hat, black & gold dress and jacket. Wedding in early evening not day; client doesn't want to look 'overdone'

Client's treatments:

Skin:	Colour:	Texture:	Type:	Sensitivity:		Problems:
Products used by client:	Cleanser:	Toner:	Moisturiser:	Mask:		Night/day creams:
Recommended products:	Cleanser:	Toner:	Moisturiser:	Mask:		Night/day creams:
	Serums:	Make-up base:	Corrective moisturiser:	Corrective treatments recommended (i.e eyebrow shape):		
Face:	Shape:	Bone structure:	Eye colour and shape:	Hair colour:		Brow colour and shape:
Make-up products used:	Foundation:	Concealer:	Powder:	Blusher:		Highlighter:
	Eye shadows:	Liners:	Mascara:	Lash curlers used:		Brow pencil:
	Lip liner:	Lipstick:	Other:			

Notes on selected make-up/application:

Client declaration: I declare the information is true and correct and that, as far as I am aware, I can undertake treatment with this establishment without any adverse effects. I am fully aware of any contra-indications: I am therefore willing to proceed and accept this treatment.

Client signature*:	*Without signature, the treatment cannot proceed	Date:
Therapist signature:		Date:

A partially completed make-up record card

TREATMENT SHEET (facials) | Date: 11/5/2010 Client ref no. 675

Any factors which need to be considered today: Client new to salon – 1ˢᵗ facial (present from husband for 30ᵗʰ bday on 15.05). Would like to buy products too.

Client's treatments:

Client: Male _____ Female ✓

Skin type: (Oily)/Dry/Combination/Mature/Young **Massage medium:** oil/(cream)

Muscle tone: Good/(Average)/Poor

Age: under 21 (30s) 40s 50s 60s over 70

Client's health: good (average)/ poor

Comments: Two small children/disturbed nights; complains of low energy sometimes (and feeling tired and irritable)

Medication taken: Occasional pain killers for period pain

Skin condition: good/average/poor specific problems/conditions to be avoided: Skin oily & a little congested, black heads along T zone. Showing as a combination skin but no dryness on cheeks. Face looking tired & a little drawn, poor colour, sallow look – could be caused by lack of sleep and wrong products

Client's lifestyle:

Sleep: Approx 4-5 hrs a night (see above) – disturbed sleep pattern	**Relaxation:** good/poor
Profession: Works from home (writer) often late pm/early am to fit round kids	**Fluid intake:** eight glasses of water taken daily? No Other drinks: Tea
Family life: Married with two children	**Smoking/drugs:** No
Exercise: None - no time & would have to organise child care	**Emotional balance:** 1-10 rating 1 being low 10 being highest:
Energy levels: 1-10 rating 1 being low 10 being highest: 1-2 (see above)	**Other:** regular mealtimes / shift work / supplements / allergies: –

Client's treatment:

Treatment chosen (and reasons):

Contra indication present: yes/no
Details:

Was client encouraged to seek medical advice? yes/no
Does treatment need adapting due to minor contra indication?: yes/no
Details:

Modifications to treatment: yes/no
Details:

Massage techniques used: Effleurage / Petrissage / Tapotement / Vibrations

Aftercare/homecare advice given (including details of recommended products):

Client declaration: I declare the information is true and correct and that, as far as I am aware, I can undertake treatment with this establishment without any adverse effects. I am fully aware of any contra-indications: I am therefore willing to proceed and accept this treatment.

Client signature*:	*Without signature, the treatment cannot proceed	Date:
Therapist signature:		Date:

A partially completed skincare record card

Obtain potential client information

Whenever you give a group demonstration, it is a good idea to ask potential clients if they would be happy to give you their personal details to be included in a mailing list for special offers and promotions. (Refer to Professional skills, page 59, for the correct storage of data under the Data Protection Act.)

For your portfolio

Devise a record card or information sheet that you could use for a group demonstration.

Providing aftercare advice

To enable the client to gain the most from the skincare and make-up instruction or application, they should be given the following information.

- Correct preparation for applying skincare products and make-up suitable for the client's skin type.
- Correct choice and application of cosmetics — colours, textures and types suitable for the features of the client and her skin type.
- Effective and hygienic use of products and equipment.
- How to keep make-up fresh by: applying pressed powder; applying a fine spray of water to keep the make-up from drying and cracking; applying more lipstick.
- Removal of make-up with products suitable for the client's skin type.
- In the event of an allergic reaction, remove all make-up, soothe with damp cotton wool and apply a soothing substance, e.g. calamine lotion.

All details should be recorded on the client record card.

Link selling and retail products

Many therapists work on a commission basis for the sale of retail products, and skincare tuition and make-up application provide the perfect opportunities to promote additional treatments and retail products to ensure the client gains the most from her visit to the salon.

Treatments could include:

- application of false lashes for special occasions
- regular facial treatment
- eyebrow treatments including brow shaping and tinting
- manicure and pedicure treatments
- waxing.

Retail products could include:

- cleanser, toner and moisturiser to suit skin type
- foundation and powder
- matching lipstick and varnish
- make-up brushes and applicator
- throat/neck cream, eye cream.

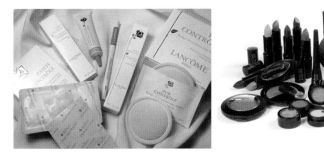

Make-up and skincare products can be purchased for the client to use at home

---

Carry out a consultation, checking for contra-indications, and skin analysis to determine which products to use

⬇

Ensure all products and equipment are close to hand

⬇

Apply moisturiser

⬇

Apply concealer and colour corrector if required

⬇

Apply foundation, check the colour on the jawline

⬇

Apply powder to set the foundation

⬇

Apply shaders and highlighters to minimise or emphasise areas as discussed with the client

⬇

Apply eyeshadow (hold a tissue under the eye to prevent flaking shadow)

⬇

Apply eyeliner or pencil (sharpen after each eye)

⬇

Apply mascara (using disposable mascara wands)

⬇

Apply lip pencil or liner

⬇

Apply lipstick

⬇

Show client the finished result and check she is happy

⬇

Record details, including products used and where applied, skin care products used and recommended

⬇

Products purchased

Apply make-up and instruct on make-up application

It is therefore important that you have a good knowledge of the products that you are recommending for home use and can demonstrate how to use these effectively. This will give the client confidence in you as a therapist. If the client purchases products, it is a good idea to record these sales on the record card, so you can assist the client on future visits if she wishes to repurchase.

Selling skills

Use open questions to aid the sale and always explain the benefits of a product when carrying out a service or demonstration.

Features and benefits of products

Many of the new age-smart products employ the latest technology, which introduces vitamins to the skin and removes dead skin cells. They have become big sellers and are directed not just at mature clientele but at all clients as preventative products.

A feature is an aspect of the product which is useful, but not necessarily part of the action of the product, such as a plastic, unbreakable bottle for travelling, or a pump action for easy dispensing. For example:

- Features of a one-to-one skincare and make-up instruction may be that it can be performed privately in the salon, and the client may not have to travel too far.
- Features of a group session are that it can be sociable and fun, and for the client who is shy, there is safety in numbers!

A benefit is the key selling point of the product to the client's advantage, such as a cream moisturising cleanser which helps keep the moisture in the skin, or a cream foundation which has a high moisture content to help a dry skin. For example:

- Benefits of a one-to-one skincare and make-up instruction may be that it can be tailor-made to suit the client's needs, and that a greater amount of understanding may take place because of the intimacy of just client and therapist.
- Benefits of a group session are that the therapist reaches a wider audience, the client may interact with friends within the audience and it provides a good opportunity for discussion with others.

My story

A satisfied client!

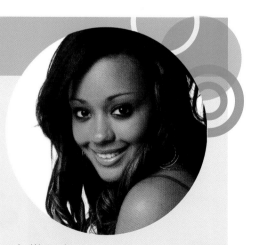

Hi, I'm Sienna. For a number of years my skin had been looking dry and sallow. A friend bought me a skincare and make-up session for my birthday and although I was very nervous I went along. My therapist Amitia was lovely, and after cleansing and analysing my skin and asking me a number of questions, she began selecting and demonstrating the products on me. She seated me in front of a mirror, showed me how to use the products and let me have a go. It was great fun and I learnt a lot. After selecting the correct skincare products for my skin type and condition, she showed me some very simple but effective day make-up techniques. The effects were stunning but not difficult to recreate. Amitia wrote down all of the products she recommended on a treatment planner, and although I could not afford to purchase all of the products in one visit I have now bought the range of products — and my skin and make-up application looks wonderful. I now regularly go to the salon for facials.

Evaluate the success of instruction

When you have carried out an individualised session or a group session you will need to evaluate the effectiveness of your treatment session with the client(s). This will enable you to work on your presentation and delivery techniques.

Asking the client to evaluate their own learning and provide support

You could ask the client what she has enjoyed and what she found difficult to master. You may need to re-cap areas and give her product samples that she can take away and practise with at home.

Asking questions and using feedback

It may be that you have devised a treatment/evaluation card specifically for skincare/make-up lessons or demonstrations, or simply added notes to client record cards. Always make a note of products used and recommended so you can follow this up with the client in the future. This feedback will allow you to make improvements to your own skincare and make-up instructional techniques, if necessary.

After the skincare and make-up instruction — whether a one-to-one session, demonstration or group session — has been completed, hold a question and answer session. Have you:

- met the objectives
- checked the finished result with the client
- been cost-effective, both with time and product use
- carried out the service in a commercially acceptable time
- filled in a client record card
- obtained the audience's details for a promotional mailing (if group demonstration)
- tidied away and left the area immaculate
- enough products for other demonstrations, or will more need to be ordered?

After the event, it is important to look at your performance and judge if you were happy with all aspects of it. Ask yourself:

- How do I think it went?
- What would I change if I could?
- Was I fully prepared?
- What would I do differently next time?
- What sort of feedback did I get from the audience? Were they interested and attentive? If not, why not?
- Did the client(s) show full understanding of my instructions, and did she (they) show interest in purchasing a product, or booking a service or treatment?

Frequently asked questions

Q Why is it important to ensure a client has the correct skincare products?

A Having the correct products for the client's skin will ensure damage does not occur and enables the client to get the maximum benefit from any other services offered. Correct products also ensure make-up that is applied looks the best.

Q What is the benefit of regularly using an exfoliator?

A An exfoliator removes dead skin cells that can clog the surface of the skin making it appear dull and lifeless. Dry, dehydrated patches also cause foundation to look patchy.

Q Why is giving samples of skincare products important as part of a good salon service?

A Samples allow the client to try the recommended products for a few days to see how they get on with the application. Also, however good the products are, some clients will still react to some products and this can prevent costly mistakes. This will give the clients faith in your treatment planning and professionalism.

Q Why is it important to do a skin analysis prior to carrying out a make-up application?

A It is important so that you can fully assess the client's skin type and select suitable products. This should be carried out on cleansed, dry skin.

Q What action should be taken if the foundations are not the correct shade?

A You can blend your own shades by mixing two or more colours together on a palette to obtain the correct shade.

Q Do I have to use a colour corrector if a concealer has been used?

A Colour correctors do just what they say — they neutralise the colour to make a more even shade — so they should only be applied where they are needed.

Q Is the lighting really that important when applying make-up?

A The more natural the lighting and the closer to daylight, the better the finished results will look. Different coloured light bulbs and shades on light fittings can give a false appearance and you may find that the application is too sparing or too heavy handed.

Q Why is it important to use the correct products on black/Asian skins?

A Because of the different colours and pigmentation of the skin, specialist products should be used so the correct skin tones and a natural look can be achieved.

Check your knowledge

1 On which bone would you try the colour of foundation?

2 Which skin type would benefit from the use of a mineral foundation?

3 On the colour star, which colour would neutralise red colouring?

4 When applying eye make-up to more mature clients, what type of product should be avoided?

5 What aspects should you consider when undertaking a special occasion make-up?

6 What should you do between each eye when using a pencil to line the eyes?

7 Why is the position of the client important when applying make-up?

8 What type of mascara is best to use on a client who wears contact lenses?

9 How would you contour a client with a round face shape?

10 Does a highlighter enhance an area or make it recede?

11 Name two benefits of a one-to-one skincare and make-up instruction session.

12 Name two benefits of a group skincare presentation.

13 When talking to clients why is it important to vary your tone and speech patterns?

14 Name three resources that you could use when carrying out a skincare instruction session.

15 Why is it important to demonstrate skincare products to clients?

Apply make-up and instruct on make-up application

Getting ready for assessment

Your assessor will observe you demonstrating practical performance to a competent standard on at least three occasions for both applying make-up and instructing on make-up application.

You need to be aware of the service times for each individual treatment.

- Day make-up = 30 minutes
- Evening or special occasion make-up = 45 minutes
- Make-up instruction = 75 minutes.

You need to show your assessor that you can cover all skin types, occasions and age ranges using the products most suitable for your client in order to create the look they wish to achieve.

It is important to remember that make-up can be very subjective. As a therapist it is vital that you consult with your client to ensure that you fully understand what they want. A therapist should, of course, make recommendations and provide advice, whilst being sensitive to any flaws in the client's facial features or skin condition.

For your make-up instruction assessments you are required to show that you can give suitable skincare advice to cover oily, dry and combination skin types as well as providing the client with instruction on how to achieve a suitable make-up look for day, evening and special occasion wear.

You will need to provide photographic or video evidence and witness testimonies, as well as written work or projects for this unit. You will also be required to sit an exam to support Apply make-up and must gain at least 70% to achieve a pass. There is no exam for Instruct on make-up.

Apply make-up and instruct on make-up application

Remove hair using waxing techniques

What you will learn

- Prepare for waxing treatments
- Provide waxing treatments

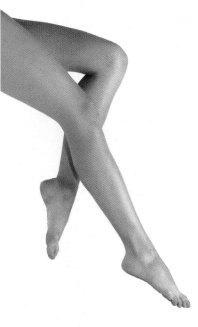

Think about it

Different cultures and religions may have different views regarding hair removal.

Key terms

Superfluous hair – unwanted body hair.

Introduction

Waxing is the temporary removal of body hair by pulling it out of the skin by the roots, using some form of bond. A hot, warm or cold wax product is spread over the hairy area, and a cotton or paper strip is used to make the hair bond stick to it. The strip is then removed in a quick, single movement. It should leave the area clean and hair-free. Hygiene, client care and lots of practice are necessary, which may mean this unit takes some patience to learn, but it is very rewarding for you and the client.

Waxing treatments always form a large part of any salon's business, and provide a salon with a steady source of income. Waxing promotions are offered in the summer to prepare clients for holidays or special occasions. It should not be forgotten that many men have chest and back wax treatments.

Before you can give the client a full consultation, then plan and prepare for the treatment, you need to understand:

- hair facts
- wax facts
- other methods of hair removal.

This knowledge will allow you to make the best treatment decision for your client, based upon a sound understanding of the choices available to suit her needs.

Benefits for the client:

- quick and effective method of removing **superfluous hair** to all areas of the body
- immediate result
- lasts 4–6 weeks depending on hair growth and colour of hair
- minimal pain
- cheaper hair removal method compared to other salon treatments, e.g. laser.

Benefits for the therapist:

- mainstay salon treatment
- treatments can often be slotted in among other longer services, therefore saving salon time
- can be offered as a promotion, e.g. summer holiday package, to increase revenue.

Prepare for waxing treatments

In this outcome you will learn about:

- preparing yourself, client and work area for a waxing treatment
- using suitable consultation techniques to identify treatment objectives
- carrying out necessary tests prior to the treatment
- providing clear recommendations to the client
- selecting products, tools and equipment to suit client treatment needs.

Preparing the work environment

Preparation for waxing is an essential part of the beauty therapist's role regardless of the treatment being carried out. Good preparation sets the whole atmosphere of any treatment, creating a calm and efficient impression. If the therapist and work area are not prepared, the client will be aware of this, which can detract from the benefits of the treatment.

In the case of waxing, preparation is vital. Most wax needs preheating so that the client is not kept waiting. All equipment and materials should be in place to avoid leaving the client alone.

Preparation of the working area

Many salons have designated rooms or areas that are permanently prepared for waxing, with heaters and all necessary products never leaving the room.

The golden rule here is to leave everything fully prepared for the next therapist to use. This means replenishing anything that has run low, cleaning and being tidy during the treatment. It would be most off-putting for a new client to find the remains of the previous client's treatment.

The preparation of the working area should include the following.

- Protective covering for the couch, so that any spillage or residue is easily removed and will not cause permanent damage.
- Where plastic sheeting is used, paper couch roll should be placed over the top. This prevents cross-infection, as the paper can be replaced easily; it also provides client comfort.
- Two waste bins, both with inner liners, should be placed behind or under the couch: one for general waste; one for wax waste – this is for contaminated materials, which will be put into a designated bin for collection by a licensed removal firm for incineration.
- The chosen heating unit for the wax type to suit the client's needs and enough wax product for the area to be treated. Obviously, a lip wax requires a small amount of product, but a full leg wax will mean the heater needs to be quite full. Remember that it may take a full half-hour to heat the wax to a working temperature, so that needs to be the first job of the day. (Many salons keep a heater on all day, in anticipation of clients dropping in without appointments.)
- Antiseptic cleaner for the skin, or the manufacturer's recommended skin cleanser.
- Talc-free powder.
- Fabric or paper strips which are compatible with the manufacturer's requirements for the wax chosen.
- Disposable gloves, usually vinyl with a talc-impregnated lining so they are easy to put on – refer to your individual professional body's guidelines for use. Wearing gloves may help to prevent contact dermatitis.
- Disposable wooden spatulas or a suitable applicator – again refer to your professional body's guidelines (there are no spatula requirements for roller waxing, of course).
- Tissues, cotton wool and a jewellery bowl for the client. (It is important that the client removes all facial piercings if you are waxing an area of the face.)

Think about it

Check to ensure that the client does not have a latex allergy before putting on gloves. Alternative gloves are available, including vinyl or nitrile powder-free gloves. These should be used if either the client or the therapist has an allergy.

- A pair of scissors and tweezers in a container soaking in suitable disinfectant to sterilise – the scissors may be required to trim the hair length prior to treatment, and the tweezers to remove the odd stray hair which has escaped the wax.
- After-wax lotion or oil.
- Aftercare leaflets for the client to take away.

Wearing suitable personal protective equipment

The personal protective equipment a therapist should wear when waxing is a disposable apron and gloves.

Checking your position and posture

When waxing, you may find that you get very close to the skin to inspect every pore and hair to make sure you have missed nothing. It is important to remember your posture to prevent back strain and repetitive strain injury. Remember to bend at the knees and keep a straight back.

Ensuring the treatment is cost-effective and minimising wastage

Cost is the price paid for something. It is measured in time, money or energy. Effectiveness means producing a result.

So how does this apply to hair removing? Imagine you own your own business and you have to pay for all outgoings, equipment, overheads, stock and products, along with staffing and wages.

How can a therapist be economical?

- Only use the amount of product needed. Do not be too quick to do a heavy application of wax – it does not give the best results.
- Do not be wasteful with disposable items. Couch roll can be split in half, cotton wool pads can be split, and smaller tissues can be used rather than 'man-sized' ones.
- Give time careful consideration. Time is money and if the treatment times are not planned carefully through the day, there may be a gap of 15 minutes per client. This adds up to an extra hour at the end of the day that could be put to good use, either with vital chores or another cash-paying client.
- Be organised and prepared. Time spent preparing the working area not only gives a professional appearance, it also saves time.
- Do not indulge in false economies. Paying to have equipment maintained and repaired makes good financial sense. If the equipment starts failing and the therapist is unable to offer some treatments because of it, revenue may be lost. Bad advertising through word of mouth will also mean lost revenue.
- Invest in good labour-saving equipment. For example, borrowing an old machine to wash all the towels may seem to cut costs, but an industrial washing machine will have low maintenance costs. Towels need to be washed at a minimum of 60°C to prevent cross-infection occurring.
- Work out overhead costs on a realistic basis, and try to gear your prices to that figure. Work out how many hours you work a week.

- Be wary of both consultation and aftercare times. Some clients love to chat, and while the therapist wants to give a quality treatment, time can slip away, and that is expensive. Giving the client a leaflet is a good time-saving technique, and the client can take it away to refer to.

- Do some research and find out what sort of prices the competition asks for waxing treatments. The salon may offer both warm and hot wax. Adjust your prices so they are about the same — they should be not so expensive that custom is lost but not so cheap that clients think there is a catch.

Disposing of hazardous waste

When waxing, you will be dealing with contaminated skin waste products from many different clients.

The following Acts require all clinical waste to be kept apart from general waste and to be disposed of to a licensed incinerator or landfill site by a licensed company:

- Environmental Protection Act, 1990
- The Controlled Waste Regulations, 1992 (as amended)
- Special Waste Regulations, 1996 (as amended).

Clinical waste includes:

- waste which consists wholly or partly of animal or human tissue
- blood or other body fluids
- swabs or dressings
- syringes or needles.

Refer to Professional skills and Follow health and safety practice in the salon for further information.

All waste products from a waxing treatment must be classed as contaminated waste: there is a possibility that blood spotting will have occurred, especially when carrying out a bikini or underarm wax, and some skin cells will be caught up in the wax. You only need to perform a wax treatment on a tanned skin to see how much of the darker skin is removed along with the hairs. Self-tanning products will also be removed when waxing; to ensure that the client maximises their self-tan they should be waxed at least two days before a tan is applied.

Put all your used strips into a lined small bin, tie the bag up and put it into the larger, lined clinical waste bin that is provided by the salon. A contractor will empty this weekly, but if a salon is a busy wax centre, then twice weekly emptying stops the bin from becoming a health hazard.

The person who empties the clinical waste bins should wear industrial gloves as added protection. The bins are usually taken to the council incinerator for burning. Large hospitals often lease out one of their own incinerators to companies.

While it would be very unlikely that your waxing waste would contain any infections, as you thoroughly check for contra-indications before treatment begins, you must follow the procedures laid down by the law and by your own professional code of ethics to protect yourself and your clients.

Think about it

It is vital that the waxing waste is not mixed with ordinary rubbish or waste from other treatments. If it is not separated, health inspectors could close down your salon as a health hazard.

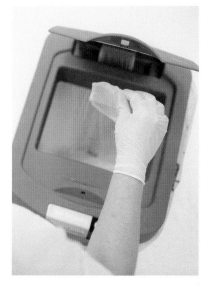

Dispose of waste such as wax strips in the correct way

Remove hair using waxing techniques

Leaving the work area and equipment suitable for further treatments

After the client has left the salon, it is time to go back to your workstation to clear up. Waxing is a notoriously messy business, especially in your early training. You will probably have dripped wax down the side of the pot and on to the floor while trying to get it from the pot to the area to be waxed. You may also have flicked some of it on to yourself. Some of this is to be expected when you first start, but your technique must get cleaner as you progress.

To avoid dripping wax on to the floor, fold up a tissue in your free hand and hold it underneath the hand holding the spatula to catch any drips. This is much easier than trying to pick wax off the floor — it never comes off completely once it has set.

Always wear a protective apron — it is much easier to throw away a plastic apron than to get wax off a new overall.

Think about your method of work. Could you have been tidier as you went along? Unless the client is the last one of the day, you will not have the luxury of plenty of time to clean and tidy the area. Get into the habit of putting all waste straight into the bin, which should be beside you. Bad habits soon form, so do not put bits and pieces on the side of the trolley, or worse still, on the couch. If your next client is in straight away, you could be in trouble with treatment timing if you have to spend a long time tidying and preparing for your next treatment.

Good habits for keeping tidy

Organise the layout of the trolley in an ordered fashion. Arrange all the products in order of use with the labels facing you, so you can easily find the one you need. Replace them into their slot when you have finished with them. They will always then be at hand, and you will look tidy and in control.

Have a space for everything. Have a system whereby all necessary tools are in a jar or pot (even a plastic beaker is easy to clean), and the tissues and cotton wool are in their own plastic bowl or tub.

Tidy as you go along — put used tissues and cotton wool into a small pedal bin (lined with a bin liner) as you finish with them, rather than leaving them on the trolley.

Have gloves and strips at the ready. Wash your hands in front of the client, although this may not be possible if you do not have a sink near the workstation — but try not to leave the client unattended.

Minimise waste by using only the amount of product required. This is not only cost-effective, it also means there is very little product left over to have to clear up.

Mop up spills as they occur and do not allow them to endanger others.

After each treatment, cover the couch with clean couch roll. The trolley should be as you would wish to find it. Do not leave a wax pot with a tiny amount of wax in it that is not enough for the next client to have a treatment. Ask the receptionist or a junior therapist to put on a second pot, or ask your technician to add some more wax pellets or sugar, so it can be heating while you clear up.

These tips prevent a major clean-up being necessary at the end of your treatment. Becoming tidy is a skill that comes with experience.

Think about it

You may share a work station or salon cubicle with other therapists, therefore it is important to tidy up after treatments to ensure you are effective with your time and do not annoy colleagues.

Ensuring the client's records are up to date and accurate

If the client is a regular visitor to the salon, a record card will be held. Each treatment will be recorded along with the area treated and any reaction to treatment.

With a new client a full consultation will take place and a sensitivity test will be carried out prior to treatment. The Habia Code of Practice for Waxing Services states that it is advisable for a sensitivity test to be carried out 24–48 hours prior to treatment. This test is usually carried out on the cleansed wrist or elbow of the client, by applying and removing a small amount of product to the area to make sure the client does not have an allergic reaction to the wax. A positive reaction will leave a red, irritated and sore area, where a negative reaction will show no change to the skin and therefore the treatment can go ahead.

A treatment plan will be needed that is mutually agreeable to both client and therapist. It will include:

- type of hair growth (coarse, thick, thin, light, short or long)
- the area to be treated
- whether it is the first or a subsequent treatment
- skin type and sensitivity
- any reaction to a previous treatment
- result of the sensitivity test
- any contra-indications present.

A record card could look something like the one shown opposite.

Complete the client record card accurately. Refer to Professional skills (pages 24–26) for client record keeping.

It is important, both for the client and yourself, that you fill out the waxing sheet details accurately to avoid any health and safety problems and to protect your professional reputation. Do not return the record card to be filed incomplete, thinking you can do it later: you will not remember and vital information may not be recorded.

Be constructive when filling out the card. Be positive and helpful in what you write, and avoid making any negative comments or personal observations about the client. Clients are entitled to view their own records under the Data Protection Act. Also avoid leaving the card lying around for anyone to read. Once you have completed the write-up, give it to the person who is responsible for filing.

For your portfolio

Devise a record card that could be used to record your waxing treatments.

Waxing treatment record card

Waxing and record of treatment client file copy

Client reference: _____

Initial consultation date:			Therapist:		

First treatment: Yes ☐   No ☐

Contra-indications checked: Yes ☐   No ☐

Contra-indications noted: _____ None ☐

Allergies:	Disorders:
Skin conditions:	Wax used:

Date and treatment no.	Area	Contra-action	Special notes Contra-indications or adaptations	Therapist	Patch test
1					
2					
3					
4					
5					
6					

NB After 6 treatments client requires new consultation and analysis

Leaflet given: Yes ☐

Aftercare – for a period of 24 hours:

- ◆ No sunbathing or sunbeds
- ◆ Avoid bathing in sea or swimming pool
- ◆ Do not take a *hot* bath or shower
- ◆ Do not use deodorant / anti-perspirant
- ◆ Avoid tight clothing
- ◆ Do not use perfumed products on the area
- ◆ No make-up or self-tanning preparations
- ◆ Do not keep touching or picking at the area

Remove hair using waxing techniques

411

Using consultation techniques to identify treatment objectives

Think about it

Regardless of the treatment chosen, all under-16s require their parent/guardian's written consent for a treatment to be carried out, and hair removal is no exception. A parent/guardian should also be present at the treatment.

Before you can effectively consult with the client, decide on their waxing needs and draw up a treatment plan, you need to have thorough background knowledge of all the products. So, look closely at hair facts (page 420) and wax facts (page 422) before deciding on your recommendations.

It is important to ensure that you treat every client equally and in line with current legislation (e.g. Disability Discrimination Act 2005 and Equality Act 2006. For details refer to Follow health and safety practice in the salon.) The service and standard of care you provide should be the same for everyone.

You should use appropriate consultation techniques, including visual, questioning and manual checks, to establish the treatment plan for the client. Remember that you should record all details on the client record card and that clients must give their signed consent before the waxing treatment is carried out.

Remember that your consultation should be carried out with sensitivity and tact to give the client confidence. You should conduct the consultation in a polite and friendly manner to find out what the client's particular needs are.

Once you have conducted the consultation, you will be able to decide on the best treatment plan to meet the needs of the client. You should always agree your approach with the client before you begin.

Identifying contra-indications to waxing

The questions that you ask need to establish if the client has a contra-indication — that is, a condition that will prevent the treatment taking place, or mean that the treatment needs adapting.

Diseases and disorders of the skin include:

- **allergy** — a reaction to one or more substances, which can cause a reaction to be seen on the skin. It can be seen as itching, swelling and redness and can vary in the degree of severity
- **dermatitis** — similar to eczema in appearance, but the cause is not the same. A reaction or allergy to something in contact with the skin usually causes dermatitis
- **uticaria (hives)** — this reaction resembles nettle rash and is usually caused by a reaction to a substance
- **impetigo** — highly infectious, this starts as small red spots, which then break open and form blisters. Most common around the corner of the mouth and, if picked, will spread. Can be spread through the use of dirty equipment
- **furuncle (boil)** — this infection forms at the base of a hair follicle. Bacteria can spread through an open scratch in the skin. The area is red, raised and painful and pus may be present
- **carbuncle** — skin infection that involves a group of infected hair follicles that occur deep in the skin — these are often referred to as a mass
- **sycosis** — this is commonly known as folliculitis — inflammation of the hair follicle
- **keratoma** — commonly known as keratosis, these are rough, raised lumps on the skin. There are a number of forms but the most common is keratosis pilaris, often seen on the upper arm

- **polyps** — sac-like growths of tissue
- **xanthoma** — a condition where fat builds up under the surface of the skin. Common in older adults or people with high cholesterol
- **steatoma** — sebaceous cysts of various sizes which are commonly found in the scalp, face and back. They are painless and easily movable
- **steatosis** — fatty deposits often associated with liver conditions
- **anhidrosis** — the absence of sweating caused by the under activity of the sympathetic nervous system
- **bromhidrosis/osmidrosis** — excessive body odour, an overpowering and unpleasant odour
- **hyperhidrosis** — excessive sweating
- **miliaria rubra** — commonly known as prickly heat. This is caused by blockages in the sweat glands
- **bulla** — a large fluid-filled blister
- **crust** — refers to a change in the surface of the skin caused by either dried blood, pus or sebum
- **fissure** — a crack in the skin which is usually narrow but deep
- **macule** — a flat change of colour on the surface of the skin
- **scale** — a dry or greasy mass of keratin on the stratum corneum
- **wheal** — a reddish purple mark on the skin that usually disappears within 48 hours
- **tubercle** — a small warty growth described as a nodule
- **vesicles** — fluid-filled blisters — similar to those seen in chicken pox or the herpes virus
- **warts** — small, compact raised growths of skin — can be light or brown in colour, present on the face and neck
- **eczema** — very dry skin, often scaly and flaky, can be red and often very itchy
- **acne vulgaris** — inflamed whiteheads, blackheads and pustules in various degrees of congestion. Mostly associated with hormones — and the presence of bacteria can make the conditions infected
- **acne rosacea** — seen as a flush of red over the nose and cheeks with a raised feel to the skin
- **dilated capillaries** — the result of loss of elasticity in the walls of the blood capillaries — the cheeks and the nose are often most affected. Exposure to weather, harsh handling and lack of protection, along with spicy foods and alcohol, can be contributing factors
- **split capillaries** — weakening and rupturing of capillary walls
- **lentigo** — also known as age spots, these are larger and more distinctive than a freckle, and may be slightly raised
- **chloasma** — hyperpigmentation — consists of irregular patches of brown pigment caused by the overproduction of melanocytes. Often appears on the face during pregnancy and is sometimes linked to the contraceptive pill
- **vitiligo** — hypopigmentation — a condition in which small patches of skin have lost their pigmentation and appear a lighter colour than the rest of the skin
- **port wine stain** — a bright purple, irregular-shaped, flat birthmark that can vary in size. It is thought to be due to damage by pressure during foetal development

Remove hair using waxing techniques

413

- **strawberry naevus** — a raised and distorted area, often on the face, bright pink/red

- **spider naevus** — a central dilated vessel with leg-like projections of capillaries. The face and cheeks tend to be most affected — can occur during pregnancy

- **basal cell carcinoma, squamous cell carcinoma and malignant melanoma** — all types of skin cancer. These conditions would be contra-indications to any type of treatment unless a GP referral is given

- **phlebitis** — inflammation of a vein — commonly seen in the legs. The area would be tender and there may be redness present

- **hyperkeratosis** — commonly seen on darker skins. Common on knees and elbows and caused by a thickening of the horny layer of the epidermis.

Refer to You and the skin, pages 208–213, to see photographs of some of these skin disorders and diseases.

Diseases and disorders of the hair include:

- **asteatosis** — refers to infections or disorders of the skin or scalp which can be caused by bacterial infection, infestation or excessive itching/scratching

- **canities** — the technical term for greying hair. This is caused by the loss of the hair's natural melanin pigment

- **discoid lupus erythematosus (DLE)** — a chronic condition that has deep red inflamed patches that look scaly and crusty. This condition affects the scalp, face and ears

- **fragilitis crinium** — brittleness of the hair. The hair tends to split or break

- **hypertrichosis** — the abnormal amount of hair growth on the body

- **monilethrix** — also known as beaded hair, this results in short, fragile and broken hair. This is a genetic condition

- **ringed hair disorder** — a rare disorder where some of the hair shafts have alternate pigmented and light bands

- **trichoptilosis** — commonly known as split ends. Poor hair care and excessive heat treatments can be the cause

- **trichorrhexis nodosa** — where the hair shaft has a weak or thickened part causing the hair to break easily

- **pityriasis simplex capitis** — shedding of dead skin cells (often called dandruff)

- **pityriasis steatoides** — a more severe form of dandruff that is characterised by waxy scales. These stick to the scalp and cause irritation

- **seborrhea oleosa** — oily secretions that can appear yellow and crusty. They are particularly found on the forehead area and around the nose

- **tinea vavosa** — ringworm of the scalp — a highly infectious disease

- **tinea capitis** — fungal ringworm that can affect all or some of the hair. The area will itch and the scalp will become red. Hair may fall out as a result of this

- **pediculosis capitis (head lice)** — a mite that lays eggs which hatch out in the hair. Common condition in children

- **alopecia areata** — often called spot baldness. Can affect the entire body but is most commonly found on the scalp

- **alopecia totalis** — when all of the hair on the scalp is lost

- **alopecia universalis** – when the hair falls out over the entire body including the pubic area
- **alopecia senilis** – age-related baldness due to the slowing down of the metabolic rate with age
- **traction alopecia** – caused by the hair being tugged or pulled too tight, e.g. in a pony tail or braid. The hair can break off or thin
- **telogen effluvium** – where the hair growth cycle is disrupted due to illness, after child birth or due to stress. When more than the normal 10–20% of hairs fall out.

It may be that an area has to be protected or avoided, for example where a mole or skin tag is present. Accurately record the client's answers and encourage them to ask questions so that you can establish any problems and take any necessary action if required.

The areas to be treated should be examined in good lighting to judge if any of the following conditions are present:

- skin diseases or disorders
- open skin, infection, inflammation or healing skin (scabs present)
- recent laser treatments within the last two weeks (it is not advisable to wax an area that is being treated with laser)
- micro-dermabrasion, dermabrasion treatments or skin peel treatments within the past two weeks
- areas where steroid cream has been frequently applied – these creams can thin the skin
- medication for acne such as Retin-A and Accutane
- bruising
- very thin or papery skin (diabetics have thin skin that does not heal very well because of poor circulation; also long-term use of steroid creams or medication can cause the skin to thin, which could cause tearing if the area is waxed over)
- sunburn – after a sunbed or natural tanning or if a heat rash is present. If the client has a self-tan application this will be removed with the waxing process
- recent scar tissue
- moles, warts or any unidentified skin problems
- varicose veins or broken capillaries on the legs
- cold sores, eye infections, styes or colds when treating the face
- urinary infections – if treating the bikini area
- unidentified lumps, breast-feeding and mastitis when treating under the arm
- previous reactions to treatment, which could be related to the products used or a known allergy to adhesive resin such as a plaster
- excessive ingrown hairs from previous treatments.

The client would also not be suitable for treatment if she had just had heat treatment, such as infrared treatment or a sauna or steam bath.

Prior to or during menstruation, clients may have a lower pain threshold and the skin may be more sensitive and react unpredictably. You can suggest clients take an over-the-counter painkiller to help, but only if they have used them before with no adverse reactions.

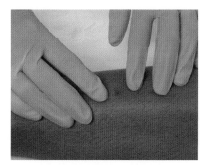

Look out for moles and skin tags which may restrict the treatment in the area

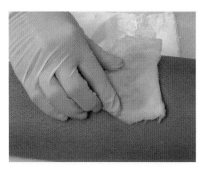

Use a pre-wax cleanser from a manufacturer to cleanse the area

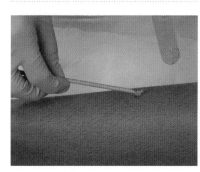

Cover the mole with petroleum jelly to prevent the wax from adhering to it – this will ensure you do not cause any damage to the mole

Remove hair using waxing techniques

Explaining possible contra-actions

Even when you have been faultless in hygiene, safety and product use, your client may react to the wax – even if she has had the same treatment for years. It could be a reaction caused by medication being taken or the result of fluctuating hormones, or it could be that an allergic reaction has developed.

Possible **contra-actions** to waxing may be immediately visible, either during or after the treatment. They may also appear when the client goes home or back to work. Either way you should act responsibly and make your client aware of what action to take.

Unfavourable skin reaction

Recognised as redness or soreness to the area, this could be caused by the wax being too hot on the skin, by an allergic reaction or from too vigorous scraping of the spatula on the skin during application. Stop the treatment, apply a cold compress to the area, and apply and give aftercare cooling lotion for the client to continue applying.

Burning or blistering

Recognised as a burning sensation, this is caused by the wax being too hot. Was it tested on the therapist, and a little applied to the area prior to treatment?

Refer to the individual waxes for first aid recommendations (pages 425–30).

Swelling in the area

Recognised as the area being tender and the skin having a puffy appearance, swelling is caused by the wax having too high a temperature or by the strips being lifted off in an upward motion rather than back on themselves.

Refer to the individual waxes for first aid recommendations.

It is also advisable to give your client an aftercare leaflet to take away and refer to, so that any potential contra-action can be avoided and maximum benefit is gained from the treatment.

Agreeing the waxing treatment and outcomes to meet the client's needs

During the consultation the therapist needs to discuss the realistic outcomes of a waxing treatment.

Unrealistic aims of waxing

It would be unrealistic for the client to believe that:

- waxing is permanent hair removal
- waxing makes the hair growth weaken
- all the hairs grow back at the same time
- waxing lightens the hair colour
- the hairs grow back with a sharp, spiky feel to them
- waxing is painless.

Realistic aims of waxing

- Waxing lasts 3–6 weeks depending on hair growth.
- As the blood supply to the hairs is increased with waxing, the hairs may grow back slightly thicker and coarser.

- The hairs grow back spasmodically as the hair growth cycle for each follicle is different.

- Waxing does not change the hair colour.

- Shaving and cutting blunt the ends of the hair, making them feel spiky; after waxing the hair grows back with its natural tapered end, feeling smooth to the touch.

- Waxing feels like a plaster being taken from the skin. Pain thresholds will vary and some clients will feel more than others.

Ensuring the client is in a suitable position to be treated

- The couch should initially be placed in an upright position to allow the client to be comfortably seated, and then placed into the appropriate position for the area to be treated. A pillow covered with a towel and protected with couch roll should be used. It is vital that the client is in the right position not only for their comfort and ease but to ensure that as the therapist you don't suffer any injuries when undertaking the treatment.

- Help the client into a comfortable and relaxed position. Offer a covered towel as a prop, should she or he require extra support under the knees or in the small of the back.

- Ask the client to place protective couch roll around the panty line if doing a bikini wax, or around the bra if doing an underarm wax, rather than just assuming the client would be comfortable for you to touch those areas.

- Remember when the couch is in a semi-reclining position and the client is having the front of the legs waxed, it is very comfortable. However, you must lower the couch head so it is flat again before you ask her to turn over, otherwise she will be in a very awkward position.

Think about it

It is important to be honest with the clients, so they know what to expect. Honesty between therapist and client is part of the ethical conduct that maintains high professional standards for all beauty therapists.

Think about it

Advise the client not to wear expensive underwear when having a wax. Protect the client's clothing with towels and tissues. If the client is having a bikini wax prior to a holiday, she should wear her swimsuit or bikini bottom for waxing to ensure the line is right. If not, an old pair of briefs with the same leg shape will give the correct line.

Remove hair using waxing techniques

My story

Salon life

My name is Nikita. When I first left college I was not very quick or confident with my waxing skills. On my first day, my manager asked me about my favourite and least favourite treatments. I had to say that waxing was my least favourite. So instead of giving me a few wax clients during my first month, my manager made sure I had mostly waxing treatments in my column. My manager was always around to give me support and guidance and although I was nervous at first, my confidence and speed quickly grew. I'm really glad I faced up to my fears and worked hard on my weakest treatment. I now enjoy waxing and have many regular clients.

Benefits to client and therapist

Benefits of waxing for the client:

- Quick and visual treatment

- Areas stay hair free for longer

- All parts of the body can be covered

- Treatment available to male and female clientele

- After a number of treatments hair growth usually becomes sparser.

Benefits of waxing for the therapist:

- Quick treatment to carry out

- Staple salon treatment that provides regular income

- Can be performed as a mobile treatment

- Good treatment to link with promotions; for example, leg wax and pedicure for the summer.

Ask the experts

Q *Do you have any tips for advice that I should give to clients to reduce the pain?*

A Firstly, remind the client that her pain threshold is at its lowest around her period and to avoid treatment at this time. Secondly, a client's pain threshold is also at its lowest if they are feeling under the weather or tired. Thirdly, suggest the application of an after-wax lotion following treatment to reduce redness and aid healing.

Q *I worry about causing bleeding when carrying out underarm and bikini-line waxing.*

A Make the client aware that as the hair in these areas is strong terminal hair there may be some blood spotting and that bleeding or spotting is a normal reaction. Use an after wax lotion which is formulated to deal with spotting.

Top tips

It is important to make sure you are confident in your own abilities as this is reassuring for the client. If you feel weak in a particular skill or treatment, make sure that you keep practising it. Practice makes perfect and treatment times will improve with experience.

Provide waxing treatments

In this outcome you will learn about:

- communicating and behaving in a professional manner
- following health and safety working practices and industry Code of Practice for Waxing Services
- positioning yourself and the client correctly throughout the treatment
- using products, tools, equipment and techniques to suit client's treatment needs, skin type and conditions
- completing the treatment to the satisfaction of the client
- recording the results of the treatment
- providing suitable aftercare advice.

Why is the human body hairy?

As the human body evolved it was extremely hairy all over for warmth; the body also laid down fat deposits to keep warm. Facial hair on men through the ages has been considered a sign of virility, strength and masculinity. Men only started shaving with razors during the twentieth century. In fact, most Edwardian gentlemen had handlebar moustaches or full beards. There has been a big change in fashion towards clean-shaven faces, except of course for the 'designer stubble' trend of celebrities.

We still retain hairs for the purpose of warmth and protection. Terminal hair (refer to Related anatomy and physiology, page 252) grows long and is often coarse in texture:

- Scalp hair – protects the head and helps keep in the heat.
- Eyelashes – protect the eyes by catching particles that may fall into the eye.
- Underarm and pubic hair – protect the delicate skin and cushion against friction caused by movement.
- Body hair – protects against heat loss.

For the anatomy of the hair's structure and the hair growth cycle, refer to Related anatomy and physiology, pages 252–254.

Factors determining hair growth

Both men and women have terminal hair, but hair growth is determined by several factors.

The number of hair follicles

A large number of follicles equals lots of hair and the hair will look very thick. This tends to be genetic, which means it has been inherited from the parents. (If a man has baldness in his family, there is a strong possibility he will develop the same hair-growth pattern.)

Cultural influences

Hair-growth patterns as well as strength, texture and the amount of hair are also influenced by geography and ethnicity. There is a higher proportion of blonde and light-skinned people in countries such as Norway and Sweden. Face or body hair on these people is light and not noticeable. However, the nearer the Equator, and hence nearer the sun, that people live, the darker their skin and hair colour is likely to become. Italians, Spaniards and Greeks usually have dark hair and skin. Their facial hair or body hair may be more noticeable. British colouring can be a mixture of light and dark — Scottish and Irish people tend to have darker colouring. Generally, it is darker-haired clients who are more concerned with superfluous hair, mostly because it is more visible.

Hair strength and texture

Again, this tends to run in families. People with a thick, strong hair growth may also have lots of follicles and a really full head of hair. Others may have lots of follicles, but the hair itself may be very fine in texture. Some people have the combination of few follicles with fine hair texture. For these people body hairs are not noticeable and they may never need the services of **depilation**.

Illness

This can have a strong effect on hair growth, usually making the hair lank and lifeless, and could affect hair styling.

Medication

Some drugs have a strong effect on hair growth. They might produce coarse, thick hair, which can be depilated, with a doctor's permission, or the follicles might weaken and wither, causing the hair to fall out. Some forms of chemotherapy for the treatment of cancer cause baldness. Often this is only temporary and the hairs will regrow.

Hormones

Hormones can also have an effect on hair growth. Women going through the menopause, when hormone levels may be erratic, may find they develop 'whiskers' of coarse hair on the face.

Emotion

A sudden shock, accident or the death of a loved one can cause hair loss, which may regrow, or may not. This is called alopecia and can mean patches of hair loss or total baldness. It is unusual for alopecia to occur on a leg or an arm.

In our society some women dislike having hairy legs and body hair. Some men may also consider having hair removed from the body. For example, some professional sportsmen such as cyclists and swimmers may wish to enhance their performance by reducing body hair.

Hair facts

Superfluous hair

This term is used where hair growth is normal, but the client feels it to be unattractive. Dark-haired clients, especially, may feel that their growth is visible, for example on the upper lip.

Removal of unwanted hair, particularly by waxing and sugaring, is referred to as depilation. This is a popular salon treatment as it provides a quick and efficient way of removing unwanted hairs in both small and larger areas.

Some clients do not want the hair removed, but like it to be lightened by **bleaching**. Other clients wish to have their hair permanently removed using more advanced methods such as epilation (electrolysis) or laser treatment.

Key terms

Depilation – any method of hair removal used on the body.

Think about it

In some European and Mediterranean countries, hairy bodies are considered the norm. Strong underarm hair or other body hair is not considered unattractive in women. Be careful not to be hasty with treatment advice.

Key terms

Bleaching – a method used for lightening the hair by removing or lifting the colour without penetrating the skin. This is a temporary method.

Additional knowledge

Epilation (sometimes referred to as electrolysis) is a specialist treatment at Level 3. It is permanent removal of the hair and requires considerable skill and training. A small needle is inserted into the hair follicle and a current is passed through the needle. If the hair is in the anagen phase of hair growth, the dermal papilla has the blood supply sealed, preventing a new hair from growing. Epilation is a permanent method of hair removal if the hair is in the correct growth stage. The client will need to be aware that a number of treatments may be required before all the hair is permanently removed.

Laser hair removal is usually carried out in specialist clinics rather than local salons, and treatments can be costly. As with epilation a number of treatments may be required for successful hair removal, but unlike epilation larger areas can be treated in one session. The laser treatment involves a laser beam being passed down a handheld instrument; the laser energy is converted into heat, this heat destroys the hair follicle and dermal papilla preventing the hair from regrowing. The treatment causes a slight stinging sensation, especially in sensitive areas.

Many hair-removal creams can be bought over the counter, as well as electric shavers for women and disposable razors with adapted shaving foams. These ensure that the skin is kept soft and moisturised.

Hair removal is very much a matter of personal choice and the client should be given all the information available, so an informed decision can be made. The client needs to know the various methods of hair removal available, with the advantages and disadvantages of each, and to be given the therapist's professional advice for her particular problem area, with consideration of the cost and time involved.

Abnormal hair growth

Two terms are used when talking about abnormal hair growth:

- hirsutism
- hypertrichosis.

Hirsutism

This is when the hair growth of a woman develops male characteristics; it is seen as a strong growth of a beard-like formation, the development of chest hair, and more prominent back hair. The pubic hairline can grow upwards towards the navel — all the hair growth patterns of a male. It is caused by hormone imbalances, usually a sensitivity to androgens, which are one of a group of steroid hormones secreted by the adrenal cortex (above the kidneys) and in the ovaries in small amounts.

Hypertrichosis

This is the abnormal growth of terminal hair in an area not normally seen in either sex, such as along the forehead.

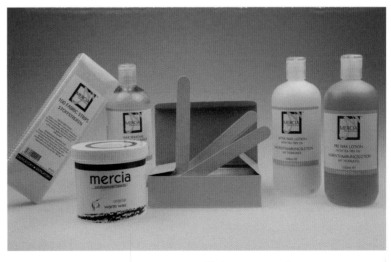

Various wax products

> **Think about it**
>
> Hair growth patterns can also depend on ethnic background. Japanese women can be virtually hairless, while women in India and Mediterranean countries often have a strong, dark hair growth.

> **Key terms**
>
> **Hirsutism** – increase of terminal hair on the body where hair is usually minimal or absent; hair growth in the male sexual pattern.
>
> **Hypertrichosis** – the abnormal growth of terminal hair.

Remove hair using waxing techniques

Key terms

Couperose – reddening of the skin associated with dilated or broken capillaries.

Wax facts

Advantages and disadvantages of the different methods of depilation and hair lightening

Method of hair removal	Advantages	Disadvantages
Warm wax	• Quick, cost-effective • Efficient over large areas • Once mastered, easy to apply	• Sticky • Can cause skin damage if reapplied over the same area • Can leave a residue, which if not fully removed can leave the client feeling sticky
Hot wax	• Good for strong hair growth • Suitable for ethnic hair types, which may have bent follicles	• Skilled technique of application may take some time to master • Because temperature control has to be accurate, application needs to be quick • Not suitable for some skin types, e.g. **couperose** skins • Can be messy when learning application
Impregnated cold wax strips	• Minimal skill needed • Less messy for home use • No specialist equipment needed • Quick	• Bruising or skin damage may occur as the strips stick to the skin and not to the hair • Painful to remove • Unsatisfactory results • Can be costly for large areas • If the hairs are not all the same length, this method may not be successful. The client would need to wait until the hairs were a similar length, as with hot or warm wax, for an effective result • If the client has bruised skin from waxing at home, this would contra-indicate a salon treatment
Strip sugaring	• As warm wax • Water soluble	• Can be less efficient than warm wax • Tricky technique to master
Manual sugaring	• Water soluble • Applied at body temperature, so less likely to burn skin • Cost-effective no paper/material strips necessary	• Difficult technique to master • More time-consuming to perform
Cutting	• Quick • No skill involved • Home treatment • No pain involved	• Short term only • Blunt regrowth, as hair removed only to skin level • Risk of cutting the skin *Effects on waxing:* Ensure that hairs are long enough to wax effectively
Shaving	• Quick • No skill involved • Home treatment • No pain • Equipment	• Suitable for all skin types • Blunt regrowth • Risk of skin damage • Not hygienic • Short term only • Only removes surface part of the hair *Effects on waxing:* Ensure that hairs are long enough to wax effectively

Method of hair removal	Advantages	Disadvantages
Tweezing	• Precise • Ideal for small areas, i.e. on the face • Equipment cheap to purchase	• Only suitable for small areas • Risk of skin damage (bruising or pinching the skin) • Breakage of hair may occur • Can be time-consuming • Not ideal as a DIY treatment for clients who wear glasses *Effects on waxing:* Can distort the hair follicle, which may cause the hair to twist and grow inwards. Also if the client wished to have epilation in the future, the hair follicle, where the needle is inserted, can become distorted, therefore epilation would not be a suitable treatment
Threading	• Cheap • No equipment needed • Suitable for Mediterranean and Asian clients as this is a common method used for many years in Asian countries • As effective as tweezing	• Skill needed to apply • Possible breakage of the hair *Effects on waxing:* Possible distortion of hair follicle, which may mean the area is unsuitable for epilation
Abrasives (mitts/pumice stones)	• No skill needed • No specialist equipment needed • Improves the skin texture as dead skin cells are shed (desquamation) • Cheap treatment for home use	• Hair breakage may occur • Hair is only removed at skin surface level • Could result in skin damage • Not terribly effective on strong-dark hair growth *Effects on waxing:* Waxing should not be undertaken directly after using an abrasive glove as the skin could be sensitised; also the hairs should be of a similar length for the treatment to be effective
Electrical appliances (e.g. electric razors, etc.)	• No skill needed • Re-usable • Ideal for home use • Clean and quick	• Only removes surface hairs • May damage the skin • Some can be expensive • Regrowth produced is blunt and stubbly *Effects on waxing:* Waxing should only be undertaken if the hairs are of the correct length. The use of electrical razors gives the same effect as shaving, where the hair is just cut off at skin level, whereas an epilator removes the hair from the root. As with all waxing treatments the result will depend on the length and the stage of hair growth
Depilatory creams	• Cheap • Quick • Ideal for home use • No skill required	• Dissolves hairs by using a chemical reaction at skin level • Some products have an unpleasant fragrance • Not suitable for allergy-prone or sensitive clients – always carry out a sensitivity test prior to use *Effects on waxing:* As with other methods, the hairs will need to grow to a suitable length if waxing is to be effective

Remove hair using waxing techniques

Method of hair removal	Advantages	Disadvantages
Bleach	• Little skill involved in application • Quick results • Suitable for facial hairs • Suitable for clients having epilation	• Not suitable for all skin types • Sensitivity test required • Not suitable for large areas, e.g. the legs • Regrowth is more noticeable when it does come through • Skin irritation can occur *Effects on waxing:* This method could be used for clients who do not wish to have waxing but are concerned by the darker hair. It can also be used between epilation treatments if the client so wishes, as to wax or tweezer the hairs would be counter-productive to the treatment
Laser treatments (including intensive pulse light)	• Can be used for large or small areas • Precise application • Suitable for most skin types	• Costly • Specialist practitioner • More than one treatment may be required • Can be painful *Effects on waxing:* If a client is having laser treatments on an area, no other method should be used while the course of treatment is being carried out as it can affect the treatment and the skin can become oversensitised
Epilation	• Precise application • Salon treatment • More than one method available to suit client requirements	• More than one treatment required • Not for clients with a needle phobia • Can be costly to clear a large area *Effects on waxing:* Waxing could be used on a client at the commencement of the treatment to attempt to put all the hairs into the first stage of hair growth (anagen) to speed up the treatment process

For your portfolio

Research hot and warm waxing products and equipment. Look at manufacturers' websites and in salon supply magazines, and evaluate which you think are the most suitable and economic products to use.

Type of wax and its working temperature (Source: Bellitas Ltd)

Properties of wax treatments

There are many excellent types of wax available, with various ingredients and different effects. Wax is classed according to its working temperature. The temperatures below are supplied courtesy of Bellitas Ltd, beauty suppliers, known for their 'Strictly Professional' waxes. Manufacturers' instructions will vary with different products, so always refer to the recommended temperatures and heating units for maximum benefit and safety.

Type of wax	Working temperature
Hot hard depilatory wax	Works best at 48–68°C
Warm soft depilatory wax	Works best at 40–43°C
Cream depilatory wax	Works best at 35–43°C
Organic wax	Organic wax varies – refer to suppliers
Cold wax	Needs no heating

Ingredients

The ingredients of a wax will determine its working temperature. The ingredients will vary from manufacturer to manufacturer, but the higher the proportion of good-quality **resin** in relation to **beeswax**, the more heat is required to get it to a manageable working consistency.

Resins are organic polymers that may be naturally occurring or synthetic. A polymer is a compound such as starch or perspex. It forms the basis for all plastics and artificial fibres. Natural resins occur in certain plants and trees. The fluid that oozes out from a wound in the plant or tree hardens into a solid resin to protect the injured part. The balsam, pine, gum and rubber tree all produce resins. The gum tree produces chewing gum resin.

Resins are used in the making of perfume, waxing and some cosmetics. Chemists can now make synthetic resins to prevent the overexploitation of plants. Large quantities of resins are produced as a by-product of the petroleum oil business, and are extracted from crude oil after it has been pumped out of the ground.

EU directive 88/379 provides information on all precautions, correct handling, storage and first aid measures.

Latest ingredient developments

Companies are incorporating rich and natural ingredients into their wax formulas to help soften and moisturise the skin. Cannabis sativa is a drug-free hemp derivative that is rich in essential fatty acids to help lock in moisture. It also has anti-inflammatory properties. For sensitive skins, tea tree wax is very soothing with antiseptic properties. Hemp wax is also very kind to a sensitive skin, and cream waxes moisturise.

Aloe vera wax has soothing, moisturising and healing properties, and is suitable for sensitive skin types. Some companies have started to add essential oils other than tea tree to their wax formulas — lavender, for example, has healing and soothing properties and has long been used to treat burns and irritations.

Types of wax

Hard depilatory wax

What is it?

It is a solid wax, sold in pellet form, which becomes molten when heated.

What is it made of?

It is a mixture of natural resins, beeswax and microcrystalline wax. Insoluble in cold water, this wax is quite soluble when hot. It has a low chemical reactivity and is stable.

What are the hazards?

Hard wax is classed as non-hazardous if used in correct professional circumstances.

What are the first aid measures?

- If used at the correct temperature and with the correct procedure for hair removal, this wax poses no hazard.
- High temperatures should be avoided, as these will cause thermal burns.
- If an overheated wax has solidified on the skin, leave it in place and consult a doctor.

> **Key terms**
>
> **Resin** – a substance used in wax products; can be solid or semi-solid, natural or synthetic.
>
> **Beeswax** – natural wax product produced by bees; used in wax preparations for its emollient properties.

Remove hair using waxing techniques

425

◉ If wax enters the eyes, they should be flushed immediately with water for 15 minutes and medical attention obtained.

What are the fire-fighting measures?

◉ This wax is stable, but it has a flash point greater than 220°C. Make sure that the thermostat controlling the temperature on the heater is working.

◉ Although not strictly classed as flammable, this wax will burn. Avoid contact with flammable fabrics, e.g. placing near curtains.

◉ In the event of a small fire, foam, carbon dioxide, dry chemical powder, sand or earth may be used to extinguish it. For a large fire, use foam or water spray.

What do I do in the event of an accident?

◉ In the event of a large spillage, any wax entering the drains will solidify and cause blockages. The local health authority will need to be notified if this happens.

◉ Allow spilt hot wax to cool and solidify, then scrape up for disposal.

How do I store it?

◉ Hard depilatory waxes can be kept for up to six months in tightly closed jars in cool dry conditions, away from possible sources of contamination.

How do I handle it?

◉ Adequate protective clothing must be worn when handling wax in a molten state.

◉ It is recommended that advice be sought from the individual Awarding Body and professional organisation that is favoured by your training establishment.

◉ To ignore their recommended guidelines may invalidate any assessments taking place, but more importantly may remove insurance protection. (Refer to You, your client and the law in Professional skills, pages 42–64.)

Warm wax

What is it?

This is a soft, thick liquid. It may vary in colour from warm honey to amber or light brown.

Soft wax is supplied in a tin or plastic tub, which fits into a special heating unit.

There are many soft waxes on the market and it is recommended that the wax be heated only in the correct heater, following the manufacturer's instructions, as the temperatures for best performance may vary slightly.

What is it made of?

It is composed mainly of refined gum resin and hydrocarbon tackifiers. This gives the wax its sticking properties.

What are the hazards?

Warm wax is classed as non-hazardous if used in correct professional circumstances.

What are the first aid measures?

◉ If used at the correct temperature and with the correct procedure for hair removal, this wax poses no hazard.

◉ High temperatures should be avoided, as this will cause thermal burns.

◉ If overheated wax has solidified on the skin, leave it in place and consult a doctor.

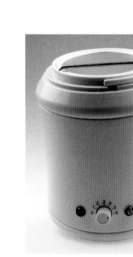

A warm wax heater

- If in contact with the eyes, irrigate immediately with large quantities of cold water for at least five minutes. Obtain medical attention.

- If inhaled, move the person away from exposure to fumes from molten products. If irritation persists, obtain medical attention.

- If ingested, no special treatment is necessary.

- If accidental skin contact with the heated product occurs, cool the affected area by plunging it into cold running water for at least ten minutes. Do not remove the adhering material. Obtain medical attention. If a limb is completely surrounded by wax, the wax should be split to avoid a **tourniquet** effect.

- If skin contact with the cold product occurs, wash thoroughly with soap and water.

What are the fire-fighting measures?

- Although not strictly classed as flammable, soft wax will burn above 200°C. Avoid contact with flammable fabrics, e.g. placing near the curtains. Ensure that the thermostat on the heating unit is in working order by regularly maintaining the equipment.

- In the event of a small fire, use carbon dioxide, dry powders or foam.

- Do not use water on soft wax.

What do I do in the event of an accident?

- When soft wax is molten, care must be taken to prevent burns by ensuring that application temperatures are kept to the minimum necessary for adequate product performance.

- At no time is it necessary to heat the product above 60°C.

- Ensure good ventilation in the working environment.

- Where accidental overheating occurs the source of heat should be disconnected and the molten product left undisturbed until cool. Make sure that all persons are aware of the potential hazard.

How do I store it?

Soft wax may be maintained as a cool liquid within its own container, or heated within the unit on a daily basis. It may keep for up to six months in cool dry conditions.

How do I handle it?

- Handle in the same way as for hard wax.

- Adequate protective clothing must be worn when handling wax in a molten state.

- It is recommended that advice be sought from the individual Awarding Body and professional organisation that is favoured by your training establishment.

- To ignore their recommended guidelines may invalidate any assessments taking place, but more importantly may remove insurance protection. (Refer to You, your client and the law in Professional skills, pages 42–64.)

- Soft waxes are unlikely to cause any environmental hazards, but do remember that all waxes are generally non-biodegradable in the short term.

Key terms

Tourniquet – tight bandage around a limb, which cuts off the blood supply to the area.

For your portfolio

Research products other than azulene that are often found in cream wax.

Remove hair using waxing techniques

427

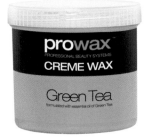

Cream wax

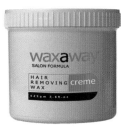

Cold wax

Cream waxes

Many manufacturers now produce a good quality cream wax. Cream wax contains ingredients such as moisturisers and azulene that help the skin's condition. Azulene is anti-inflammatory and soothing, and is suitable for more sensitive skin types. (Azulene is the ingredient that will turn the cream a blue colour.)

Cream wax also works on slightly lower melting and working temperatures, thereby enhancing client comfort during waxing.

Cream wax has enhanced sticking properties, which means that it can be spread thinly and is thus very economical to use.

Refer to the warm waxing information on the previous page.

Organic waxes

Organic waxes are very popular as they contain natural ingredients such as honey as well as the chemical ingredients they need to keep them stable. Organic waxes do not set when cold but become very liquid when heated.

Cold waxes

Some cold waxes, such as pre-coated wax strips, are available over the counter; others are supplied to salons by the manufacturer.

Retail strips

- These can be purchased from most large chemists and come in packs of 6–10 strips.
- They are usually made by the companies that produce hair-removal creams.
- The pre-coated strips are double layered — one piece of wax paper is a non-stick backing strip from which the coated strip peels away to be placed on the skin.
- They contain hydrocarbon resins so are sticky, but as they are cold, the adhering properties are not as effective as warm or hot wax.
- Most manufacturers recommend the strips be warmed between the hands before splitting and applying.
- The wax coating is quite fine and may not be sufficient to grip strong hair growth, so the strips are only suitable for light growth. They are not normally recommended for facial use, elderly people, diabetics and people with skin irritations.
- They can be used as a stopgap for quick removal of a light growth between waxing, and for special occasions should the client not be able to visit for warm waxing.
- Follow instructions on the individual packaging.

Roller waxing

Many manufacturers provide complete systems with disposable roll-on heads. These are proving very popular in salons and with therapists offering a mobile beauty therapy service. This system is suitable for warm wax application.

The applicators look a little like a roll-on deodorant stick, and come in various roller head sizes for different parts of the body. They can be disposed of after use. Alternatively, the head can be stored in a sealed bag and only used on a specific client to prevent cross-contamination occurring. Otherwise, refill cartridges can be used and the head attachments taken off for cleaning and sterilisation. The applicators are heated in a specially designed self-contained heating cabinet, which is portable and easy to clean. City & Guilds will require candidates to have knowledge of, and use, this equipment as part of their criteria for assessment.

Other products used in waxing

Pre-waxing lotion

What is it?

This is a cleansing lotion applied to the area before treatment to cleanse and remove any grease or dirt on the skin that may prevent good hair removal.

What is it made of?

The product usually contains ethanol and camphor oil in a cosmetic lotion. The ethanol is an alcohol for cleansing, and the camphor has antibacterial and anti-inflammatory properties as well as being antiviral. It is also a counter-irritant.

What are the hazards?

If used properly, this product has no hazards.

What are the first aid measures?

- If ingested, drink milk or water.
- If it goes into the eyes, wash well with water. If irritation persists, seek medical advice.

What do I do in the event of an accident?

If spillage occurs, clean up with an absorbent material, then wash with detergent and water to avoid a slippery floor.

How do I store and handle it?

No special precautions are considered necessary.

Purified talc or talc-free alternatives

Purified talc or talc-free products are products that contain no additives or fragrance. They are used to prevent allergies and respiratory conditions when used regularly.

What is it?

It is a dry powder that is used as a light dusting over the area to be waxed. It ensures the hairs have a covering for the wax to adhere to and that the hairs stand away from the skin.

What are the hazards?

All dry powders can give respiratory problems if precautions are ignored and they are inhaled. Avoid excessive use, especially near the nose and mouth.

This product is non-flammable.

What are the first aid measures?

- If ingested, drink milk or water.
- If inhaled, move the person to the fresh air and keep her warm.
- Avoid prolonged skin contact as this can lead to dry skin.
- If it goes into the eyes, wash well with water.

What do I do in the event of an accident?

Sweep or vacuum up the powder, avoiding dust.

How do I store and handle it?

Store in a cool, dry place, keeping containers tightly sealed.

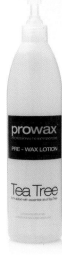

Pre-waxing lotion

After-wax lotion

What is it?

This is a soothing lotion used after treatment to help cool and calm the skin and prevent irritation.

What is it made of?

The product contains an emulsion of oils, waxes, water, water-soluble ingredients, emulsifiers, fragrance and preservatives.

What are the hazards?

If used properly, this product has no hazards.

What are the first aid measures?

- If ingested, drink milk or water.
- If it goes into the eyes, wash well with water. If irritation persists, seek medical advice.

What do I do in the event of an accident?

If spillage occurs, clean up with an absorbent material, then wash with detergent and water to avoid a slippery floor.

How do I store and handle it?

No special precautions are considered necessary.

Wax equipment cleaner

What is it?

This is a liquid with a very strong smell!

What is it made of?

It is a hydrocarbon solvent and a very powerful cleaner.

What are the hazards?

It is highly flammable and is hazardous. It should not be used in an enclosed space as the fumes are highly noxious.

What are the first aid measures?

- If it goes into the eyes, irrigate immediately with large quantities of cold water for at least five minutes. Obtain medical attention.
- Do not inhale as this may cause dizziness. If it is inhaled, move to fresh air.
- If ingested, drink plenty of milk or water.
- Avoid prolonged contact with the skin. If irritation occurs, seek medical advice.

What are the fire-fighting measures?

The cleaner is highly flammable. Evacuate the area and inform fire-fighters of the hazards.

What do I do in the event of an accident?

- Clean the contaminated area with lots of detergent and water to avoid slippery floors.
- Do not absorb on to combustible material such as a tissue.

How do I store it?

Store in a cool place away from direct sunlight. Large quantities should be kept in a fire-resistant store.

Benefits and effects of waxing

Type of wax	Benefits	Effects	Possible drawbacks
Hot wax	As hot wax needs to be heated to a high temperature it is extremely effective on strong hair growth.	The solid wax turns into a liquid when heated and when applied to the skin, it coats the hairs, gripping them firmly. The wax is applied with a disposable spatula in a thick layer. A lip of wax is then lifted to allow a firm hold to take the whole patch off.	Only really suitable on longer hair growth – results not good if the hair is shorter. Hot wax may cause a slight skin reaction, so not suitable for sensitive skin, or sensitive areas. Application is a skill that needs a lot of practice to master. The wax needs to be applied quite thickly, so it can be quite costly in materials. Wax should not be applied over the same area twice, as the skin may burn. Can be messy to apply so it is hard to keep the equipment clean. These considerations need to be thought about when choosing hot wax.
Warm wax	More comfortable on sensitive skins than hot wax, and can be reapplied over the same area. Even short hairs can be successfully removed with warm wax. The equipment is easy to maintain and keep clean.	Warm wax is applied with a disposable spatula, in a very thin coating and a fabric or paper strip is applied over the top of the wax for easy removal – rather like a plaster coming off. The wax and hairs adhere to the strip. A single strip can be used over again until it reaches saturation point.	There is some risk of infection, as loose skin cells may also be lost during waxing, leaving hair follicles open to infection. As the wax is applied quite finely, it may not remove all strong growth in one go. Strips have to be used with warm wax, and may add to the cost of the treatment if not used economically.
Cold wax	This treatment can be done at home for a top-up treatment, and is therefore convenient.	Hairs are removed by an impregnated strip, with no heat.	Not very economical if using on large areas as lots of strips will have to be purchased. Not suitable on large areas of strong hair growth. As it can be applied to oneself, there is more pain and discomfort than when a trained therapist does it. For self-administration the angle of removal may not be correct for a swift, clean taking off, and that may be another reason for it to hurt.
Roller wax	Very little possibility of cross-contamination from the rollers. Very quick, clean and easy to use. Very economical. Safe – no possibility of spillage as the wax is contained within the cartridge.	Precise application of the wax can be achieved because there is a variety of roller head sizes, allowing more accuracy.	Very few, except that the initial outlay may be high for purchase of the heaters and cartridges. The units are specially made to fit each manufacturer's make of cartridge and therefore are not interchangeable if the type of wax proves to be unsuitable.

Remove hair using waxing techniques

Suitability of hair removal products for different parts of the body

Method	Eyebrows	Facial hair	Legs	Bikini line	Forearms
Warm wax	✓	✓	✓	✓	✓
Hot wax	✓ Depends on skin sensitivity	✓ Depends on skin sensitivity	✓	✓	✓
Sugaring	✓	✓	✓	✓	✓
Hair removal creams	✓ Care required	✓	✓	✓	✓
Tweezing	✓	✓	✓ Only for stray hairs after depilation	✓ Only for stray hairs after depilation	✓ Only for stray hairs after depilation
Mechanical depilators	✗	✗	✓	✓	✓
Cutting/shaving	✗ Only to shorten brows	✓	✓	✓	✓
Shaving	✗	✗	✓	✓	✗
Creams – using any depilatory cream will depend on the results of a skin sensitivity test.	✗	✓	✓	✓	✓
Epilation – more suited to smaller areas.	✓	✓	✗	Could be used for smaller area.	✗
Laser – use will depend on skin sensitivity and pigment of the hair.	Due to goggles being worn, this area is not usually covered. Often between brows and above the brow line.	✓	✓	✓	✓

Waxing at a glance

	Legs	Eyebrows	Upper lip	Armpits	Brazilian	Bikini
Waxing facts	Waxing really does slow down the hair growth after several treatments.	Waxing gives a nice clean finish to the eyebrows – any stray hairs can be tweezed out.	A good way of getting a tidy upper lip with no shadow. It does hurt but the result is really clean.	Hot wax is still the favourite for underarm hair – several strips may be needed if the hair growth is circular or in different directions.	This does not render you completely bare between the legs (that's a Hollywood). A thin strip of hair is left, so thongs can be worn. Often called the landing strip.	You can keep underwear on for this as they become the guide line for your treatment.
How long it takes	Half leg 30 mins; full leg including bikini 45–60 mins	10 mins	5 mins	10 mins	15–20 mins	5 mins
How long it lasts	4–5 weeks depending on hair growth	3–4 weeks	About 3 weeks	2–3 weeks	4 weeks	4 weeks
Pain ratio	5/10	8/10	9/10	8/10	10/10	7/10

Additional knowledge

Bleach can be used to lighten hair instead of removing it. It is suitable for clients who wish to avoid waxing or as a temporary solution between treatments. A sensitivity test should be carried out before use.

Conducting a skin sensitivity test

A sensitivity test should be carried out on a clean, dry area of skin, usually on the forearm as this is hair free. Consult with your own Awarding Organisation and professional therapies federation, as they may insist you carry out a sensitivity test on the area you are treating. The test should always be carried out at least 24 hours prior to the treatment and recorded on the client record card.

Having heated the correct type of wax to be used for the client, test it on yourself for the correct temperature, then apply a small circle of wax to the client's forearm. Remove as for hair removal and note any immediate reaction on the skin.

Put the details on to the client's record card and ask her to monitor the result for the next 24–48 hours.

You must be tactful when informing the client that she is not suitable for treatment if there is an adverse reaction to the sensitivity test. Be discreet, too, and tell her somewhere private, rather than in the middle of reception where everyone can hear.

Warm wax and roller wax operate at much lower temperatures than hot wax, so an alternative product might prevent a reaction from occurring. Another sensitivity test will be required using the different product. If that proves satisfactory, and the client is happy, then the treatment can go ahead.

Establishing hair growth pattern before application

The direction of your wax application will depend upon the way the hair is growing, which varies in different areas of the body.

Closely examine the direction of the hair, from the point where it comes out of the skin to its tip. Always work in the direction of the hair growth and you will get great results.

The legs

Most hair on the front of the leg along the shins grows downwards towards the foot. However, the hair along the calf muscle (gastrocnemius) often starts to grow across the leg, going sideways and downwards. This is often dictated by the pressure of clothing on the hairs.

Along the top of the thigh the hair starts to grow inwards towards the inner thigh, but the bikini line tends to grow down and inwards.

Think about it

If a reaction occurs, it will be noticeable as redness in the area of the sensitivity test, which may also be itchy. This will indicate either that the wax type is unsuitable for the client, or that waxing cannot take place at all.

Think about it

Not all methods of hair removal are suitable for all clients. A full consultation will be needed to establish which method is suitable and agreeable to you both. Remember a sensitivity test would be advisable to people with sensitive skin.

Think about it

A good tip to pass on to the client who has booked for a waxing treatment is to take a couple of over-the-counter pain killers prior to the treatment. This helps to block the pain killing nerve endings in the skin, therefore the treatment will be less painful. The pain killers must be ones the client has used before with no adverse reactions.

a) front of legs   b) back of legs

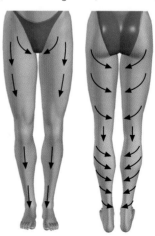

Direction of hair growth on the legs

Remove hair using waxing techniques

433

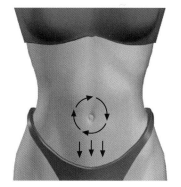

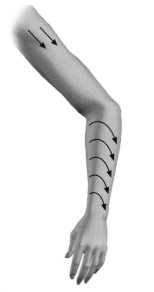

Hair growth pattern on abdomen

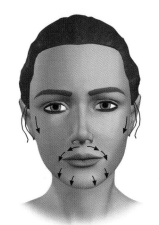

Direction of hair growth on the arm

Direction of hair growth on the face

The abdomen

The hair around the navel grows upwards from the pubic hairline, and then forms a circle around the navel. You may need several small strips to completely remove the circular pattern. Be careful if the client is menstruating – she may wish to avoid the area because of pressure. Do not wax a client on the abdomen if there is a possibility she may be pregnant.

The arm

The hair on the forearm tends to grow sideways across the arms, rather than downwards towards the hand and wrist. It usually grows from the inner to the outer sides.

Underarm hair varies – some clients have perfect circles of hair around the pit of the arm, some have downward hair and some have hair growing sideways. Very often more than one strip is required to remove underarm hair.

The face

Hair on the upper lip tends to grow in the male pattern of a moustache, that is downwards from the nose towards the upper lip, with some longer hairs growing down on the side of the lip.

Chin hairs often grow straight outward or down, depending on the strength of the hair.

Using methods of application correctly

Check this list before you apply the wax.

- Is the working area fully prepared and the wax pre-heated?
- Are you fully prepared with protective clothing and gloves?
- Have all safety and hygiene precautions been observed?
- Are the manufacturer's instructions being adhered to?
- Has a full consultation been carried out?
- Can the treatment proceed with no contra-indications present?
- Has a sensitivity test been carried out before the treatment?
- Has the client had a full explanation of the treatment so she knows what to expect?
- Has the client been fully informed with regard to aftercare and home care?
- Has a record card been filled out for the client, or the existing one updated?
- Has the area for waxing been examined in a good light and the best method of waxing decided and agreed between the therapist and client?
- Has the area to be waxed been cleaned so it is grease-free, has it been talced, and has pre-wax lotion been applied?

My story

The importance of good waxing techniques

Hi, my name is Martine. When I left college, waxing was the treatment I really enjoyed doing, and the salon I worked for had a lot of regular waxing clients. As many of the clientele wanted intimate waxing, the manager sent me on a course to learn the correct techniques to use. It was a little strange at first, but I soon mastered the different methods. The course made me aware of what could occur when treating clients in this delicate area. I now feel confident and have many regular clients. It's worth remembering that if you are not properly trained, your insurance will be invalid.

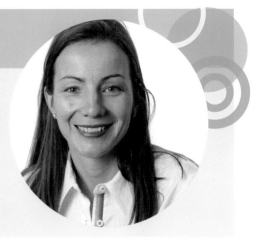

Health and safety

Health and safety information for the different types of waxes used in a salon is included on pages 425–30, along with potential hazards and first aid measures.

Refer to You, your client and the law in Professional skills, pages 42–64, for legislation affecting all beauty treatments.

Below are general precautions for safe practice when waxing.

- Do not have any naked flames near waxing preparations or equipment as the ingredients make them very inflammable.
- Do not have heating units near anything flammable, e.g. curtains, in case the thermostat breaks and the wax ignites.
- Do not have the heater on a glass-topped trolley, in case the glass breaks and molten wax spills.
- Do a thorough consultation, check for contra-indications and carry out a sensitivity test prior to treating the client.
- Firmly stretch and support the skin in fleshy areas to avoid bruising, especially in the bikini and underarm areas.
- Be aware of your own professional guidelines regarding insurance cover and the use of gloves and protective clothing.
- Thorough moisturising after waxing can help to avoid the problems of ingrown hairs, which is when the hair grows back under the skin causing infection. This is always a problem with continual waxing.
- When hot waxing, never allow the wax to become too cool on the skin as it will be too brittle to remove effectively, and may cause the client a great deal of discomfort.
- With hot wax always test the temperature on yourself and carry out a small patch test on the client to avoid giving a burn.
- With organic wax do not allow too much of a build-up on the muslin strip as this can cause undue lifting of the skin during removal.
- With organic wax it is important to keep the angle of pull on the muslin strip horizontal to the skin's surface, as the hairs can break off at the skin's surface and bruising can occur in fleshy areas.

Think about it

Follow all electrical precautions: ensure there are no trailing wires to fall over, carry out regular maintenance checks for efficient and safe working of machines, follow manufacturers' instructions and follow health and safety guidelines.

A thin layer of wax is more effective than a thick layer on a strip. Too much wax builds up on itself and does not coat the hairs. It is therefore less effective.

For maximum comfort and minimum embarrassment give the client lots of towels to protect her modesty, especially with a bikini wax. Plenty of protection will make the client feel more secure and means that the therapist can manoeuvre her into good positions for easy and effective removal. Ensure that the waxing area has adequate ventilation, especially with hot wax, which can give off fumes when first heated.

Safe working practices for hot and warm wax equipment

Refer to Follow health and safety practice in the salon and Professional skills to make sure your own actions reduce risks to health and safety. As a therapist you should ensure that you follow health and safety legislation and salon rules and procedures when carrying out a treatment. All therapists should follow the Habia code of practice for waxing and adhere to their professional body's code of ethics for professional practice. Therapists should also be insured to carry out treatments and follow manuacturers' directives and COSHH regulations relating to the products they use.

Remember: As a therapist you are not insured to carry out intimate waxing treatments unless you are suitably qualified.

Applying and removing the product

Leg wax

The lower leg is a simple area to treat as the hair growth can be seen easily. The hairs usually grow towards the ankle on the front of the leg but may go slightly sideways on the calf. Hair growth may be coarse if the client has shaved the area and results are usually good as the hair growth in the area is strong. Moving the leg around slightly will allow access to the ankle hair if the growth pattern is not straight down. The client may ask for the toes to be waxed too.

1   The client can be lying down, or sitting up for the front of the legs. Remember, though, to put the couch back into a flat position before the client is turned over for the backs of the legs.

2   It is important that the client's clothing is protected, so provide a towel for cover. Be aware of protecting the client's modesty if repositioning is required.

3   Cleanse the area and prepare for waxing following the usual sanitising procedure.

4   Start from the ankle and work up the leg systematically.

5   To keep the skin taut at the knee, ask the client to bend it.

6   Turn the client over (lowering the couch) and follow the same routine with the back of the leg. Pay special attention to the hair growth, which may not be straight down.

7   Do not apply wax to the back of the knee. There are usually no hairs present here, but if there are a few, then tweeze them.

8   If completing a full leg wax continue up the thigh at the front and then turn the client over, again paying attention to the direction of growth.

Step-by-step warm wax application for legs

1 Clean the whole area to be waxed with a suitable antiseptic cleanser on damp cotton wool.

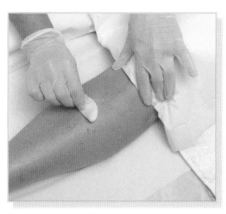

2 Blot the area with a tissue to ensure the skin is dry and grease-free.

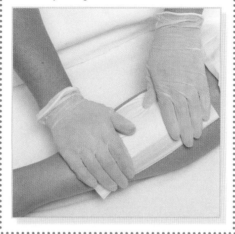

3 Test the wax on your inner arm to make certain you will not burn the client.

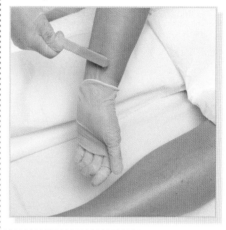

4 To avoid cross-infection drizzle the wax on to another spatula — it will also help you to check that the consistency is workable.

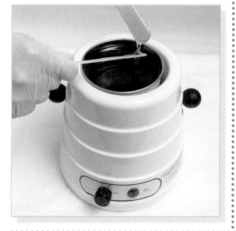

5 If the temperature is acceptable to you, apply a small area on to the legs to check with the client that the temperature is tolerable for her.

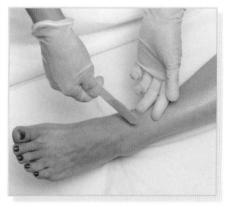

6 Following the hair growth, i.e. downward, apply a thin even strip of wax to the leg, approximately the width of the paper strip.

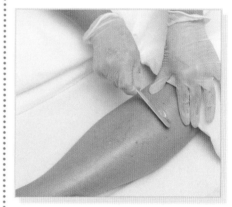

7 Press down firmly over the wax strip, to ensure all the hairs are fully attached to the strip.

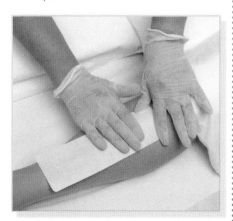

8 Peel back a small edge of the strip to hold on to.

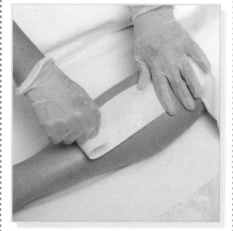

9 Holding the leg, grip the wax strip edge and pull the strip off. It is almost a peeling back of the strip, but it must be quick, to minimise pain.

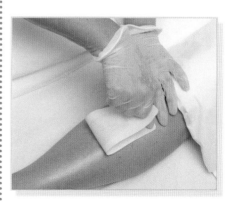

Remove hair using waxing techniques

10 Any missed hairs, too short for the wax to pick up, can be tweezed out. Sterilise the tweezers first.

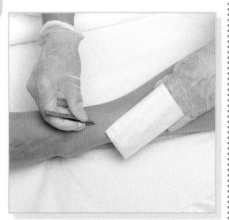

11 After-wax lotion will remove any wax residue.

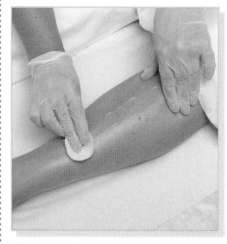

12 The finished result should be a moisturised, hair-free front of leg.

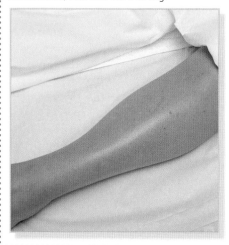

13 Ask the client to turn over — remember to ensure you put the back of the couch down first. Repeat the cleansing and blotting process.

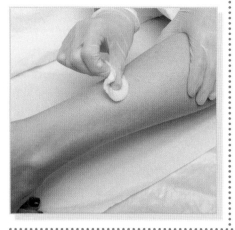

14 As the hairs grow in different directions, you will need to cut the wax strips into manageable sizes.

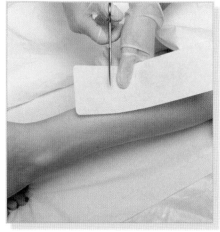

15 Check the direction of the hair growth, which may be diagonal as shown here. Remember to test the wax again — first on yourself and then on your client.

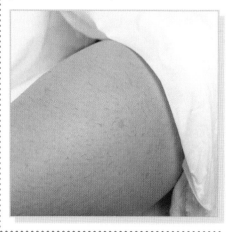

16 Apply a thin even strip of wax to the leg, following the hair growth, i.e. diagonally as shown here, and repeat the process as for front of leg.

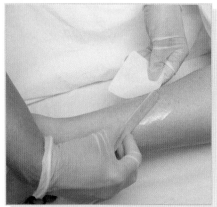

Think about it

Check with your own professional body with regard to the use of spatulas. Most state that once a spatula has come into contact with the skin, it has become contaminated and should be thrown away and a new one used for the next application. Refer to Habia codes of practice for waxing.

Note: Some Awarding Organisations only expect gloves to be worn if there is a danger of drawing bodily fluids, for example, underarm or bikini line. Therefore, it may be permissible to wax legs without gloves.

Warm wax is applied in a thin film using a spatula in the direction of hair growth with a firm press, without hurting the client.

1   Test the wax prior to use on the inside of the wrist. If it is at a comfortable temperature for the therapist, it should be fine for the client, but also test a small patch on the wrist or ankle of the client depending upon the area to be waxed.

2   Take up a manageable amount of wax on the spatula and twist it so that it stays on the end. Remove any excess on the side of the pot. In the other hand have a folded tissue covering the palm to catch any drips from the spatula and any spillage during the transfer from pot to client.

3   Transfer the wax onto the skin following the hair growth, holding the spatula at a 90-degree angle, and spread a strip-sized width of wax on to the hairs. (As skill levels increase and practice is gained, you will be able to apply and quickly remove longer strips.) Support the skin with the free hand.

4   Firmly press the fabric or paper strip and rub down several times to bond the wax to the hairs in the direction of the hair growth. Leave a small flap free at the end of the strip with which to grip the strip for removal.

5   Using the flap, grip firmly, stretch the skin slightly with the free hand and pull the strip away from the skin, going back against the hair growth, with the strip almost going back on itself, in one swift movement. Try not to lift upward as that may cause skin damage. The swiftness of the hand really does make a difference to the pain the client will feel. Do not hesitate, or stop halfway through, as that is just prolonging the agony.

6   Apply a little pressure to the area with your hand to help reduce the tingling and pain, which occurs after strip removal.

7   Work in a logical sequence over the whole area to be treated taking care not to miss any hairs, but avoid overlapping the strips as that will mean the skin may be sore in that area.

8   The strip will last for several removals before it becomes too laden with wax to pick up any more hairs. When that stage is reached, fold the wax strip in on itself so that the clean side is on the outside and place it in the bin with a liner that is designated for contaminated waste. Use a fresh strip for the next removal and continue.

9   After the waxing is complete, if any stubborn, stray hairs remain, they should be tweezed out with a sterile pair of tweezers. With warm wax it may be possible to reapply a strip over an area with lots of hairs remaining, as there is little skin reaction at low temperatures. This is not advisable with the higher temperature of hot wax.

10 Apply after-wax lotion liberally and go over aftercare with the client.

11 Clearing up can now take place. This is as important as the rest of the treatment as cross-infection can occur through the contaminated waste. Dispose of used spatulas, wax strips, gloves and couch roll in the appropriate bags (unless the strips are to be used again).

12 Clean the equipment with the recommended manufacturer's cleaner and clean the plastic couch covering. Wash hands and begin with the next client.

Remove hair using waxing techniques

Step-by-step warm wax application for eyebrows

1 Cover the closed eye with a damp cotton wool round and cleanse the eyebrow area with suitable cleanser. Cut up some small pieces of paper or material strips.

2 Decant petroleum jelly onto a spatula, using a covered orange stick; apply to hairs you do not want to remove. This barrier stops the wax sticking to the hairs.

3 Remember to test the wax on your forearm, before applying to the client. You do not want to burn the delicate eye area.

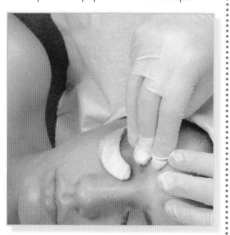
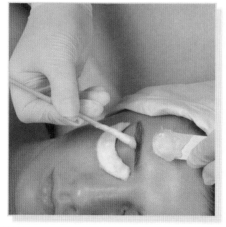
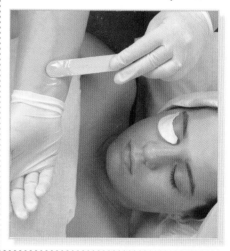

4 Apply a small amount of wax to the area under the eyebrow, working in the direction of the hair growth. Take care not to dribble wax on to the client's face.

5 Using a small piece of wax strip, press on to the arch, under the eyebrow. Smooth over with your finger, to ensure all of the hairs are stuck to the strip.

6 Stretch the eyebrow. Remove hairs against the hair growth, that is working inwards towards nose. The movement needs to be quick to avoid pain, and it is like peeling back on the strip. Apply after-wax lotion.

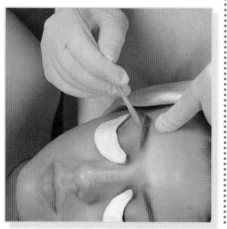
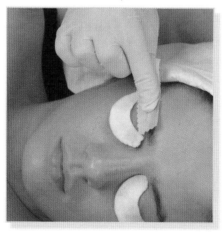
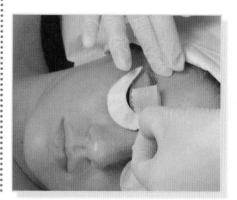

1 Cleanse the eyebrow area, having removed make-up, and follow all the usual sanitising procedures.

2 Cut a large wax strip into smaller manageable strips.

3 Discuss the shape required with the client taking into account face shape and the direction of hair growth.

4 Apply a suitable barrier cream to the hairs not being removed – this will prevent the wax adhering to them and avoid accidental total eyebrow removal.

5 Apply a small amount of wax to the hairs being removed, following the direction of hair growth (an orange stick may be a more suitably sized applicator than a spatula).

6 Press the small strip firmly to the skin.

7 Remove the strip against the hair growth and continue to shape the eyebrow as required.

8 Use a hand mirror to consult the client at every stage, and be flexible to client suggestions.

9 Follow aftercare and home care routines.

Step-by-step warm wax application for the lip and chin

1 Cleanse the upper lip area. The skin should be clean and grease-free. Blot if necessary.

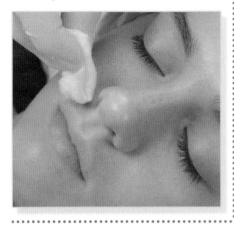

2 Decant petroleum jelly onto a spatula, using a covered orange stick, and cover the lip up to the lip line.

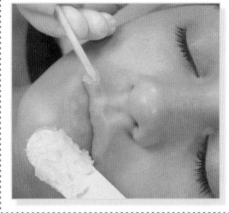

3 Remember to test the wax on your forearm, before applying to the client.

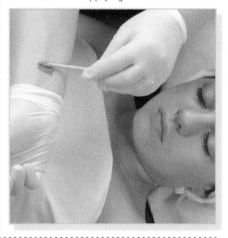

4 Carry out a sensitivity test. Use a small drop of wax near the area, to test the temperature is acceptable to the client.

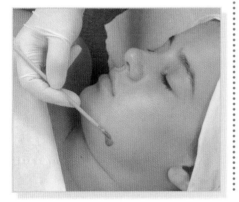

5 Build up a good layer of wax on upper lip. Ask the client to smile slightly to help stretch the skin. Remove as for warm wax application and apply after-wax lotion.

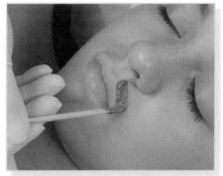

6 The finished result.

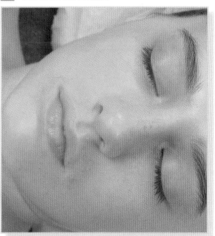

Lip wax

- Cleanse the area and follow the usual sanitising procedures.
- Protect the upper lip with barrier cream.
- Apply wax to one side of the upper lip using a small spatula or orange stick and following the hair growth.
- Apply and remove a small strip back on itself, pulling the skin as taut as possible but being careful of the nose.
- Repeat on the other side.
- Being careful not to re-wax the sides, apply wax to the centre panel working down to the centre of the lip.
- Apply aftercare and discuss home care routines.

Chin wax

- Remove make-up and cleanse the area, following normal sanitising procedures.
- If the hairs are very long, trim with scissors, but not too short for waxing.

> **Think about it**
>
> Do not to press too hard on the jaw area, especially if the client is wearing dentures.

Remove hair using waxing techniques

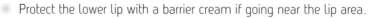

- Protect the lower lip with a barrier cream if going near the lip area.
- Apply the wax following the hair growth.
- Stretch the area and remove the hair with a small strip against the hair growth, keeping the skin as taut as possible. The client can help by jutting out the lower jaw and placing the tongue over the lower teeth.
- Repeat until all hairs are removed.

Step-by-step warm wax application for the bikini and thigh area

1 The client should be in a reclined position with either a pillow for support or resting the leg on the couch.

2 Pay special attention to both client modesty (provide a towel) and protecting the client's undergarments with tissues or couch roll.

3 If the hair growth is long, trim with scissors, but not too short.

4 Hold the skin tight when applying the wax. If the area is fleshy, the client may help by stretching the leg as wide as possible.

5 Pay attention to hair growth patterns. Several directional strips may need to be applied rather than one big one.

Think about it

Make the client aware that as the hair in this area is strong terminal hair, there may be blood spotting, and that it is not unusual for this reaction to occur. Cold compresses can be applied and careful aftercare and home care must be adhered to.

1 Protect the edge of the client's underwear with couch roll. You can avoid embarrassment by asking the client to tuck the couch roll in.

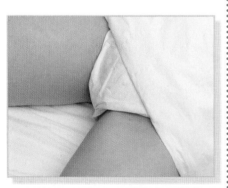

2 Clean the area with suitable cleanser, leaving the skin clean, dry and grease-free.

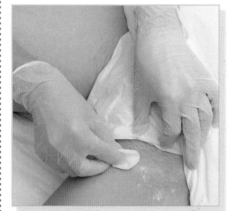

3 After testing the temperature on yourself, apply the wax with the hair growth, in a firm pressing motion. Usually this is a downward direction towards the inner thigh.

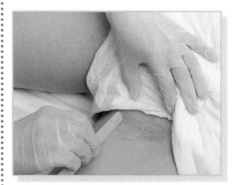

4 Apply the wax strip and press onto the hairs. Ask the client to help stretch the skin, to minimise pain, and remove the wax strip against the direction of hair growth.

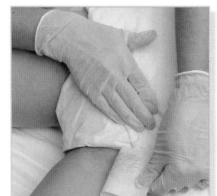

5 Should any blood spots appear, apply light pressure with a clean tissue and then wipe them away. Apply after-wax lotion.

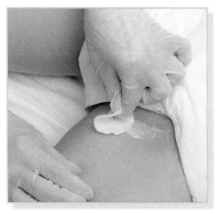

Forearm

1 Apply wax following the hair growth pattern.

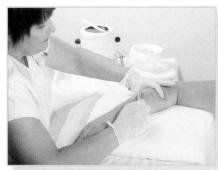

2 Press wax strip firmly onto arm, stretching the skin.

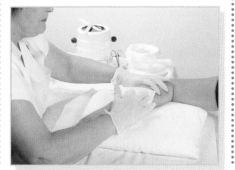

3 Remove against the hair growth, stretching the skin.

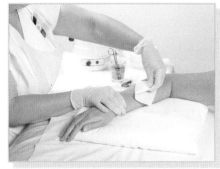

1 The client can be semi-reclined, or if this is the only area of the body to be waxed, the client could sit opposite the therapist across the couch.

2 If the client's sleeves are rolled up, remember to protect the clothing.

3 Follow the usual pre-wax preparation and cleansing routine.

4 Wax is applied in the same way as on other parts of the body; that is, following hair growth.

5 The skin can be kept taut by grasping the underside of the skin not being worked upon.

6 Follow aftercare and home care routines.

Step-by-step warm wax application for underarms

1 Protect the client's clothing with couch roll and cleanse the area. A light dusting of talcum powder or talc-free product will absorb any residue perspiration and make the hair stand out from the skin.

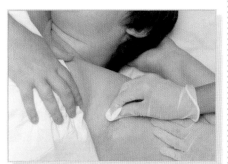

2 After testing on yourself, apply the wax, going with the hair growth. If hairs are diagonal, then go in that direction.

3 Firmly press the strip down to bond the hairs to it.

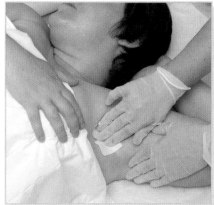

4 Stretch the armpit area and, if necessary, ask the client to help, with her free hand. Grip the edge of the strip and quickly and firmly remove the strip against the direction of hair growth.

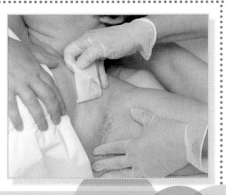

5 Should any blood spots appear, apply light pressure with a clean tissue and then wipe them away. Apply after-wax lotion.

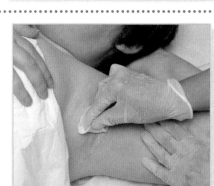

Remove hair using waxing techniques

Area	Time
Eyebrows	15 minutes
Facial (lip and chin)	10 minutes per area
Full leg	45 minutes
Half leg (up to knee)	30 minutes
Underarm	15 minutes
Bikini	15 minutes
Forearm (wrist to elbow)	20 minutes (not a prescribed range)

Treatment time guide for warm wax in line with the VRQ guidelines

1   The client's armpit should be stretched and extended as far as possible.

2   The client should be in a semi-reclining position or flat down on the couch, depending upon client preference.

3   Follow the standard procedures for cleansing and hygiene.

4   Study the hair growth carefully as underarm hair can be very diverse in its growth, and some underarm hair can grow in circles.

5   Small strips should be used, and the hair may need trimming before treatment.

6   Remember to protect the bra with couch roll or tissues.

7   The skin can be extremely delicate and there is a danger that infection may occur, causing glands to swell.

8   Never treat the underarm if mastitis is suspected.

9   Aftercare and home care are extremely important for underarm treatment.

The above is a guide only – the time it takes to complete a wax treatment will depend upon the amount of hair growth, how strong the growth is, and how experienced the therapist is. In time and with experience, timings can greatly improve as the confidence and judgement of the therapist improves.

However, it is important to remember to be cost-effective when waxing with both time and use of materials.

Hot wax application

Hot wax application is a skill that needs more practice than warm waxing, but many beauty therapists trained in hot wax prefer to use it. As the temperature is higher, the removal of strong, coarse hairs is very effective and it gives a nice clean finish.

Additional knowledge

The abdomen is also suitable for warm wax hair removal, although it is not a range in this qualification. The same application techniques would apply.

Unlike warm wax, hot wax is applied as a thicker layer, which is built up by firstly going with the hair growth and then against the hair growth, until sufficient thickness for removal has been achieved. The procedure is as follows.

1   Test the wax on yourself on the inner wrist. Then, if the temperature is comfortable, test a small patch on the client on the area to be worked upon. If the client confirms that she is happy with the feel of it, commence the treatment.

2   Look closely at the hair growth in the area, as this affects both application and removal.

3   Gather a manageable amount of wax on to the spatula, and keep twisting the spatula to avoid drips, wiping any excess on to the edge of the heater. A tissue in the free hand, held underneath the spatula, will catch any drips on the way from heater to couch.

4   The wax should be the consistency of icing ready to go on a cake: spreadable but not too thick. Apply the wax, and build up several layers, working firstly against and then with the hair growth. Ensure that the edges are quite thick too, as when the wax is removed, the edges may break off if too thinly applied.

5   Try not to make the strips too large as this makes them difficult to remove. Two or three applications should give a covering about 3 mm thick. Avoid the temptation to apply too many layers, as the wax will just build up on itself and not adhere to the hairs.

6   The trick is to be quick, and apply several patches in one go. As the first patch is setting slightly, the second and third can be applied. Do not let any of them dry out totally on the skin, as they will become brittle and break off, and will hurt the client when removed.

7   A thick lip on the edges of each patch will allow a firm grip when removing.

8   As each strip starts to set slightly, press with the fingers. It should feel dry but still supple to the touch, and the lip can be flipped up.

9   Grip the lip you have created and with the other hand pull the skin slightly away from the wax patch to minimise client discomfort. Be quick and firm, and swiftly remove the wax against the direction of hair growth.

10 Immediately soothe the area by applying pressure to it. Quickly move on to the next patch as that will be setting.

11 Fold each wax strip in on itself, with the hairs inside, and put them into the lined bin for disposal into the collectable waste bin.

12 Should there be any small remains of wax, press the larger patch over the area and the remains should be picked up easily.

13 Work methodically all over the area to be waxed in a pattern, so that all hairs are removed, but avoid overlapping and therefore over-waxing.

14 Any hairs that have escaped may be tweezed away, and the result should be clean and clear. The skin will be slightly pinker than with warm waxing because of the higher temperature.

15 Aftercare and home care advice can be given. A soothing after-wax lotion can be applied, and a nice gesture is to provide the client with a sample-size aftercare lotion to take away and apply at home.

16 Clearing up can now take place. This is as important as the rest of the treatment, as cross-infection can occur through the contaminated waste. Dispose of used spatulas, wax, gloves and couch roll in the appropriate bags.

17 Clean the equipment with the manufacturer's recommended cleaner and clean the plastic couch covering. Wash hands and begin with the next client.

Area	Time
Eyebrows	10–15 minutes
Facial (lip and chin)	10–15 minutes
Full leg	45–60 minutes
Half leg (up to knee)	20–30 minutes
Underarm	15 minutes
Bikini	15–20 minutes
Forearm (wrist to elbow)	20 minutes

Treatment time guide for hot wax – as a practised therapist the treatment times for the application of hot wax should be the same as warm wax but on larger areas a salon and your assessor may give you a few minutes longer. These are approximate service times per treatment for hot wax

Think about it

This treatment guide is dependent upon the skill of the therapist. Hot wax needs to be nurtured up to the correct working temperature and consistency, and then used. Temperature control is vital when using this method and this can affect the treatment timings. The application of hot wax requires more training and a higher skill level.

Remove hair using waxing techniques

Step-by-step hot wax application for legs

1 Cleanse the area with a suitable cleanser, to make sure that the skin is dry and grease-free. Apply a light dusting of talcum powder or talc-free powder – this will make the hairs stand up.

2 Test the hot wax on your forearm before applying any to the client.

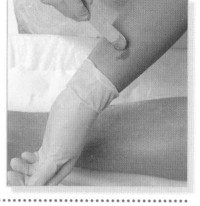

3 Decant a good amount of hot wax from the pot on to another spatula, to avoid contamination. The consistency of wax should be like soft treacle.

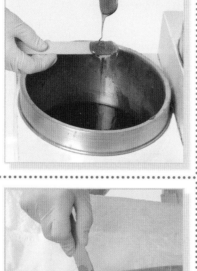

4 Test a small patch of wax on the client, to avoid burning the skin.

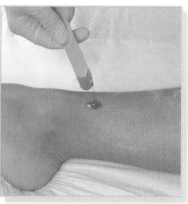

5 Working against the hair growth to begin with, apply the wax in a figure of eight shape. As you keep applying, you will build up a thick patch of wax.

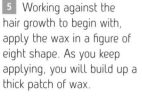

6 When the wax layer looks set, pressure from the knuckles will help bond the hot wax to the hairs. The wax takes on a matt finish as it cools.

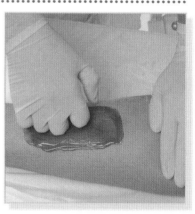

7 Using the same techniques as with a wax strip, flick a lip up, and gripping firmly, quickly remove the patch of wax – against the direction of hair growth.

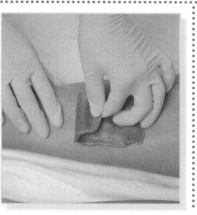

8 The hairs should be clearly visible, embedded in the wax strip you have removed.

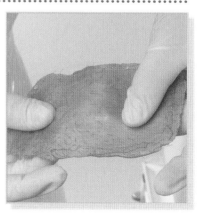

Ensuring the client is satisfied with the finished result

The client will appreciate it if you discuss the finished result with her. You can make sure the client is satisfied, and that the agreed treatment plan has been met.

Carefully check the area over. If necessary, tweeze the odd hair away using sterilised tweezers.

Check the results before applying the aftercare lotion, as this makes the skin quite slippery so the odd hair is more difficult to pick up with the tweezers.

A mini-massage while applying the aftercare lotion is always very soothing to the nerve endings, and finishes the treatment with a pleasant feeling for the client. You do not have the time for a full massage routine, however.

Once you've completed the treatment, take time to fill out the client record card.

- Were there any reactions during the treatment that will affect the future treatment plan? Remember, it may not be you doing the next treatment.
- Did the client express any preferences or dislikes for waxing mediums?
- Would you leave something out next time?
- Did the client feel much pain? An over-the-counter painkiller could be taken prior to the next treatment.
- Were products purchased?
- How was the skin reaction? Were there contra-actions?

Giving aftercare and home care advice

It is important that you discuss aftercare and home care with your client during the consultation, so that her skin reactions and contra-actions can be explained and understood.

A leaflet to take away is ideal for your client to refer to, as she may not take in all the information, especially if she finds the treatment painful.

Immediate aftercare

Your client should realise that the waxed area will be red and there may be some blood spots, especially where the hairs are strong, i.e. on the bikini line or underarm. The after-wax cleanser should be applied to remove any sticky remains on the skin followed by after-wax soothing lotion to help cool the skin and keep it moisturised.

Preparation — you, your working area and the client.

⬇

Two waste bins with liners.

⬇

Choose wax most suitable for client and area. Heat it up half an hour before appointment.

⬇

On the trolley:
- antiseptic cleaner
- talc
- fabric/paper strips
- disposable gloves
- wooden spatulas
- tissues and cotton wool
- jewellery bowl
- scissors and tweezers
- after-wax lotion
- record card.

⬇

Consultation, with record card. Fully explain treatment.

⬇

Wash hands.

⬇

Test temperature on self and on client.

⬇

Area to be clean and grease-free. Commence treatment.

⬇

After wax — wash hands.

⬇

Aftercare and home care.

⬇

Dispose of used spatulas, etc. Clean working area.

⬇

Wash hands.

⬇

Start again with next client.

Waxing

Home care

Your salon may like to devise a home care card like the one below:

Aftercare – for a period of 24 hours:

◆ No sunbathing or sunbeds	◆ Avoid tight clothing
◆ Avoid bathing in sea or swimming pool	◆ Do not use perfumed products on the area
◆ Do not take a *hot* bath or shower	◆ No make-up or self-tanning preparations
◆ Do not use deodorant / anti-perspirant	◆ Do not keep touching or picking at the area

Waxing home care card

Think about it

For 24 hours after waxing, advise the client to avoid:

- tight clothing
- hot baths/showers, or swimming
- sunbeds, sunbathing or other heat-related treatments
- applying perfumed products, including deodorant, and make-up to the area
- applying fake tan products.

Think about it

When giving treatment advice and recommendations for other treatments, be accurate and constructive. Consider what you and the client can realistically achieve.

For your portfolio

Devise an aftercare or information leaflet that you can give to a client following a waxing treatment. Consider both the short- and long-term aftercare that will be appropriate. Produce the leaflet on a computer.

Long-term home care advice

◉ Encourage your client to look after the skin on her body as she would the skin on her face.

◉ Lots of moisturiser will stop the skin becoming too dry, especially in the winter months when legs are kept under trousers and tights.

◉ Sloughing the skin with a loofah in the shower will help keep the blood circulation stimulated, bringing lots of oxygen and nutrients to the skin to keep it in good condition.

◉ Massage will help remove the build-up of toxins in the skin and keep the area both nourished and smooth. Instruct your client to always work towards the lymph nodes to help the body's natural lymphatic drainage.

◉ Exfoliating the skin will help to stop the hairs becoming ingrown.

◉ Gentle exercise, regular sleeping patterns and eating plenty of fruit and vegetables, while cutting down on smoking and alcohol, and drinking lots of water really do work, and not just for the face.

Before leaving the salon, the client should be encouraged to make a repeat appointment, usually in 4–6 weeks. However, this will depend upon the colour and density of the hair and the area. It is important to stress to the client that for effective waxing the hairs should be at the correct length.

My story

Never ignore aftercare advice!

Hi, my name is Nicola. I won't forget my first leg wax! It was a lovely, sunny day and I was looking forward to going on holiday. I was telling the therapist all about it. She advised me not to sunbathe or to apply any products to the area for 24 hours after the treatment. When I got home, I wanted to show off my beautiful hair-free legs! So, forgetting the therapist's advice, I put on sunscreen and went and sat in the garden for a couple of hours. I really wish I hadn't – by early evening my legs were so painful. I learned my lesson the hard way and now always listen to the aftercare advice I'm given.

Frequently asked questions

Q	What would happen if grease is left on the skin?
A	The skin has a barrier of grease or oil on it which will prevent the wax getting a grip on the hairs. Always clean the skin thoroughly to prevent this barrier building up.
Q	Can waxing take place on any length of hairs?
A	If the hairs are too short, they will not stick to the wax.
Q	What would happen if the wax is not hot enough?
A	The removal of the hairs will not be effective and the wax could matt, making removal difficult.
Q	What would happen if the wax is applied too thickly?
A	The wax will not be able to get a grip on the hairs, and will congeal on itself.
Q	What would happen if the wax is applied or removed in the wrong direction?
A	The hairs will not be removed and this can cause pain and discomfort to the client.
Q	What would happen if the skin is not pulled taut when waxing?
A	The skin will be too slack, and the wax will set into the body's natural creases – very common when first attempting underarm waxing. Pull the skin so it is taut and ask the client to help. This makes it easier to apply the wax, and it is also less painful. This method should be adopted when waxing all areas.
Q	What would occur if the wax was not removed quickly enough?
A	This will result in an ineffective removal of hair, and pain for the client. Try not to lift upwards when removing the strip; always try to bring the strip back on itself. Be bold and confident, and it will be less painful and give a better result.
Q	What would occur if hairs are not trimmed when too long?
A	Hairs should be trimmed to prevent tangling and ineffective removal (especially on the bikini area).
Q	What should you do if the skin is red after the first strip is removed?
A	This could indicate that the wax is too hot. You should test it on yourself and the client before application. The pressure that has been applied with the spatula may also have dragged on the skin, so ensure that the wax is of the correct consistency before application.

Remove hair using waxing techniques

Check your knowledge

1 Waxing is a:
   a) permanent method of hair removal
   b) temporary method of hair removal
   c) long-lasting method of hair removal
   d) short-term method of hair removal.

2 Hot wax is most suitable for use on:
   a) strong hair growth
   b) weak hair growth
   c) bent follicles.

3 Hair removal creams are:
   a) suitable for all skin types
   b) not suitable for all skin types
   c) a painless method of hair removal
   d) a permanent method of removal.

4 Warm wax is:
   a) most suitable for all areas
   b) easy to apply
   c) not easy to apply
   d) a temporary method of removal.

5 Hot wax works best at a temperature of:
   a) 48–68°C
   b) 20–30°C
   c) 60–80°C
   d) 15–20°C.

6 Warm wax works best at a temperature of:
   a) 40–43°C
   b) 20–30°C
   c) 60–80°C
   d) 15–20°C.

7 The main ingredients used in hair removal wax are:
   a) resins and beeswax
   b) starch and flour
   c) sugar and water
   d) crystals and polish.

8 Pre-wax lotion must be used to:
   a) dry up the skin
   b) cleanse the area
   c) make the area smell nice
   d) make the hairs stand on end.

9 Talc or talc-free products are used to:
   a) make the skin smell nice
   b) provide a coating for the wax to stick to
   c) make the hairs stand away from the skin
   d) make the skin white.

10 After-wax lotion helps:
   a) soothe the skin
   b) stop the area going pink
   c) make the skin smell nice
   d) calm the client down.

11 Tests must always be carried out to:
   a) try out the heat of the wax on the client
   b) see if the client is suitable for treatment (i.e. no reaction occurs)
   c) let the client know it hurts
   d) give the client a bald patch on her arm.

12 Aftercare is important because:
   a) it ensures the client understands how to look after the area
   b) it stops you from being sued for poor treatment
   c) it's just part of the job
   d) it stops the client from picking at the area.

Getting ready for assessment

Your assessor will observe you demonstrating a treatment to a competent standard on at least three occasions on three different clients. It will be important to demonstrate that you can use both hot and warm wax correctly and know the areas that may benefit more from the use of hot wax. Where the practical criteria do not occur naturally your assessor may choose to ask oral questions or cover this knowledge with written evidence in the form of portfolio work or witness statements from formative work that you have undertaken. You will also be required to sit a mandatory written paper in which you have to achieve at least a 70% pass mark. Subsequent portfolio work will be used to support your underpinning knowledge so that the unit can be successfully signed off by your assessor.

As well as performing the treatment and leaving a good clean result, the assessor will be checking that you have:

- used all consultation techniques
- carried out waxing treatments on all areas with hot and warm wax
- have dealt with the necessary actions in the range (if applicable)
- covered all the criteria for effective work techniques to ensure the client has a pain-free treatment
- provided suitable aftercare and home care advice.

Remember that waxing is a skill that requires a lot of practice to improve both your technique and cleanliness. Before attempting an assessment, make sure you have had sufficient practice to feel confident and self-assured in your knowledge of what to tell the client.

Although the areas of the body are specified, you may be able to cluster your assessments. One client may have several areas waxed in one treatment, and they all count.

Be careful that the length of hair is right. If the hairs are too short, the wax does not have enough of the hair shaft to adhere to, so the results will be patchy. If the hairs are too long, it will be advantageous to trim them down with scissors before starting. Otherwise the hair will become tangled and again the results will not be clean.

Be very careful to check the direction of hair growth, as that will dictate the direction for your wax strips. Show that you understand the relevance of hair growth even if it means using smaller strips, say for a circular direction of underarm hair growth.

Be clean and hygienic, and check with your professional body about when to use gloves. The best clean results on the skin will be spoilt by an unhygienic treatment approach and a messy workstation with wax on the floor.

Do not forget to test the wax on yourself and to carry out a small patch test on the client before you begin — burning the client's skin will not gain a competent assessment.

The assessor is looking at the whole approach, including client care, hygiene and a good result.

Remove hair using waxing techniques

Provide manicure and pedicure treatments

What you will learn

- Prepare for manicure and pedicure treatments
- Provide manicure and pedicure treatments

Key terms

Manicure – treatment performed on the hands and lower arm, working on improving the condition of the nails, skin and cuticle.

Pedicure – treatment performed on the feet and lower leg, working on improving the condition of the nails, skin and cuticle.

Top tips

When a client books in for nail extensions, either ask them about the condition of their nails, cuticle and skin or, if in person, make a visual analysis. If they are in poor condition, recommend a manicure treatment or series of treatments. This will improve the condition of the nails before having nail extensions, creating a better finish and generating more profit for the salon.

Introduction

Together, **manicures** and **pedicures** are the foundation of the professional beauty therapist's skills, on which they can build more advanced techniques. Both treatments are very popular in nail bars, spas and salons, for both male and female clients, as they can be performed to improve the condition of the nails, cuticle and skin or purely as a relaxation treatment. Also, for clients who intend to have nail enhancements such as fibreglass nail extensions or nail art, nails in good condition, with healthy cuticles, are a perfect base to work upon.

There are other reasons why a client will choose to have a manicure or pedicure – for example, they may want to stop biting their fingernails or prevent the occurrence of ingrowing toenails. It is the responsibility of the therapist to perform a thorough consultation and analysis to determine the client's needs, then design an individual treatment plan. This unit also looks at how to turn a basic treatment into a luxury treatment by incorporating additional products and equipment that enhance the effects of a manicure or pedicure.

Manicures and pedicures offer the client a range of benefits.

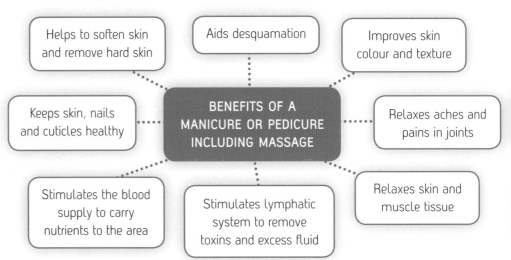

Helps to soften skin and remove hard skin

Aids desquamation

Improves skin colour and texture

Keeps skin, nails and cuticles healthy

BENEFITS OF A MANICURE OR PEDICURE INCLUDING MASSAGE

Relaxes aches and pains in joints

Stimulates the blood supply to carry nutrients to the area

Stimulates lymphatic system to remove toxins and excess fluid

Relaxes skin and muscle tissue

Prepare for manicure and pedicure treatments

In this outcome you will learn about:

- preparing yourself, your client and work area for manicure and pedicure treatments
- using suitable consultation techniques to identify treatment objectives
- carrying out a nail and skin analysis
- providing clear recommendations to the client
- selecting products, tools and equipment to suit client treatment needs, skin and nail conditions.

Salon requirements for preparing yourself, the client and the work area

Preparing yourself

Before a client arrives at the salon to have a manicure or pedicure treatment, the working area and therapist must be prepared fully to ensure the treatment runs smoothly. As a therapist, you have a professional image to maintain and this is vital to your success and that of the business. When training to become a therapist, you are assessed on your personal presentation and hygiene. These standards are set by the Awarding Organisations. Your assessors must follow these standards during your assessment. You will be expected to continue these high standards throughout your career.

To learn more about professional presentation, see Essential professional knowledge, page 9.

Think about it

Before leaving for work, have a look at your appearance in a full-length mirror and ask yourself, do I look professional? If you do not follow the designated dress code, you instantly create a poor image of your workplace, your colleagues and yourself. These basic guidelines are vital to the success of any business.

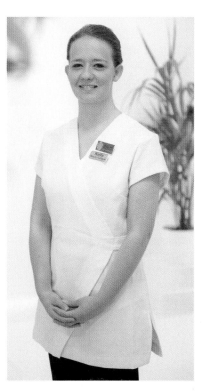

Maintain a professional image

Preparing the client

When a client has a manicure and/or pedicure treatment they need to be positioned correctly. This will depend upon the size of the nail studio, salon or spa and if the client is having additional treatments at the same time. When a client has a pedicure, always remember to provide a towel for their lap to protect their modesty and their clothing from the products used. To learn more about the importance of health and safety as part of client preparation, see Follow health and safety practice in the salon, page 67.

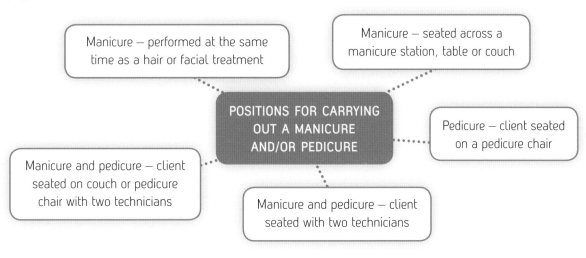

Manicure – performed at the same time as a hair or facial treatment

Manicure – seated across a manicure station, table or couch

POSITIONS FOR CARRYING OUT A MANICURE AND/OR PEDICURE

Pedicure – client seated on a pedicure chair

Manicure and pedicure – client seated on couch or pedicure chair with two technicians

Manicure and pedicure – client seated with two technicians

Provide manicure and pedicure treatments

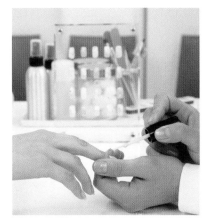

Good preparation helps to ensure a successful treatment

Preparing the working area

The location of the treatment will influence how you set up the work area. However, always begin by sterilising all your tools and sanitising the working area – to learn more, see Essential professional knowledge, page 34.

When performing a manicure it is ideal to perform the treatment across a manicure station, where all your products and tools can be neatly and safely stored. However, if you are working across a table or alongside another treatment, then a trolley can be used as an alternative. Remember, if the manicure is being performed alongside another treatment, you will need to support the client's arm and wrist, either on the arm of a pedicure chair or use a rolled-up towel on your lap (make sure the client is comfortable). When setting up your station or trolley ensure you have all your products and equipment; then you will be prepared for every eventuality.

Environmental conditions suitable for manicure and pedicure treatments

It is important to create a perfect environment for the client's treatment so that they feel totally relaxed and to enable you to perform the treatment effectively.

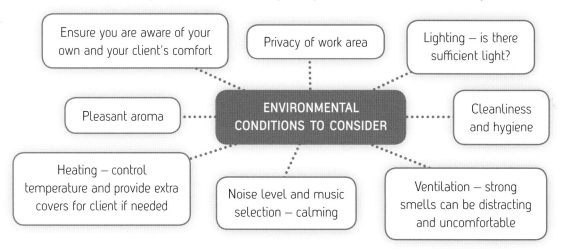

Ensure you are aware of your own and your client's comfort

Privacy of work area

Lighting – is there sufficient light?

Pleasant aroma

ENVIRONMENTAL CONDITIONS TO CONSIDER

Cleanliness and hygiene

Heating – control temperature and provide extra covers for client if needed

Noise level and music selection – calming

Ventilation – strong smells can be distracting and uncomfortable

To learn more about suitable environmental conditions in the workplace, see Essential professional knowledge, page 20; and for information on the Performing Rights regulations, see Essential professional knowledge, page 59.

My story

Salon life

My name is Alex and I work as a beauty therapist in a busy city-centre nail studio. I have 15 years' experience and have worked on many different clients, some with very specific needs. I am passionate about my line of work and have had many happy clients over the years.

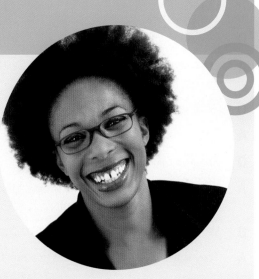

Unfortunately, because I have had a really successful career, I recently let down my professional guard and my attitude became a little too relaxed. A client came in for a pedicure treatment during a very busy Saturday morning and I was too busy to perform a full consultation. The client, who had never had a salon treatment before and had never worn enamels, had her toenails painted. Shortly afterwards, she had a mild allergic reaction to the enamel and after I talked with her she disclosed that she had very sensitive skin. Usually she would avoid most products, including enamels, make-up and perfume. If I had completed a full consultation I would have discovered this earlier and performed a skin test with certain products such as mask and creams. I would have also chosen alternative enamels, as I could have used solvent-free, water-based products that are free of ingredients like toluene or formaldehyde. This was a very difficult lesson to learn and thankfully the client gave me a second chance. I learned to always remain professional and put the needs of the client first in order to uphold the reputation of the salon and the quality of the services we provide.

Ask the experts

Q *How do you perform a skin test?*

A Select the products that might be a possible allergen, like creams for instance, and apply a small amount on the inside of the arm or near the wrist and leave for 24 hours. The client must monitor the area; if it feels warm and itchy, or if there is redness or blistering, then they have had a reaction.

Q *Is there anything else that I can do to minimise the chances of a client having a reaction?*

A Yes, choose products that do not contain known allergens, like lanolin or formaldehyde, and try to have a range of products for a more sensitive skin.

Benefits of offering the service for the therapist:

- Excellent retail opportunity for recommending products: cream, scrub, enamel remover, nail files
- Repeat business, recommending and booking in clients for their follow-up treatments and promoting additional services
- Can be a promotional offer where a manicure and pedicure treatment could include nail art or as a course of treatments to prepare nails in poor condition to be ready for artificial nails
- Can be promoted with additional treatments like paraffin wax or electrical heat treatments

Benefits of the treatment/service for the client:

- Softens and nourishes the skin, cuticles and nails
- Improves the colour and condition of the skin and nails
- Relaxes tired muscles and achy joints
- Visually improves appearance of hands and feet, showing latest enamelling techniques
- Provides individual treatment plans

Provide manicure and pedicure treatments

Frequently asked questions

Q How short should I cut toenails if the client wants a French polish?

A Leave a slightly longer free edge. This will produce a nice effect, but if you leave the nails too long they could press against the skin and cause discomfort.

Q What if a client wants a really short free edge?

A Do not cut or file below the flesh line or you will expose the hyponychium and the area will be prone to an infection.

Q Should I buff toenails?

A If the nails are not ridged or stained and are a healthy length then do not buff as it will stimulate nail growth and clients do not want to keep cutting their toenails.

Q Why should I recommend aftercare products to every client?

A They maintain the effects of the treatment and will increase the salon's profits.

Q Why do I need to learn about the ingredients of manicure and pedicure products?

A If you recognise an ingredient and learn about its effects, you can understand how a product works. Also you need to understand the side-effects, to prevent damage. For example, most chemicals are harsh and if they are left on too long they could cause dryness to the nail and skin area.

Top tips

It is important to perform an allergy test. Remember to ask your clients when they book an appointment whether they have any known allergies or very sensitive skin. It takes less time to perform a skin test than it does to deal with an unhappy client who has had a reaction.

Top tips

Between clients, sterilise and wash your tools and refresh and sanitise the working area. Aim to keep the area tidy during treatments. This will prevent cross-infection and present a professional image, which will give your clients confidence in your performance.

Consultation techniques used to identify treatment objectives

During the consultation process, perform visual and manual checks of the area and ask questions to determine if there are any contra-indications with the client's skin, cuticle or nails. Performing a good consultation will help you to decide if the treatment needs to be adapted and what the client's expectations are, which will enable you to create an individual plan. You will also need to discuss whether the nails need cutting and the required shape of the nail.

To learn more about consultation techniques, see Client care and communication in beauty-related industries, page 99.

The importance of carrying out a nail and skin analysis

To learn more about the importance of nail and skin analysis, see page 147.

How to select products, tools and equipment for manicure and pedicure treatments

There is a vast range of manicure and pedicure products, tools and equipment available to suit a variety of needs. Whether you are in industry or education, you will be trained to use these items and you will need to understand how, when and why to use them so you have the necessary knowledge to create suitable treatment plans for individual clients.

Manicure and pedicure tools and equipment

Some of the following tools, which are usually made of metal, plastic or rubber, can be washed, sterilised and reused. There are also disposable items made of wood or plastic.

Trolley or manicure station

A manicure treatment is usually performed on a manicure station, which should be of the correct height and width for safe use. A trolley or manicure station can be used to store products and tools ready for use – it usually has drawers for storage and a wrist support for the client.

Manicure or pedicure soaking bowl

Nail soak or pedi soak with warm water is added to the bowl. The nail bowl has specially designed finger holes, so that the client can comfortably and effectively soak their nails in the bowl. Pedicure bowls are much larger in size in order to fit both feet in comfortably. They usually have a flat bottom so they are safe and secure while the client's feet are soaking. Soaking their nails will cleanse the area and prepare the nails for further work.

Nail brush

Nail brushes are used when soaking the client's nails in a manicure bowl, either to remove dirt and debris from under the free edge or to remove oil from the nails before enamelling.

Rubber hoof stick

A plastic or wooden tool, with a flat rubber end that is used to gently push back overgrown cuticles, to aid removal of excess cuticle.

Nail buffers

There are three different types of buffer, which are used to stimulate the blood supply to improve nail growth, create a healthy colour, produce a shine and smooth out any surface lines or ridges.

- A chamois leather-covered pad with a plastic handle is used with buffing paste but does not create a high-shine finish.
- Three- or four-way buffers or buffer blocks do not require a buffing paste. They create a high shine and are more effective at producing a smooth nail than the leather pad.
- Electric nail buffers are used as a quicker option. They create the same effects as the manual buffers but again the leather pad creates the least shine.

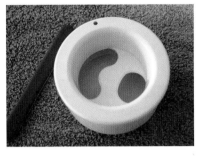

Manicure bowl

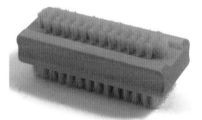

Nail brush

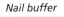

Hoof stick

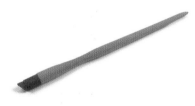

Nail buffer

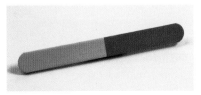

Three-way buffer

Provide manicure and pedicure treatments

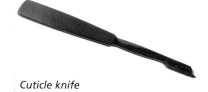

Cuticle knife

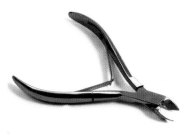

Cuticle nippers

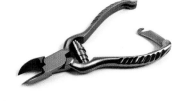

Toenail clippers

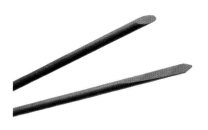

Orange sticks

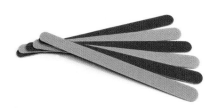

Emery boards

Cuticle knife

A metal tool, used to remove the eponychium and lift overgrown cuticle ready for removal with the nippers.

Cuticle nippers

A metal tool, used to remove excess cuticle and any hangnails.

Manicure scissors

Designed to cut fingernails, they can be straight or curved in shape.

Pedicure toenail clippers

Designed to cut strong toenails, they are much more effective at cutting than scissors.

Callus shaver, foot rasp, foot file, ceramic foot file or pumice stone

These are all used to remove hard skin from the feet by gently grating it away. They can be used on either dry or pre-soaked feet but are more effective when the skin is dry.

Orange sticks

Orange sticks are multi-purposed and can be used either as they are or tipped with cotton wool. They can be used to apply cuticle products to the nail or when tipped with cotton wool they can remove enamel that has accidently been applied to the skin. They are made of wood and, for hygiene reasons, are disposable.

Emery board

An emery board has two sides: a fine side to file fingernails into shape and a coarse side to file toenails. It can also be used to file fingernails to shorten them. However, it is advisable to cut the nails with scissors, as too much filing using the coarse side can create friction, which produces heat that can dry out the nails.

The grit quantity determines how coarse or fine a file will be:

- 80 grit – extra-coarse
- 100 grit – coarse
- 180 grit – medium
- 240 grit – fine.

Emery boards can only be cleaned using special cleaners and then sterilised in the UV cabinet, but ideally they should be disposed of after use, as it is difficult to clean them fully.

Spatulas

These can be made of wood (disposable) or plastic (reusable) and are used to remove products from their container, either to be dispensed or as a palette/surface to work from.

Barbicide jars

These contain a **disinfectant** solution and are placed on the workstation to store pre-sterilised metal tools, including scissors, cuticle knife, nippers and clippers.

Key terms

Disinfectant – a chemical solution that will destroy most micro-organisms.

Wrist support cushion

A cushion or a rolled-up small towel is used to support the client's wrist during a manicure.

Waste bin or rubbish bowl

A lined, pedal waste bin or a lined waste bowl is placed next to the therapist to maintain hygiene standards.

Lined dishes or bowls

Dishes or bowls containing consumables such as cotton wool are placed on the workstation. A further bowl can be used for the client's jewellery if applicable. Bowls can also be used to warm oil for cuticle treatments.

Towels and couch roll

These can be used to protect trolleys from damage that can occur from manicure or pedicure products such as enamel remover. They can also be used to protect the client's clothing, the working area and therapist. Towels or face cloths can either be dampened with hot water or dampened with cold water and warmed in a towel heater, and then used to remove products such as exfoliators or massage oil.

Cotton wool or tissues

Cotton wool is used to apply or remove products, for example nail varnish remover and antiseptic. Both can be used as an alternative method for separating the toes when enamelling.

Gown

A gown can be worn by the client to protect their clothing.

Protective arm tissue

Protective arm tissues are used to protect the client's clothing.

Clingfilm or foil

Clingfilm or foil can be used with a paraffin wax treatment. Once the wax has been applied, the area is wrapped in clingfilm or foil to retain the heat and enhance the effects of the treatment. They are also used to prevent the wax breaking up and making the working area untidy.

Thermal mittens and bootees

Thermal mittens, used during a manicure treatment, and thermal bootees, used during a pedicure treatment, are electrical heat treatments. Heat enhances the effects of products applied to the skin, allowing them to penetrate deeper. Heat is also relaxing for sore muscles and joints.

Paraffin wax

Paraffin wax can be used during a manicure or pedicure treatment to soften the skin, nourish the nails and relax the muscles and joints. The wax can be heated to an average temperature of 49°C in a paraffin wax bath. It is applied to the skin by a brush from the wax heated in a bath or from a cartridge containing the wax that is warmed in a heater, and is sprayed onto the skin's surface.

Top tips

There are other more durable and easy-to-clean nail files on the market, including glass, crystal and ceramic stone files. These files can be washed to ensure complete removal of nail particles and can be used on natural or artificial nails, creating a smoother, damage-free nail. Invest in better quality tools and you will benefit financially and professionally.

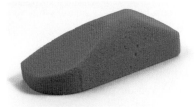

Pumice stone

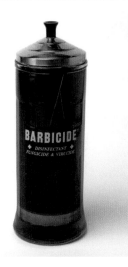

Barbicide®

Top tips

To reduce the salon's outgoings, always be aware of ways to be cost-effective. Here are some suggestions:

- Split tissues, cotton wool pads and couch roll.
- Use reusable tools that can be washed and sterilised, instead of disposable tools, for example plastic spatulas and glass nail files.
- Use the correct amount of product.

Provide manicure and pedicure treatments

Key terms

Oil-in-water mixture – a product that has more oil in it than water.

Lanolin – oil found on sheep's wool.

Cocoa butter – a yellow-white fat from cocoa beans.

Liquid paraffin – mineral oil.

Emollient – moisturiser that contains oil and water to nourish skin and prevent water loss. Contains either an oil-in-water solution or water-in-oil solution. More oil makes it a heavier product (cream). More water makes it a lighter product (lotion).

Beeswax – wax produced by bees in a hive.

Emulsifying agent – allows hand to glide/slip along skin during massage.

Alkaline – measure of alkalinity on a pH (potential of hydrogen) scale.

Caustic – a chemical substance that destroys living tissue.

AHAs – alpha hydroxy acids, from sources such as fruit. They cause the skin to produce new cells faster, exfoliating the skin.

Talc – a fine-grained white, greenish or grey mineral.

Kaolin – a fine clay.

Stannic oxide – a white powder that is insoluble in water.

Solvent – a liquid that dissolves other substances such as enamel. When added to enamel it helps the enamel to dry and to keep the correct consistency (not too thick or thin).

Manicure and pedicure products

Remember, never waste products. Be cost-effective and always use the correct amount, or it will affect your salon's profits.

Cuticle massage cream

The cream is applied to the cuticles and then the nails are placed in the manicure or pedicure bowl containing warm water and nail or pedi soak, to soften the cuticles for easy removal.

Ingredients: **oil-in-water mixture** – **lanolin, cocoa butter, liquid paraffin (emollients); beeswax (emulsifying agent)**

Cuticle oil

Cuticle oil, or massage oil that has been warmed over a bowl of hot water, can be used as a cuticle treatment to nourish and soften dry cuticles.

Cuticle remover

The main purpose of a cuticle remover is to loosen and release the cuticle for further cuticle work. The remover may contain harsh chemicals such as potassium hydroxide or sodium hydroxides which are **alkaline** and also **caustic**. When the cuticle remover is applied to the cuticles it softens and breaks down the cuticle. If left on too long, it will irritate and dry out the cuticle. There are milder formulations that contain **AHAs**, derived from plants that break down the skin cells.

Ingredients: 2.5% solution of potassium hydroxide or sodium hydroxide and glycerine (emollient)

Buffing paste

Used with a chamois leather buffer to remove surface ridges and produce a shiny nail plate, creating a smoother nail for enamelling.

Ingredients: **talc, kaolin, stannic oxide**

Lotions and creams

Lotions and creams are emollients that soften the skin and cuticles and can be used to perform the massage during a treatment. They may contain other benefits, including anti-ageing properties such as sunscreen to prevent age spots, AHAs to minimise wrinkle depth, collagen to make the skin plump or, for the feet, peppermint to cool the skin.

Massage cream or oil

Oil or cream media have a high oil content so that they remain on the skin surface during massage. They help the hands to glide over the area, and are especially good for very dry skin.

Nail varnish remover or enamel remover

The remover is a **solvent** that dissolves enamel. It is applied to cotton wool and then wiped over the nails. It usually contains acetone, but acetone-free removers can be purchased for clients who wear artificial nails. Acetone is also used to remove artificial nails, as it is a strong and effective chemical, but it can be very drying to the nail plate.

Ingredients: solvents (acetone, ethyl, butyl acetate), glycerol, mineral oil

Nail enamel thinners or solvents

Thinners are used to dilute old enamel that has become too thick to use.

Ingredients: ethyl acetate

Nail varnishes or enamel

Enamels carry colour within them and are applied to the nail to add colour, either in a matt or shiny finish.

Ingredients: nitrocellulose and resin (**film formers**), ethyl acetate, butyl acetate (solvent), isopropyl myristate (**plasticiser**)

Base coat

This protects the nail plate, as it is applied before enamel to prevent the enamel staining the nail plate. It also provides a smooth base to apply enamel on to and helps the enamel last longer.

Ingredients: **resins**, nitrocellulose, plasticisers

Ridge filler

This has a thicker consistency than base coat and is used to fill ridges so as to create a smoother finish when enamelling.

Ingredients: nitrocellulose, plasticisers, resin, **fibres**

Top coat

This protects the nail plate and is applied over the top of an enamel to give a shiny finish and to help prevent the enamel from chipping.

Ingredients: nitrocellulose, plasticisers, resin

Nail strengtheners and hardeners

Applied like a base coat, these strengthen/harden weak nails.

Ingredients: aluminium potassium sulphate (film-forming plastic resin), formaldehyde (film-forming plastic resin), resins, glycerols

Quick-dry spray

This is sprayed over the enamel to reduce drying time and harden the enamel.

Ingredients: mineral oils, silicone (**lubricant**), natural oils, alcohol

Hand or foot cleansers

Antiseptic cleansers are used on cotton wool to wipe over the skin to remove dirt, sebum, sweat and body products.

Hygiene spray

An antiseptic that is sprayed over the area to sanitise it.

Nail bleach

This is used to whiten the nail plate and surrounding skin.

Ingredients: **hydrogen peroxide**

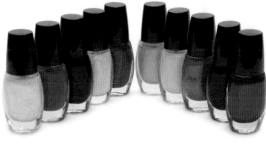
Nail enamels

Key terms

Film formers – hold the colour of the enamel.

Plasticiser – provides flexibility to reduce chipping of enamel.

Resin – gives enamel its flexibility and helps it adhere to the nail plate.

Fibres – make the ridge filler thicker in consistency.

Key terms

Lubricant – provides a smooth or slippery surface.

Hydrogen peroxide – a chemical that bleaches the nail.

Provide manicure and pedicure treatments

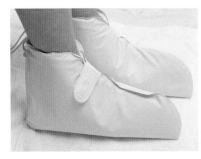

Thermal bootees

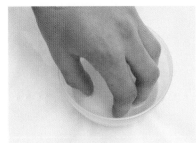

Warm oil treatment

White pencils

Used under the free edge to create a whiter tip and reduce staining of the free edge.

Ingredients: aluminium potassium sulphate, formaldehyde, resins

Hand/nail soak

Hand/nail soak is added to warm water in a manicure bowl to cleanse and nourish the area. It also enhances the effects of the cuticle massage cream and aids removal of excess cuticle.

Ingredients: vary between manufacturers – may include essential oils such as lavender, camomile or peppermint (soothing aroma and antiseptic)

Foot soak (pedi soak)

Foot soak is added to warm water in a foot bowl to cleanse, sooth, cool and revitalise the feet.

Ingredients: vary between manufacturers – may include herbs such as peppermint oil extracts (cooling, reduce odour and revitalising) or green tea (an anti-oxidant to cleanse body of toxins), avocado oil (moisturising), essential oils like lavender, vanilla or jasmine (soothing aroma), Epsom or Dead Sea salts (contain mineral magnesium to soothe aching muscles, reduce inflammation and swelling)

Manicure and pedicure specialist treatments

To turn a basic treatment into a luxury manicure or pedicure, a therapist can use any of the following equipment.

Thermal mittens and bootees

To use mittens or bootees:

1 Apply either a cream, lotion, oil or mask to the hands or feet.
2 Wrap the hands/feet in plastic liners or clingfilm before inserting into the mitts or bootees for 10–15 minutes.
3 Remove the hands/feet and remove the plastic liners.
4 As the massage is performed, the tissues are softened and the joints are relaxed, which will enhance the effects of the massage and the cuticle work.

Warm oil treatments

Warm oil will soften and nourish dry nails, cuticle and skin. Various types of vegetable-based oils can be used, for example olive oil. Pour a small amount of oil into a small bowl, then place the bowl into a larger bowl of hot water to warm the oil. Remove the small bowl and place the fingertips into the oil for five minutes, then continue with the treatment.

Exfoliators (foot/hand scrubs)

Exfoliators contain abrasive particles, which are either synthetic or natural, such as salt scrubs. They exfoliate the skin's surface by removing dead skin cells, especially hard patches found on the soles and palms. Use a large circular movement, as small movements will cause skin irritation and damage.

Hand mask

Usually applied after exfoliating to soften, nourish and revitalise the skin, a hand mask may also have anti-ageing benefits.

Ingredients: vary between manufacturers — may include AHAs (to thin the skin to minimise wrinkle depth), collagen (to plump the skin), plant extracts (to lighten age spots), rosemary (to moisturise and protect), vitamin A (to aid cell renewal), aloe vera and camomile (to soothe), nut oils (to soften), vitamin E (to moisturise)

Foot mask

Usually applied after exfoliating to soften, nourish, cool and revitalise the skin.

Ingredients: vary between manufacturers — may include peppermint oil (reduces odour, revitalises and cools), kaolin clay (to deep cleanse), cocoa butter (to soften)

Paraffin wax

To use a paraffin bath:

1 Line a plastic bowl with foil and use the ladle to dispense the melted wax into the bowl.

2 Quickly distribute a rich cream over the skin and place the client's hand, palm up, over a large piece of foil that has a small towel underneath. Then test the wax on your wrist first to check the temperature and next on the client's wrist, as they could be more sensitive to the heat than you are.

3 Quickly apply the wax to the client's hand and wrist area — do not use too many brush strokes, as the wax will now begin setting. Turn the client's hand over and apply to the opposite side.

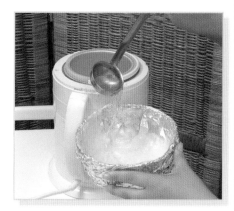

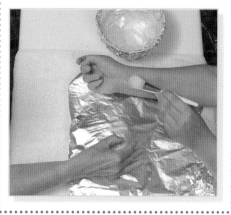

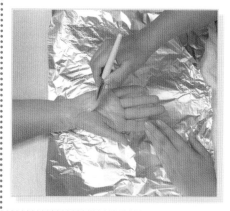

4 Wrap the hand in the foil to retain the heat and maximise the effects of the wax.

5 Now wrap the hand in a towel to slow down the cooling of the wax.

6 Once the wax has set, uncover the area and peel off the wax to reveal soft, smooth skin and relaxed muscle tissue and joints.

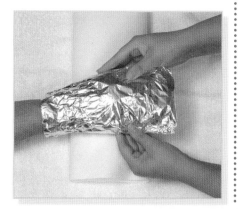

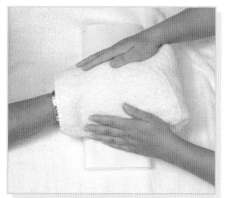

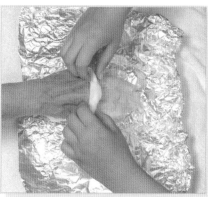

Provide manicure and pedicure treatments

Top tips

Promote additional treatments, such as paraffin wax, warm oil and thermal mittens and bootees, to enhance the effects of your treatments, improve the client's satisfaction and to make more profit for the salon.

Nail and skin conditions and contra-indications

See You and the skin on page 181, to learn more about:

- nail and skin conditions
- diseases and disorders of the nail and skin that prevent or restrict manicure and pedicure treatments.

Structure and functions of the nail, skin, muscles, bones, arteries and veins and lymphatic vessels of the lower arm, hand, lower leg and foot

To learn more about the anatomy and physiology of the lower arm, hand, lower leg and foot and their relevance to manicure and pedicure treatments, see the Related anatomy and physiology unit, page 227.

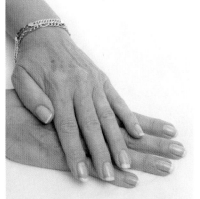

Provide manicure and pedicure treatments

In this outcome you will learn about:

- communicating and behaving in a professional manner
- following health and safety working practices
- positioning yourself and your client correctly throughout the treatment
- using products, tools, equipment and techniques to suit clients' treatment needs, nail and skin conditions
- completing the treatment to the satisfaction of the client
- recording the results of the treatment
- providing suitable aftercare advice.

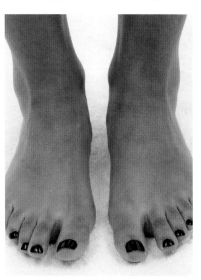

How to communicate and behave in a professional manner

To learn more about the importance of communication and professional ethical conduct, see Client care and communication in beauty-related industries, page 99.

Health and safety working practices

To learn more about health and safety in the workplace and legislation that affects working practices, see Follow health and safety practice in the salon, page 67.

The importance of positioning yourself and the client correctly

This was briefly considered in Salon requirements for preparing yourself, the client and the work area (see page 455). To find out more, see Follow health and safety practice in the salon, page 67.

The importance of using products, tools, equipment and techniques to suit the client's treatment needs, nail and skin conditions

First, you must understand how to perform a basic manicure or pedicure treatment — either of these treatments will take 45 minutes. A luxury treatment with extras such as an exfoliator and paraffin wax will take an hour.

Toenail shapes

To prevent ingrowing toenails, cut the nails straight with clippers, then file them straight with curved corners just above the flesh line to leave a short free edge. If the nails are incorrectly cut and filed, they will begin to grow into the skin and an infection may occur. In this case, the client should see their GP for treatment.

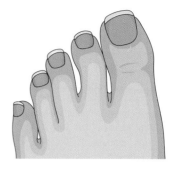
A square nail with curved corners

> **Top tips**
>
> Never presume to know what fingernail shape a client wants. During the consultation, discuss shapes. You can recommend a shape that would best suit them, but if a client specifies a different shape, you will have to do what the client wants, to ensure a happy outcome.

Fingernail shapes

Round	*Squoval*	*Square*	*Oval*	*Pointed (tapered)*
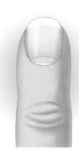	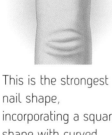	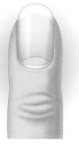	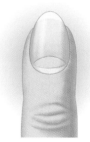	
A short and neat shape that is ideal for professionals such as nurses or cooks, who need a strong short nail.	This is the strongest nail shape, incorporating a square shape with curved corners. It is very popular, especially for those who have long nails or artificial nails.	The shape produces very straight sides and a blunt straight line at the free edge. This is a strong shape but looks so blunt that it can make fingers look short and wide and is not very flattering.	The nail is filed into an egg shape (oval), producing a slightly weaker nail, although it is more flattering to short fingers with wide nails and gives a more feminine appearance.	This is a very old-fashioned shape that is weak and prone to damage — it is best not to recommend it.

Claw (or hook)
The nail naturally curves and becomes very thick — this condition is known as onychogryphosis The nail should be kept short to minimise the appearance of a claw shape.

Fan
The nail is much wider at the free edge than the nail attached to the nail bed and creates a fan shape. Corrective filing is required — the nail should be filed to create an oval shape.

Provide manicure and pedicure treatments

Provide manicure and pedicure treatments

Basic manicure procedure

Once your treatment plan has been created and you have sterilised your tools, prepared your working area and the client is positioned comfortably, then you can begin.

1 During the consultation, discuss the client's needs. You should include the preferred nail length, shape, type of varnish, etc. If there are no contra-indications, you can begin the service.

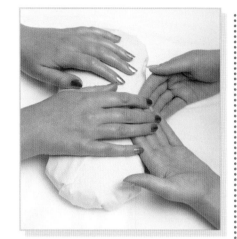

2 Ask the client to choose the varnish she would like. Provide a wide range of colours for the client to choose from including clear, light, dark, matt, frosted and French polishes.

You should recommend a varnish that is suitable for the client.

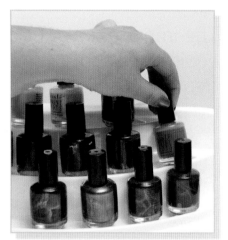

3 Remove any existing nail enamel from both hands and check the condition of the nails and cuticle in their natural state. Sanitise the hand to prevent cross-infection while you carry out a manual contra-indication check.

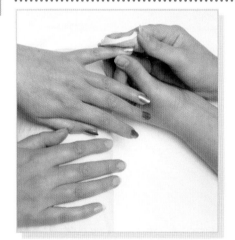

4 If the nails require cutting to shape, use the nail scissors and dispose of the nail cuttings from both hands.

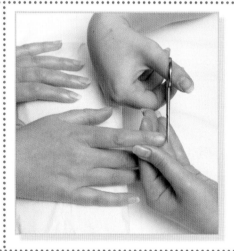

5 Use an emery board to file the nails into the desired shape, using the correct movements at a 45° angle and holding the end of the file. File from the outside in, then change sides and repeat – do not use a sawing action (going back and forth would create friction, which produces heat and dries out the nail, causing it to split and peel). File only the nails on the right hand.

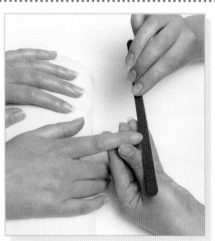

6 After filing the nails into the correct shape, perform upward strokes with the emery board to seal the free edge layers and prevent dehydration of the nail. This technique is known as bevelling.

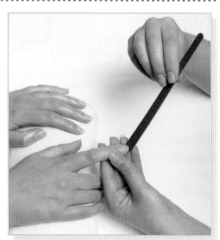

7 Using a spatula, remove a small amount of cuticle cream from the pot and then use an orange stick to distribute to each nail of the right hand.

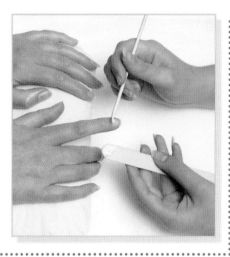

8 Massage the cream into the nails and cuticles of the right hand, two fingers at a time. This will aid absorption of the product.

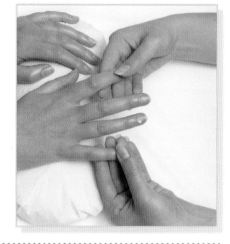

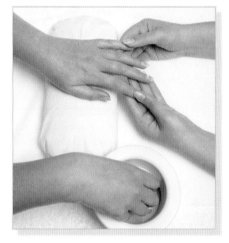

9 Dispense nail soak into a manicure bowl and add warm water. Now soak the right hand to soften the cuticles further and repeat steps 5–8 on the left hand.

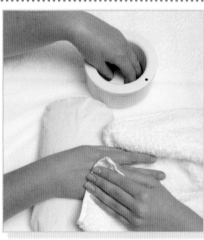

10 Remove the right hand and dry thoroughly with a towel.

11 Using either a cotton bud or a cotton wool tipped orange stick, apply cuticle remover to the cuticle area. Do not re-dip the cotton bud or orange stick, as this will contaminate the product.

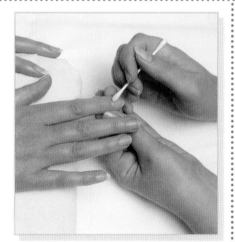

12 Using a hoof stick, perform small circular movements and gently ease back the cuticle.

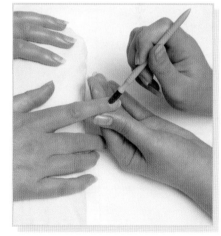

Top tips

Remember – do not cut too much cuticle or it will bleed and it will create access for infection.

Top tips

To produce more effective results, when working on each nail, support each finger securely to prevent damage and enhance stability.

Provide manicure and pedicure treatments

13 Use the cuticle knife flat at a 45° angle and perform circular movements from the outside in to ease the excess cuticle away from the nail plate. Then flip over the knife and repeat on opposite side of nail plate. Also keep the knife damp, so it glides along the nail plate without scratching the nail.

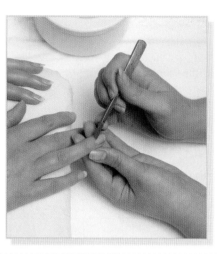

14 Use the cuticle nippers to trim any excess cuticle. Do not pull or you will damage the cuticles.

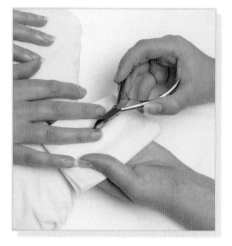

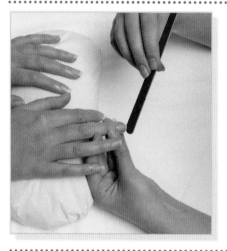

15 Repeat the bevelling movement again and repeat steps 9–15 on the left hand.

16 Choose the appropriate massage medium – this could be oil, cream, hand lotion or talc – and begin the massage (see Different massage techniques and their benefits, page 475).

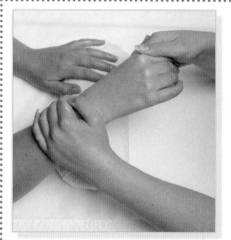

17 Use soapy water and a nail brush to remove the oil from the nail plate. If you do not, this will act as a barrier when enamelling.

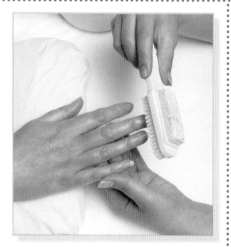

18 If the client chooses to have enamelling, first apply a base coat, nail strengthener or ridge filler.

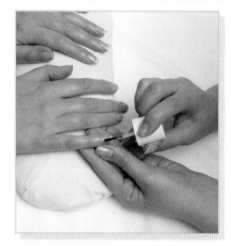

Top tips

Buffing the nails – this can be done either after filing (step 5) or at the end of the treatment (step 17) if the client does not want enamelling but a natural sheen. Use either the chamois buffer (with or without paste) or the four-way buffer, depending upon the desired effect.

19 Apply two coats of coloured enamel, with minimal brush strokes and without flooding the cuticle or staining the skin. If you apply enamel to the skin, use either a cotton bud or orange stick tipped with cotton wool soaked in enamel remover and carefully remove enamel. Apply a top coat to prolong the life of the enamel and quick-drying spray.

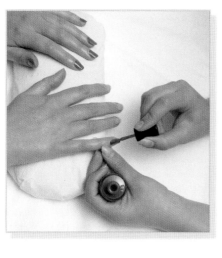

20 Check your client is happy with the results..

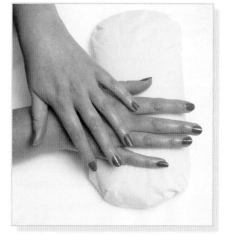

Basic pedicure procedure

The procedure for a pedicure treatment is essentially the same as a manicure treatment, so what has been performed on the hands is repeated on the feet with some minor differences. Buffing would not be performed on the feet unless there were ridges, discoloration, problems with nail growth or the client did not want enamelling but did want a natural sheen to their nails. Buffing stimulates nail growth and clients do not want their toenails to grow as fast as their fingernails. Also, feet tend to have more hard skin, known as calluses, so the technician would work more on the problem areas.

Top tips

A rasp can also be used before soaking the feet, which is often more effective as the skin is dry.

1 During the consultation, discuss the client's needs and check for contra-indications. Once you are ready to begin, wipe over the area with a sanitiser or antiseptic lotion and remove old enamel, if present, with enamel remover on a cotton pad.

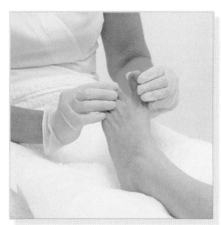

2 Cut the toenails on the left foot straight across if they are too long.

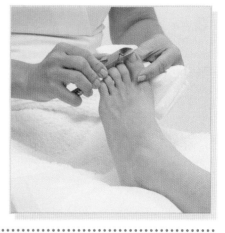

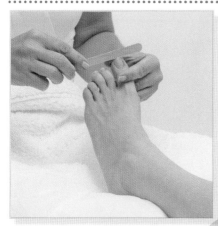

3 File the toenails on the left foot straight with curved corners, to prevent ingrowing toenails.

4 Using a spatula, remove a small amount of cuticle cream from the pot and then use an orange stick to distribute to each nail of the left foot. Massage the cream into the nail and cuticle of the left foot, two fingers at a time. This will aid absorption of the product.

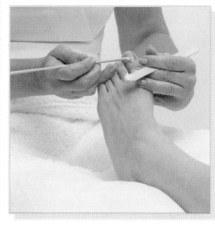

Provide manicure and pedicure treatments

5 Dispense foot soak into a pedicure bowl and add warm water. Now soak the left foot to soften the cuticles further and repeat steps 1–5 on the right foot.

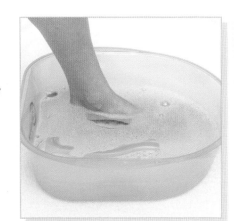

6 Remove the left foot and dry thoroughly with a towel. Then, using either a cotton bud or a cotton wool tipped orange stick, apply cuticle remover to the cuticle area. Do not re-dip the cotton bud or orange stick, as it will contaminate the product.

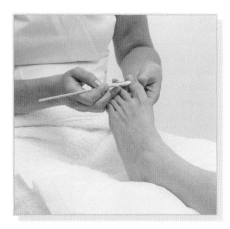

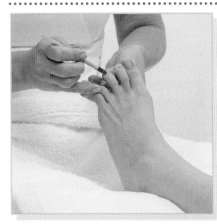

7 Using a hoof stick, perform small circular movements and gently ease back the cuticle.

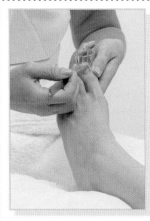

8 Next, use the cuticle knife flat at a 45° angle and perform circular movements from the outside in to ease excess away from the nail plate. Then flip over the knife and repeat on the opposite side of nail plate. Keep the knife damp so it glides along the nail plate without scratching the nail. If the cuticles are very overgrown then use the cuticle nippers to trim any excess cuticle but do not pull or you will damage the cuticles. Do not remove too much as the toenails do not require it.

9 A foot scrub can be used to help remove any calluses. Remove the product from the tub with a spatula then apply to the skin using large circular movements to lift away the dead skin cells. A rasp can be used if the calluses are very hard and require further work.

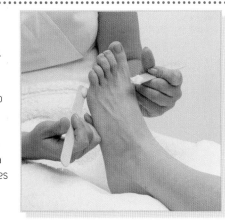

10 Choose the appropriate massage medium – this can be either oil, cream, lotion or talc – and begin the massage (see Different massage techniques and their benefits, page 475).

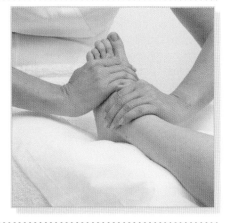

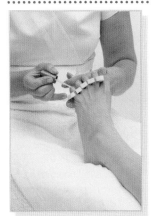

11 If enamelling is required, use soapy water and a nail brush to remove any oil from the nail plate (as oil will act as a barrier). Place cotton wool or tissue between the client's toenails. Before enamelling, apply a base coat, nail strengthener or ridge filler. Apply two coats of coloured enamel, with minimal brush strokes and without flooding the cuticle or staining the skin. If you apply enamel to the skin, use either a cotton bud or orange stick tipped with cotton wool soaked in enamel remover and carefully remove enamel. Lastly, apply the top coat to prolong the life of the enamel and quick-drying spray.

12 Check your client is happy with the results.

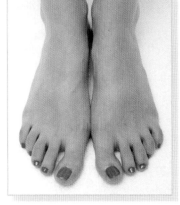

Nail finishes and techniques

Application of enamel

There are many tips that can help to produce a smooth application of enamel, with long-lasting results that will not chip, peel or look streaky.

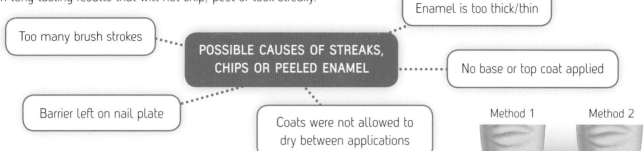

Too many brush strokes

Enamel is too thick/thin

POSSIBLE CAUSES OF STREAKS, CHIPS OR PEELED ENAMEL

No base or top coat applied

Barrier left on nail plate

Coats were not allowed to dry between applications

Clear or coloured enamelling

There are two methods of applying clear or coloured enamel either with three or four strokes that must not be too close to the cuticle or too close to the sides of the nail. Method 1 with four strokes is better for clients with a larger nail plate.

French polish enamelling

There are different methods of application and colour intensities with French polish kits, from very natural tones, including beige, pink or peach bases, and from natural whites to bright whites for the free edge.

To carry out a general application:

1 Apply a base coat.
2 Apply the white enamel to the free edge, either free-hand or by using special guide strips.
3 Peel off the guide strips (if used), then apply the flesh-coloured enamel.
4 Lastly apply the top coat.

There are also new versions of the original French polish design, as originally the French polish had very white tips with a flesh-toned sheer base.

American French polish

A more natural effect is created with a white and flesh-toned base.

Reverse French

A dark colour like black is applied to the whole nail and then a light colour like white or silver is applied to the free edge.

Reverse French with double French

This is the same as a reverse French but the lunula is also painted the same colour as the free edge.

Funky French

This is where a clear or natural base is applied with glitter, metallic or holographic polish on the free edge.

Chevron French polish

White tip is applied from the left-hand side downwards and across on an angle, then repeated from the right-hand side.

Method 1 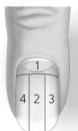   Method 2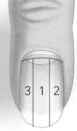

This is the better method for wide nails

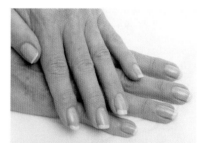

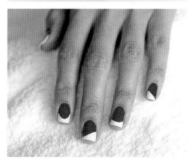

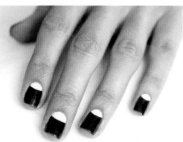

Variations on the traditional French polish – the top image shows an American French polish, which uses more natural bases

Think about it

Once you have mastered a basic French enamel, why not try out a funky French?

Using the correct products, tools, equipment and techniques to avoid adverse effects

With everything you do, it is important to have excellent knowledge of the treatment procedure and understand what the effects are. This includes the correct use of tools, equipment and products, as what you decide to do during a treatment can either have positive or adverse effects. If the desired effects are not achieved, a number of issues can arise.

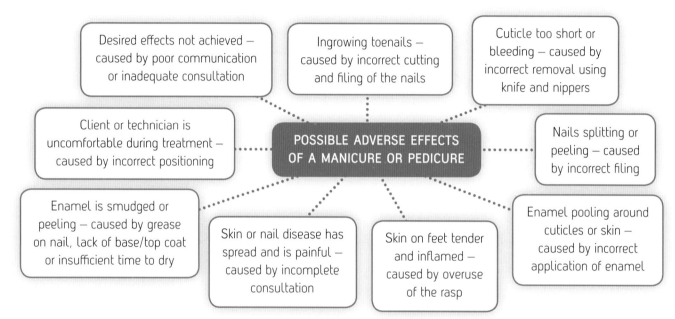

Desired effects not achieved – caused by poor communication or inadequate consultation

Ingrowing toenails – caused by incorrect cutting and filing of the nails

Cuticle too short or bleeding – caused by incorrect removal using knife and nippers

Client or technician is uncomfortable during treatment – caused by incorrect positioning

POSSIBLE ADVERSE EFFECTS OF A MANICURE OR PEDICURE

Nails splitting or peeling – caused by incorrect filing

Enamel is smudged or peeling – caused by grease on nail, lack of base/top coat or insufficient time to dry

Skin or nail disease has spread and is painful – caused by incomplete consultation

Skin on feet tender and inflamed – caused by overuse of the rasp

Enamel pooling around cuticles or skin – caused by incorrect application of enamel

How treatments can be adapted to suit the client's needs

When performing a manicure or pedicure, you will need to assess which products, tools and equipment to use, depending upon the client's individual requirements. This is where you need to learn how to adapt a basic treatment.

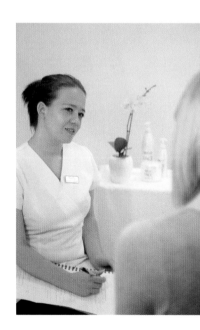

Considerations	How to adapt
The cuticles are healthy and not overgrown	Do not use the cuticle nippers – use the cuticle knife instead
Male client	No enamel Buff the nails Firmer massage Extra work on overgrown cuticles
Clients who are very thin and bony	Perform lighter massage movement or the client will feel uncomfortable
Larger clients with more adipose or muscle bulk	Perform deeper massage movement or the client will not feel the benefits of the massage

Considerations	How to adapt
Bruised nail	If it is not tender, then a manicure can be performed with the application of a dark enamel to disguise the bruise
Severe eczema of the skin	If area is not infected but excessively dry, perform a nourishing treatment, e.g. paraffin wax or an intensive mask. Exfoliators will irritate the skin which is already very thin. Usually the cuticles will be dry and short, so no cuticle work should be performed
Split nail	Will require a nail mend, using a fibreglass or silk wrap
Old false tan	If it is a patchy tan, it can be removed with coarse exfoliators
Arthritis	Be gentle when massaging and use paraffin wax or mittens/bootees to help relieve aches and pains. Make sure the client has sufficient support when performing a treatment
Very short nails	Gently file any uneven areas to prevent further damage
Overgrown cuticles	Spend extra time working on the cuticles with the knife and nippers
Very dry skin and cuticles	Use products that contain more oil to nourish the skin and nails, e.g. rich hand cream or cuticle oil
Mature skin	Use more nourishing products with anti-ageing properties
Poor circulation	Spend more time massaging to increase circulation and any of the heat treatments
Nails with an old set of artificial nails or damaged from wearing artificial nails	Time must be added to remove the old set effectively before the manicure can begin. Also the nails will probably be damaged and thin, so no buffing (nails already too thin) or enamelling (would highlight nails)
Calluses	Extra time needed to remove hard skin and a heat treatment, e.g. paraffin wax, would soften area
Ridges on the nails	Buff to remove them and produce a smooth shiny nail
Thin and weak nails	Cut the nails short, massage with a rich cream to nourish the nails and increase blood supply
Discoloured nails and skin	Either bleach the nail, use white pencil or use a four-way buffer to remove the stain

Top tips

Never provide the same treatment for every client, as they will all have different needs and requirements. You must maximise the effects produced, while making the client feel extra special.

Think about it

Use the guidance given in the table opposite to practise creating individual treatment plans. Then imagine a client with several of the considerations listed in the table and create a treatment plan for them: for example a thin, bony client with arthritis, very dry weak nails and cuticles. What would you do? Try a few more combinations to help you prepare for your next practical assessment.

Assess your client's needs and adapt the treatment

Different massage techniques and their benefits

Massage is one of the most important parts of any treatment, as it induces relaxation and enhances the effects of the treatment. There are different massage media that can be used, including cream, oil and talc (talc is used more on a lower leg and foot massage, if the client has very hairy legs and feet).

Massage classification

There are different types of massage movements, but the three main types that can be used during a manicure or pedicure treatment are effleurage, petrissage and tapotement.

Top tips

Once you have learned the basic massage routine, you can adapt it to suit your client. If a client wants a longer massage with no enamelling then this is acceptable, as the treatment will not take any longer and will not affect your timings or profit.

Effleurage

This is a stroking movement, where the hands glide smoothly over the area; it can be performed either with light or deeper (but not very deep) pressure. Effleurage is used at the beginning and end of a massage and also to link movements together, to prevent the technician from breaking contact with the skin. The movement introduces the technician's touch to the skin, helping to induce relaxation, and also helps the technician to end the massage without a sudden stop. Effleurage is so versatile that it is even used to distribute the massage medium over the area.

Petrissage

Petrissage can consist of kneading, friction, knuckling, pinching, rolling and scissor movements, where the skin and muscle tissues are lifted then compressed away from underlying structures. The movements work at a much deeper level than effleurage, aiding relaxation of tense tissue fibres and improving muscle tone.

Tapotement or percussion

This movement consists of hacking and cupping, which produce a quick, stimulating, rhythmic effect, where the fingers break contact with the skin. This movement will improve muscle and skin tone, as it stimulates the area.

Manicure massage routine

Begin with an effleurage movement and start with light movements getting deeper each time. Use a wrist support for the client and support the area.

1 Effleurage from the hand up the right arm, over the elbow and back down towards the hand, repeat six times.

2 Perform circular thumb movements up the inside of the right forearm and slide back down, repeat four times.

3 Perform circular friction movements over the back of the hand, up and down each metacarpal.

4 Move the fingers and thumbs in a circular movement to the right and then left, while supporting the hand.

5 Support the client's hand and place the client's finger between your first and middle finger, then gently pull and twist the client's finger.

6 Support the client's forearm with one hand and interlock your fingers with the client's fingers and move the wrist back and forth.

7 Perform circular thumb movements on the client's palm.

8 Repeat step 1 but begin with a deep effleurage movement and finish with a light movement.

9 Finally, with one hand on top of the client's forearm and the other directly below, slide your hands down the arm over the hands until you slowly remove your hands from the client's fingertips.

10 Repeat the massage to the left hand and forearm.

Pedicure massage routine

Begin with an effleurage movement and start with light movements getting deeper each time:

1 Effleurage the whole foot and lower leg. Repeat four times.

2 Hold the foot with one hand and with the other hand perform petrissage movement from the foot up the calf, slide back down. Repeat four times.

3 Place the hands on top of each other and place on the calf, with thumbs positioned on the front of the leg. Using both thumbs perform thumb kneading up the front of the leg and slide back down. Repeat four times.

4 Perform thumb frictions to the upper foot by criss-crossing thumbs from the toes to the ankle. Slide back down and work from one side to the other.

5 Thumb friction to sole of foot.

6 Thumb friction to the heel of the foot.

7 Support the ankle with one hand and rotate the foot one way then the other way.

8 Rotate each toe one way then the other.

9 Support each toe individually between the thumb and first finger then pull downwards. Repeat on each toe.

10 Massage the whole foot and lower leg with deeper movements, finishing with light pressure. Repeat four times.

11 Finally, with one hand on top of the client's lower leg and the other directly below, slide your hands down the leg over the foot until you slowly remove your hands from the client's toes.

12 Repeat the massage to the left foot and lower leg.

Contra-actions that may occur during and following treatment and how to respond

A **contra-action** is a reaction that has occurred from a treatment being performed and affected the area that has been treated. It could include an adverse reaction, known as an allergic reaction, where the skin and nail become red, swollen and itchy, with blisters.

During the consultation, you must ask the client if they have an allergy, then use this information to make any necessary changes to the treatment plan. If the client has very sensitive skin but is unaware of an allergy, then a skin test can be performed 24 hours before the treatment. The client may react to a number of products, such as enamel or hand cream, so when aftercare advice is given, you must inform the client of what they must do.

A contra-action could also occur if a treatment was not correctly performed and health and safety procedures were not followed, for example:

- infection in the cuticle or nail area from excessive removal of the cuticle or cutting and filing the nail too short

- faulty equipment – not checking whether the thermal bootees or mittens were working correctly; if they are too hot this could cause deep **erythema** burns to occur

- paraffin wax too hot could cause deep erythema burns

- incorrect product choices, such as exfoliating a client with eczema (skin already very thin).

Key terms

Contra-action – an adverse physical reaction during or after the treatment. This should be recorded on the record card.

Erythema – where blood circulation is stimulated by an increase in temperature, resulting in blood capillaries rising to the skin's surface to expel excess heat, causing the skin to redden.

Provide manicure and pedicure treatments

The importance of completing the treatment to the satisfaction of the client

To learn more about the importance of client feedback, see Client care and communication in beauty-related industries, page 109.

The importance of completing treatment records

To learn more about record cards, see Client care and communication in beauty-related industries, page 103.

Provide suitable aftercare advice

Providing the correct aftercare advice is essential so that the client can maintain the effects of the treatment and knows what to do in the event of a contra-action. It will also encourage the client to make any necessary changes to how they look after their hands and feet, especially if they have any concerns such as bitten nails or calluses. The client will also need to know what to do if something happens for the first time, for example a hangnail.

It is important that you inform the client of what to do should they suffer from a contra-action after the treatment. They must:

- remove products immediately and apply a cold compress
- remove any enamel applied with enamel remover on a cotton pad – not pick it off with their nails
- if irritation persists, see their GP
- inform the therapist so it can be documented on the record card.

You should also advise the client:

- when to return for their next treatment
- to wear protective gloves when using any household or industrial cleaners at home or at work, or when gardening or performing any outside work such as cleaning the car
- to use nail scissors to remove damaged nails and file correctly with an emery board
- not to bite nails or surrounding skin
- not to use nails as tools, for example to pick off old enamel
- not to use sharp objects to clean under the nails – instead use a nail brush with hot soapy water
- not to wear ill-fitting shoes
- for those who suffer from feet odour, wash feet regularly, change socks or tights daily and apply a deodorising foot powder or foot spray
- to ensure feet are completely dry after bathing, to prevent the skin becoming inflamed and split
- to avoid wearing high-heeled shoes, as this can cause calluses and will also affect posture, causing joint and muscular pains.

The client can maintain the effects of the treatment and improve the condition of the skin, nails and cuticle by:

- using hand cream or lotions throughout the day
- using cuticle cream
- applying a foot and body cream every day after bathing
- using a foot scrub or hand scrub weekly
- applying base coat and top coat when using enamel at home
- for those with weak nails, using a nail strengthener
- using a buffer.

To learn more about providing the client with clear advice and recommendations, see Client care and communication in beauty-related industries, page 106.

For your portfolio

Use the computer to create an aftercare leaflet that incorporates all different kinds of aftercare advice that you can provide at the end of your treatment to ensure you have covered all areas. This could act as a prompt to gain further assessment, when selling and promoting products and services.

Check your knowledge

1   What are the benefits of a manicure or pedicure?

2   What are possible contra-actions to a manicure or pedicure treatment?
   a) Direct cross-infection
   b) Indirect cross-infection
   c) A reaction that happens as a result of the treatment or an allergen

3   What type of movement is effleurage?
   a) A kneading movement
   b) A stroking movement
   c) A tapping movement

4   By what other name is the tapotement movement also known?
   a) Percussion
   b) Psoriasis
   c) Paraffin

5   What shape should toenails have?
   a) Round
   b) Oval
   c) Pointed
   d) Straight with curved corners

6   What is the strongest fingernail shape?
   a) Squoval
   b) Round
   c) Oval
   d) Pointed

7   What is the average temperature of paraffin wax?
   a) 23°C
   b) 44°C
   c) 49°C

8   Name an ingredient in cuticle remover.
   a) Potassium hydroxide
   b) Hydrogen peroxide
   c) Alpha hydroxy acids

9   What is the effect of a solvent?
   a) Thins very thick enamel
   b) Provides flexibility
   c) Nourishes the nail plate

10   What is the effect of plasticiser?
   a) Lubricates
   b) Provides flexibility
   c) Acts as an emollient

Provide manicure and pedicure treatments

Getting ready for assessment

Your assessor will observe your performance on at least three occasions for both manicure and pedicure treatments. Remember clients often come in for both treatments at the same time, especially if they are about to go on holiday or as part of their preparation for a special occasion, so you would be able to count these appointments as assessment for both units (a minimum of six treatments all together). Although the range does not stipulate treatment on men, male treatments are becoming increasingly popular in both salons and spas.

You will need to show your assessor that you can:

- carry out suitable consultation techniques, including a check for any contra-indications
- select the most suitable treatment for the client
- use the correct tools and equipment to meet the treatment objectives
- deal with any contra-actions that may arise
- select a suitable varnish or buff finish
- provide the client with appropriate aftercare and home care advice, along with recommendations for future treatments.

Evidence can also be provided though witness statements, written work or projects, or photographic or video evidence. **You will also be required to sit a mandatory external examination set by your Awarding Organisation in both manicure and pedicure and gain at least 70% to achieve a pass.**

Create an image based on a theme within the hair and beauty sector

What you will learn
- Plan an image
- Create an image

Introduction

This unit looks at the planning and research that goes into creating an image based on a theme, from first ideas to the final result, and all the work that takes place in between. This process will help you to develop your career, not only on the practical side but also by providing you with the skills required to communicate with others in the industry.

You will need to demonstrate a variety of skills in the planning stage, including independent research skills using media and whatever interests you. From here, you can find something that you are passionate about that will come across in your image. Without this passion, it will be hard to grab the attention and imagination of your target audience.

Throughout the unit, you will need to demonstrate that you can work safely, following your training establishment's and the manufacturers' guidelines to create the image. It is easy to get carried away with ideas and forget the simple health and safety procedures that must be adhered to.

Mood boards will help you to plan and coordinate the creations and theme that you put together during your research. They should be exciting and filled with ideas, colours, textures and techniques that you want to express in your image. Mood boards are a very **visual** tool, used in many industries, which may help to sell your idea to your audience as they get drawn into your artistic creation.

When going through the process from planning to creation of the image, **self-evaluation** is the key to further personal development. You should be constantly assessing your plan and ideas until the final image has been created. The whole process should then be evaluated to see if the image fitted its purpose and followed the ideas laid out in the planning stage. This will help with future projects and refining your skills when creating an image.

Key terms

Visual – something to be seen; being stimulated by such an experience.

Self-evaluation – appraisal of one's work, involving an evaluation of the process.

Plan an image

In this outcome you will learn about:

- creating a mood board based on a theme
- outlining how to identify media images to create a theme
- outlining the purpose of a mood board
- outlining how to present a mood board to others
- describing the concepts of advertising to a target audience
- describing the salon's requirements for client preparation, preparing yourself and the work area.

How to identify media images to create a theme

Media can play an important part when deciding on the theme for your image. We are influenced more than we think by what we see in magazines, adverts, TV and on the internet. When researching, it is a good idea to collect images that attract your eye and fit with your theme. You can get inspiration from a wide range of media.

Many people base their image around **media styling**, sometimes combining different aspects to create one overall look. **Cultural and ethnic influences** might inspire you too. To be even more creative you may decide to follow a fantasy theme where anything goes, and you could draw on many different influences to create something unique.

The target audience

You need to decide who your target audience is – who you want your image to appeal to. You can then select the forms of media that are appropriate for the age range. Younger audiences will be influenced by television adverts, the internet, magazines and current music, while an older audience may be more interested in television documentaries and newspapers. There is a variety of radio and television programmes to suit all ages; some will be more appropriate than others.

Recording initial ideas

The beginning of the process, when you start your search for a theme, can be very daunting, as sometimes too many ideas come at once or you may have no ideas at all. When asked to put together an idea it is not uncommon at first to have a mental block.

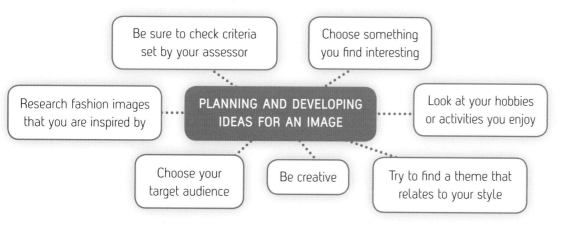

Planning and developing ideas

Normally, we can become creative and imaginative with a theme or topic that interests us. Without the interest, you will find it hard to sell your image to the target audience. The final image should be a reflection of your personality, so first take a look at your own lifestyle and sense of style.

Mind maps are an excellent tool to start jotting down initial ideas. All ideas that you think of should be recorded, even if they are very different. Once you have recorded some initial ideas, it is a good idea to leave the project for a while and come back to it later. This will give you time to think and you may find you are drawn back to one particular idea. The break allows you to work through the **concepts** and develop them further. If you have too many ideas, continually trying to develop them all into a theme may mean that the concept is lost.

At this stage you may find it better to work with other members of your group as you can bounce ideas off one another. Sometimes it only takes one person to plant a seed and the ideas then come rushing through and take the concept to another level.

Every person likes to work in different ways. The table on page 484 looks at the advantages and disadvantages of working within a team or on your own. Your salon may dictate how you work for this unit, so check with them before you start.

Create an image based on a theme within the hair and beauty sector

Individual planning	Group planning
You can explore more personal themes that interest you	You may have to settle on a theme you are not enthusiastic about
It may be more challenging to develop your original ideas further	You can bounce ideas off each other to take the concept to the next stage
You can work at your own pace	One person may influence the group too much
It may be harder to stay motivated	
The reward is greater when the final image is created	The rate at which you work may be quicker as each person can have a different job role
All responsibility lies with yourself	The buzz of working in a group can keep you motivated

The purpose of a mood board

A mood board is a visual tool to present your ideas. It should be bright, colourful and attract the eye and show the journey you have taken to reach your final theme. It will aid the planning process for your image and will tie together themes and concepts in the early stages.

Creating the mood board

Collecting resources

When creating your mood board you will need to have a wide range of resources to hand. There is no right or wrong way of making a mood board — it should just consist of your ideas and inspirations. A3 paper is a good size to use, as anything smaller will not have the same impact. It is also advisable to lay out the materials to show how they work together. Anyone looking at the mood board should immediately be able to identify what your theme is going to be.

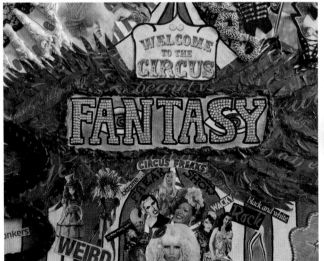

Example of a mood board

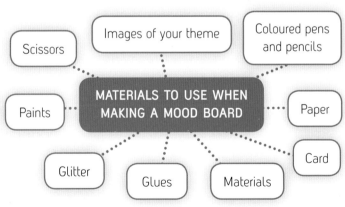

Scissors

Images of your theme

Coloured pens and pencils

Paints

MATERIALS TO USE WHEN MAKING A MOOD BOARD

Paper

Glitter

Glues

Materials

Card

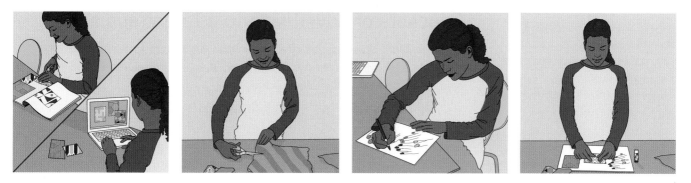

Creating a mood board

During your research, try to collect examples of everything that has influenced your theme. These will need to be evidenced on your mood board, but try to avoid putting too many different ideas on to the mood board, as they may confuse both you and the target audience of your overall theme.

Following health and safety guidelines

Protecting yourself and your working area is important at this stage — it can get very messy! Be careful where you work, as certain pens and paints may stain. Any spillages should be cleaned up immediately — you will risk spoiling your work if an accident were to happen. Keep the area organised so you can find the materials you need. There may be other people working in the same area, so avoid spreading your materials all around as they may be a trip hazard.

You may need to protect your clothing. Old clothes may be more suitable as it would not matter if they became stained. Aprons and overalls could be worn to protect them. Your main focus is creating your mood board, so keeping yourself and your working area neat and tidy will make the process simpler and more efficient. You can still be creative while following health and safety guidelines.

Evaluating the mood board

Although you will evaluate your final theme, it is also important to evaluate throughout the process. You may find ideas you placed on the mood board do not work as well as you first thought. This is the whole idea of the process — you can constantly change and update your theme. It will not be perfect at the first attempt.

Ask yourself these questions:

- Does the mood board fully express the concept of the theme?
- Does it identify colour schemes and materials you will use?
- Does it have a range of images relating to the theme?
- Is there a wide range of resources used on the mood board?
- Do the materials and colour schemes complement each other?
- Have you explained your choice of resources?

At this stage, you may wish to gather the views of your target audience in the form of **market research**. Handing out a **questionnaire** to the target audience will help you to gather their thoughts and ideas. It can help with decision making if you are unsure of any elements of your image.

Key terms

Market research – gathering of information and data before introducing new products or concepts.

Questionnaire – set of questions given out for people to complete. Helps to gather information and opinions on a variety of topics.

For your portfolio

Provide evidence when you make changes, so your assessor can see you have continually assessed and evaluated your theme. This could be in the form of a written paragraph identifying and explaining the changes you are going to make.

Top tips

Even though the image you create may not be promoting a product for sale, you are promoting your creativity and passion for the beauty services industry.

Think about it

You will need to present your image to your peers. Even if they are not your target audience you must demonstrate how you would adapt your presentation to appeal to them. Your assessor and peers may then ask questions about your image and how it came about.

Concepts of advertising to a target audience

Advertisements have a greater effect on us than we imagine, partly because the effect can often be subconscious. This section looks at how you can use advertising to promote your image to the target audience.

The mood board will be your main advertising tool. However, there are many other resources that you may wish to use to promote your image. As discussed earlier, your advertising tools must clearly outline the theme of your image and how it relates to the industry. Once you have decided on the target audience for your image, you can then choose suitable promotional tools.

Without advertising, companies would not be able to generate sales of their products, and audiences would be ill informed of the choices available. When promoting your image you will need to be able to communicate to your audience – they should be intrigued by your design – and convince them to give positive feedback.

- Positive advertising: this form of advertising will promote sales of a product and have the desired effect on the target audience. Examples of positive advertising include clients recommending the salon to friends and family, an advertising campaign that increases sales, professional working relationships with other professional organisations, and advertisements in trade magazines.

- Negative advertising: inappropriate advertising methods may fail to have the effect you had planned and not allow you to connect with the target audience, which can lead to poor or negative feedback. Unfortunately, if your method of advertising does not appeal to the target audience, they may be left uninterested and unlikely to be inspired by your theme. Examples of negative advertising include an advertising campaign that fails to increase sales or even reduces business.

Nowadays anything can be used to advertise, and we are constantly bombarded with images wherever we go – from traditional methods, such as television adverts, to modern techniques such as mobile phone apps. The diagram below suggests ways to promote your image.

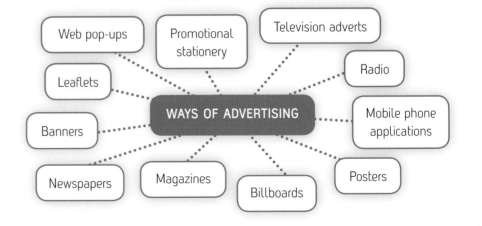

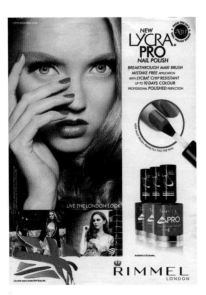

Sample advertisement

How to present a mood board to others

Once you have designed your image and carried out your research, you are ready to promote it to the target audience. For your qualification, you may be asked to carry out a role-play to create a realistic environment to carry out your promotion. Usually in the form of a presentation to your peers, it is your chance to communicate with the audience and take them on the journey of how your image was created. Along with the mood board, you may find it helpful to produce a chart showing each stage in your planning. Your chart will need to cover the following:

- Areas of interest and inspiration
- Initial ideas jotted down
- Shortlist of ideas
- Why you selected your theme
- What factors influenced your choice
- Who the theme is aimed at – target audience
- What textiles/colours/tools will help create the image
- How you will create the image – what skills are needed
- Creation of the mood board.

From the many methods of advertising available to you, it is advisable to select only a few of them to use in your promotion. Too many different methods may mean your message is lost and your target audience is confused about what you want to achieve.

Presentation skills

Many people find the thought of having to do a presentation daunting – it can make them feel anxious and under pressure. If you are unsure about your topic, you may feel even more nervous. Having good knowledge and understanding of what you are going to talk about can increase your confidence levels. The positive aspect of presenting your image is that it is your chosen topic and one you feel passionately about.

Setting up the presentation

When setting up your presentation consider the following:

- Location – ensure there are no distractions or anything that may create too much background noise, for example radios, that the working area is well lit and there is plenty of room for people to sit comfortably.
- Preparation – ensure you have everything you need before commencing. Having to stop halfway because you have forgotten something is not professional.
- Display – check that your mood board and any other props you will be using can be seen clearly by your audience.

If your preparation is thorough it will make you feel more confident before the presentation begins. Remember your audience wants to hear about your ideas and inspirations, and they want to feel inspired too. Lack of preparation will make you feel tense and anxious, which will come across in your presentation.

Think about it

Can you think of any other advertising methods to add to the list on page 486? Highlight the ones that you find particularly effective.

For your portfolio

Produce a chart showing your planning stages, using the areas suggested opposite. You may wish to include more details and other areas as appropriate.

Create an image based on a theme within the hair and beauty sector

Making the presentation

When making your presentation follow the suggested guidelines below.

- Speech – talk clearly and loudly enough for everyone to hear. Do not rush as your audience may not be able to understand you.

- Time – rehearse so you know roughly how long your presentation will take. Your training establishment may define how long it should take. Too long and your audience may start to switch off; too short and you may not have given them all the necessary information.

- Feedback – invite the audience to ask questions at the end. There may be areas of your image they want explained further. This shows they are interested in your image and not that they weren't listening properly.

- **Body language** – it is advisable to stand up during the presentation, as this looks professional. Sitting down inhibits the projection of your voice and it may appear that you are uninterested.

- Posture – stand up straight and use arms/hands as you talk, as this emphasises the points you are making.

The salon's requirements for preparing the client, yourself and the work area

After the research and planning, you are now nearly ready to start creating your image. This will take place within a professional area of your training establishment and often with other learners around. You may all be participating and creating your image at once.

Your professional environment may become a buzz of excitement as you prepare your tools and equipment. It is not uncommon for people to become overexcited and this can have a detrimental effect on the whole atmosphere. This is out of your control, so just keep focused on the task in hand to avoid being distracted.

Remember that you will be under assessment during your preparation, not just when you are actually creating your image. Stay professional and calm and listen carefully to your assessor, who will be giving you instructions of their expectations and how to meet the assessment criteria. When receiving these instructions you should briefly stop your preparations so that you can pay full attention and not risk missing important points.

As you will be working closely alongside your peers, teamwork is still vital. Help each other in your set-up and respect other learners' working areas and equipment. Do not borrow items that are not yours unless you have asked permission.

During your preparation it is a good idea to write down a step-by-step guide as to how you will create your image on the day. This will ensure you carry out the steps in the correct order.

Choosing your model

Your model, who will act as the client, will play an important role in helping present your image and bring all your research and planning to life.

Top tips

It is a good idea to get together with your model to discuss the concept of your image and then have a run-through. Even if you do not have access to all the equipment at home, you can still practise elements of your image. This will also give your model a chance to see what will be expected of them on the day and ensure they feel comfortable about how they will be presented.

Here are some points to remember when selecting your model:

- Can they commit to the day and any rehearsal days?
- Select someone who fits the theme of your image.
- As the image will be photographed, good skin, bone structure, healthy hands and nails are essential.
- Check the condition of the skin on the body if this is going to play a part in creating your image.
- Ensure they help to prepare themselves for the day – skin, hair, nails, etc.
- Choose someone who is enthusiastic about the theme, as this will help to convey it.

On the day, give your model clear guidelines on what they need to wear while the image is being created. It may be advisable to protect their clothing in case products come into contact with it. Advise them not to wear any of their own jewellery unless it will form part of the image. This means you do not have to worry about the security of these items while you are working.

Preparation of your working area

In all the excitement of preparation of the working area, it is easy to forget about health and safety and general organisation. Remember, you will be continually assessed throughout the process, so good preparation will ensure that the creation of your image will go as smoothly as possible. Not having the correct tools and equipment on hand may prevent you from being able to create a part of your image.

On the day, remember to have with you:

- plans of your image
- rough step-by-step procedure
- products
- clean equipment
- mood board
- clothing, if applicable
- consumables – tissues, cotton wool, etc.

It may take you some time to create your image, so your working area should be comfortable for both you and the model. Only have the tools you need to create your image – store anything else in a separate area. There is also a risk that clothing could get products on it, which could spoil it. The less cluttered your working area is at the start, the easier it will be to maintain it during the process.

There may be other members of your team in the professional environment and your untidy area could be a hazard to them. Your assessor will also need to walk around watching the images being created, so it must be safe for them also.

It is essential that the preparation of your area is carried out in a suitable amount of time. Your training establishment may insist that all learners start creating their image at the same time, so it would be unfair to hold other people up while you continue your set-up. Be logical when preparing your equipment and products – this will help you to avoid visiting the dispensary several times to get a selection of products. Keep focused on the task in hand and don't be distracted by the other people in your area.

Top tips

Remember to carry out **patch tests** on your model before the day of the presentation, as you will be using a variety of products on them. You must ensure they are all suitable for application on your model.

Key terms

Patch test – testing of products (for example body paints or hair colour) to ensure client is not allergic to any of the ingredients. Should be carried out 24–48 hours before treatment and recorded on the client's record card.

Create an image based on a theme within the hair and beauty sector

Due to the types of products used, you must demonstrate that you can set them up safely and in accordance with the relevant legislation. Your working area will be busy and full of a variety of products. These must be stored in suitable containers that follow your training establishment's requirements. It may not be possible to have out all the products that you wish, due to their nature – check where would be the most suitable place to keep them until they are required. Your assessor may decide to retain certain products which learners can access when required. Apart from any health and safety issues, this will help to ensure that learners do not keep products to themselves and that everyone has access to them.

To learn more about health and safety guidelines, see Follow health and safety practice in the salon, page 67.

Preparing yourself

Finally, do not forget to prepare yourself for the activity ahead.

- Ensure you are in correct uniform, including suitable shoes.
- Secure your hair up and away from your face – this not only looks professional but will ensure your hair does not contaminate products or spoil your image.
- Protect your clothing with aprons and, if applicable, wear gloves to protect your hands, as some of the products you use may stain.

Create an image

In this outcome you will learn about:

- communicating and behaving in a professional manner
- using technical skills to create a theme-based image
- evaluating the effectiveness of the theme-based image
- following safe and hygienic working practices.

How to communicate in a salon environment

During the activity, you will need to show that you can use the following methods to communicate:

- Speaking – to your assessor, model (client), peers and audience.
- Listening carefully to any instructions you are given and any questions asked by the audience at the end of the presentation.
- Body language – promoting yourself as a professional beauty therapist.
- Reading – following assessment criteria, manufacturers' instructions and relevant health and safety guidelines.
- Recording – showing your mood board and chart of planning stages.
- Following instructions – from your assessor and from manufacturers.
- Using a range of beauty-related terminology – showing your professionalism and your knowledge of the subject.

Top tips

As you will be carrying out practical treatments, you will still need to complete a detailed consultation plan to ensure your client (model) has no contra-indications that may prevent or restrict the treatment.

Technical skills required for creating a theme-based image

When creating your image you will be using a wide variety of beauty skills. All aspects of your model will come together to represent your theme, so you will need to be creative in all areas: fashion, hair, make-up and nail art/enhancements.

Fashion

From your research you will have selected fabric and materials that represent your theme. It does not necessarily mean you have to completely dress your model, but having clothes to match the theme will strengthen your image. It could be dressing of the hands and hair, if these are going to be the main aspects of your image.

Hair

You are not expected to be a hairdresser. However, if you are creating a complete look, the hair will need to be dressed in a way that complements the theme. It is your chance to be creative and experiment with styles that match your theme. In your rehearsal ensure your model's hair is suitable for the style you want. Keep it to a style that is straightforward to create on the day and make sure you allow enough time.

Make-up

Once again, you can be creative and experimental with products and application methods. There is a wide range of products available on the market to suit all themes, from high-street brands to more specialised theatrical brands. Patch testing will highlight if any of the products are not suitable for your model. During the rehearsal, plan a step-by-step guide to how make-up will be applied and in what order — use a picture from your research to help guide you.

Nail art and enhancements

You alone will know what your skill level is like for this area. Some people have a real flare for nail art while others can struggle with the application methods. Work within your own abilities, to ensure you feel confident in the application methods. Stretching yourself will add extra pressure on the day and may make you feel anxious as you create your image. Being comfortable in what you are creating will keep you relaxed and focused on the task in hand.

For your image you may wish to use all, one or a variety of the skills highlighted above. Whichever you choose, ensure they complement each other and when viewed together express the same theme. If you decide to make one area your key feature, keep others subtle so they do not distract from the main image.

Safe and hygienic working practices

During the creation of your image, you must demonstrate that you can work safely and adhere to your training establishment's health and safety guidelines. If you fail to do this, you could be putting yourself, your model (client) and any other people in your working area at risk.

Here are some important points to remember:

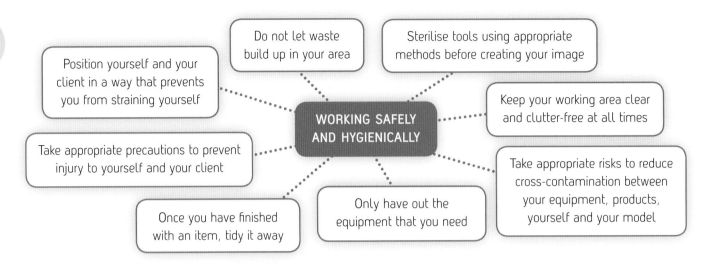

Methods of sterilisation

All tools and equipment need to be sterilised before you begin. Throughout the presentation, ensure they are kept sterile wherever possible. Avoid dropping them on the floor – if this happens, re-sterilise them. Have a sterilising solution such as Barbicide® in your working area if appropriate.

Use disposable consumables and brushes where appropriate.

Disposal of waste

Waste left in your working area will increase the risk of contamination. Place all disposable materials in a waste bin and empty if it becomes full – do not let it overflow.

If you have left-over products, follow your training establishment's policies for disposal. For example, do not pour acetone down the sink. If there is any contaminated waste, ensure it is placed in the yellow bins so it can be disposed of appropriately.

COSHH

You will need to adhere to COSHH regulations and store products appropriately. The working area must be kept well ventilated to avoid a build-up of fumes, and fans should be turned on if appropriate. Ensure all products are returned to their appropriate storage place when you have finished with them.

Personal protective equipment (PPE)

Protect yourself and your model throughout the session by wearing appropriate PPE. Your establishment will expect you to be in uniform and your client's clothes to be protected. When working with nail enhancement materials, wear a mask to prevent inhalation of dust and goggles to prevent products coming into contact with your eyes.

My story

Salon life

My name is Jenny and I have just finished my qualification in beauty therapy. As part of our course we had to create an image based on a theme. During the process we had to make presentations and create a mood board of ideas before creating the final look.

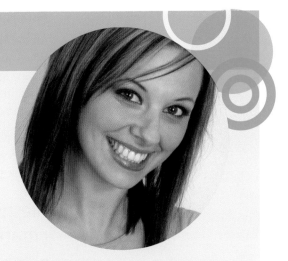

I found this experience quite daunting, as it seemed such a large project and I did not know where to start. There were so many areas to think about and all my other peers seemed to be racing ahead of me. My first hurdle was choosing a theme. I had so many in my head that I was not sure what direction to go in. After sitting down and discussing the project with my tutor I began to start whittling down my choices. We started to look at my hobbies and interests and a common theme appeared, which was dance. I had always been a keen dancer and took classes from when I was little until a teenager. Ballet had always been my main passion, so I started to explore famous productions. Eventually I came up with the concept of Swan Lake.

After deciding on my theme I still felt quite daunted about the work ahead of me, so my tutor helped me come up with a series of steps to work through. This really helped me break down the project into smaller, more manageable tasks. As I worked my way through each one I gathered ideas and evidence to place on my mood board. Before I knew it, it was full up. I was really proud of my mood board and I couldn't have been more excited to create my final image. My feedback from my tutor was very positive, as she could see how much passion I had put into the project. From feeling quite overwhelmed at the beginning I turned it completely around by using my own background to guide me.

Ask the experts

Q *Hairstyling is not one of my strengths. Will this have a detrimental effect on my image?*

A No – everyone has strengths and weaknesses. Ensure your final image shows off areas that you have greater skills in. Opt for a hairstyle that is fairly simple to achieve but still complements your theme. If you choose something too adventurous, there is a greater risk of it going wrong.

Top tips

Do not worry if you find the process daunting; just be sure to ask for help. It can sometimes be hard admitting that you need help when the rest of your peers are progressing well. Remember that everyone learns and develops their skills at different rates.

Create an image based on a theme within the hair and beauty sector

Finalising your image

All the hard work in your preparation will pay off when the final image is created. When you have carried out the necessary application take time to check your image for any improvements before it is presented. Small errors such as excess product left on the skin or uneven application could have a detrimental effect on your assessment. It is also a good idea to check that you have not forgotten to apply anything to your model that will complete the entire image.

Tidy up your working area so that when your image is viewed it shows a clean and hygienic place – untidiness could detract from your image.

Methods of evaluating the effectiveness of the creation of a theme-based image

During the planning stages, you constantly evaluated your image, developing new ideas and changing your concept until the final image was created. Many people do not even realise they are evaluating their work. They believe they are just changing their mind, but this is evaluation.

Verbal feedback

This can come from many different people in your working environment. Your model will comment on how well the process has gone and give their opinion of the final image. Your peers may also express opinions of your work – remember that your image and concept will not appeal to everyone. You have created an image that is based on your creativity and everyone has their own personal taste. Your assessor will give you verbal feedback on your final image and what you have achieved from an assessment perspective. Take the time to listen to everyone's comments, as it will help towards personal development.

Written feedback

This may take the form of a questionnaire that you hand out (see the example below), asking for feedback from your peers and any other people viewing your image. When completing the project this process may help you to assess how successful it has been and which areas could have been improved. Your assessor will give you written feedback to form part of your portfolio. This will show how you have covered the assessment criteria and in some cases which areas need more work. You should take time to read through the comments and ask questions if there is anything you do not understand or are unsure of.

For your portfolio

Your completed questionnaires can be kept as portfolio evidence. They should be anonymous, that is they should not ask for the names of people who fill them in.

Example of a feedback questionnaire

Date:	
What are your favourite aspects of the created image?	
What are your least favourite aspects of the image?	
Does the image clearly represent its theme?	
If not, what could be changed?	

Photographic evidence

For your portfolio you will need to have photographic evidence of your final image. It will need to clearly translate the creativity and work that has gone into the whole process. The diagram below shows some tips on taking photographs of your work.

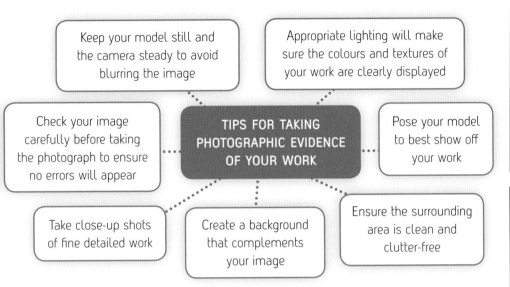

> Keep your model still and the camera steady to avoid blurring the image

> Appropriate lighting will make sure the colours and textures of your work are clearly displayed

> Check your image carefully before taking the photograph to ensure no errors will appear

> **TIPS FOR TAKING PHOTOGRAPHIC EVIDENCE OF YOUR WORK**

> Pose your model to best show off your work

> Take close-up shots of fine detailed work

> Create a background that complements your image

> Ensure the surrounding area is clean and clutter-free

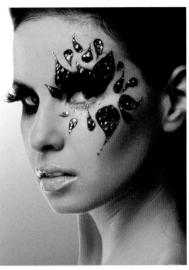

Your training establishment may wish to use your photographs to form a presentation of their learners' work, so make sure they are stored appropriately. This is an excellent way to show new and potential learners the exciting work they can be part of.

Self-evaluation

Your training establishment will encourage you to give your thoughts and opinions on your final image based on a theme. They may provide you with an evaluation form or you could create one yourself for your portfolio (see example overleaf). You need to look at the whole process from start to finish and perform a **critical analysis** of each step. Some people find it hard to evaluate their own work, so perhaps take a step back and look at it as if it were someone else's piece of work. You will find there will be elements of the image you love and some you are not so keen on. Actually creating the image and using your technical skills will highlight what you found difficult and what areas you felt you excelled in. Given another chance, would there be anything you would do differently or change about your final image? This way of thinking shows self-evaluation, as you are identifying potential improvements to your work.

Why evaluation is so important

The process of evaluation may seem insignificant after the final image has been created, but it is important to highlight what you have gained from the whole experience. The experience you have in your training establishment will help form your future career and the areas you wish to specialise in.

The evaluation process should include negative areas as well as positive. What would we learn if we were always told there was no need to improve? There would be nothing for you to work towards and achieve. You need to be able to deal with positive and negative feedback whether it comes from yourself or someone else.

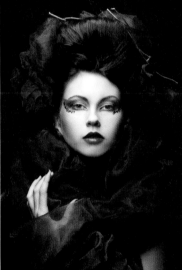

Photographs of final images

For your portfolio

Take care when taking your photographs, as this will be the only evidence of your image once everything is removed from your model. Ensure photos are saved electronically so they can be printed for your portfolio.

Key terms

Critical analysis – objective analysis of your work and performance.

Create an image based on a theme within the hair and beauty sector

Example of a self-evaluation form

Date:	Theme of image:
Was your preparation sufficient for creating the image?	
Was your final image exactly as planned?	
If not, what was different?	
What did you find challenging about the process?	
What was your favourite part of the process?	
If you were to create this image again, would you do anything differently?	
Learner's signature:	Tutor's signature:

Positive feedback

This will give you a rush of confidence and make you feel proud of what you have created. It gives the whole process a purpose and makes you feel that all the hard work and frustrating times were worth it. It will highlight what your strengths are and ascertain your skill level in the beauty industry. Listen carefully to the feedback given, as it is easy to be carried away with the rush of excitement that praise gives.

Negative feedback

This is always harder to deal with and accept than positive feedback but is equally important. Without negative feedback we would have no determination to improve and achieve more in our careers. If you find negative feedback hard to accept, it is best to review it at a later date when you have more of an open mind. Have the feedback written down and read through it later when you can take on board what the other person is saying. Never take the feedback as being a personal attack – it is purely about the work that has been created. Constructive criticism should help you to improve your skills and give advice on ways to improve your work. It should help you progress further in your training and give you something to work towards.

Personal development

The beauty industry is competitive and therapists are always trying to find new and creative ways to show off their skills and artistic side. This unit should help you to show your passion for the industry and the many different elements of your talent.

The evaluation of others and your self-evaluation will help determine the next stages of your career. Positive comments will highlight where your strengths are and what areas you could specialise in. This works well if your positive feedback matches the areas that you are interested in. When you do not feel passionately about something it is difficult to see yourself using the skill in the future, but the evaluation process should open your eyes and mind to areas of the industry you may not have considered before.

Similarly, negative feedback can highlight areas that need to be improved, which could be worked on in your training establishment, or push you to develop your skills further by attending external training courses. It can give you the motivation to improve on your weaknesses, showing you are driven – and that is a personality trait employers will want to see. Throughout your training and career you may find some tasks too challenging, but then, through sheer determination, you can succeed, and use your determination as a strength.

The diagram opposite shows how a continual cycle of evaluation will keep you on a path of improving your skills. This can be applied in all areas of your training and education, even when carrying out treatments on your client.

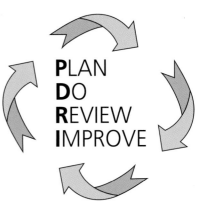

1 Plan your client's treatment.

2 Carry out your client's treatment.

3 Evaluate the treatment and how the procedure went; seek feedback from your client.

4 Improve your skills – the more you do something, the better you will become at it and the more chance you will have of achieving a high-standard result.

Plan, Do, Review, Improve model and personal development flow chart

Frequently asked questions	
Q	What material should I create my mood board on?
A	You will need a large piece of strong card. Too small and you will not be able to fit much on. You will need to be able to transport it, so the card will have to be durable.
Q	If my model does not completely fit my theme will it matter?
A	A model that will complement your theme is best, otherwise you will have more work to do when creating your image. You will have to use more styling techniques to change the model's appearance, which could take up more of your valuable time.

Think about it

Give more examples of how the Plan, Do, Review, Improve model is used in your training.

Check your knowledge

1 What is the purpose of a mood board?

2 List five different media images that could be used to create your image.

3 What advertising methods would most appeal to a younger audience?

4 Compare the benefits and downfalls of working individually or within a group.

5 What legislation is linked to creating your image?

6 Why is positive body language important when making a presentation?

7 What may happen if you have not fully prepared for creating your image?

8 What combination of skills can you use to create your image?

9 List three methods of evaluating your image.

10 Why is evaluation so important for your personal development?

Getting ready for assessment

There are no maximum service times that apply to this unit.

Evidence requirements

It is strongly recommended that evidence be gathered in a realistic working environment and simulation is avoided where possible. You should also ensure that you meet the required standards, i.e. that all outcomes, assessment criteria and range statements have been achieved. This unit is **internally assessed only** – but because of this it will almost certainly be internally verified, and the external verifier may also want to view the portfolio. This is standard when there is no external paper – the Awarding Organisation just want to double check evidence is full and well rounded.

Practical outcomes are achieved two ways:

1 The practical criteria covered when doing the assessments

2 Knowledge and understanding of task through oral questioning.

Your assessor will observe your performance of practical tasks on **at least three occasions** – maybe more if the evidence is not all there within the three assessments. If practical criteria are not covered your assessor will make a judgment through oral questioning. So, when designing your project and making mood boards make them as full as possible. Also, do not be surprised to be asked a lot of oral questions on how and why you picked your themes as this is how you achieve competency in this unit.

Index